Family Doctor
Good advice for better health

E.R.W. Fox, M.D.

Forward by M. Roy Schwarz, M.D.
  Senior Vice President,
  American Medical Association

Gatewood Press
Malden-on-Hudson, New York

Second edition, 1994

Copyright © 1993 by E.R.W. Fox, M.D. All rights reserved. No part of this publication may be reproduced or transmitted in any form or by any means, electronic or mechanical, including photocopy, recording, or any information storage or retrieval system, without permission in writing from the publisher.

All the stories in these essays are true. All the names of the patients are not.

Gatewood Press
Old Malden School
Malden-on-Hudson, New York 12453
914•246•1361   fax: 914•246•1378

ISBN 0-9639027-3-3

TABLE OF CONTENTS

Forward

Introduction

1 - Toward a More Healthy Life
   No Pain, No Gain — Why Hurting Can Make You
      Feel Good • 2
   Diet Fads and Frauds: How to Keep Pounds Off Forever • 5
   Slim and Thin Isn't "Normal" If You're Starving • 9
   Cholesterol Facts, Including a Few Good Yokes • 12
   Mellow Out To Save Your Life • 15
   Naturally Regular • 18
   Ironing Wrinkled Skin • 22
   More Advice for Sun-Worshippers • 26
   Chemicals in Our Lives • 28
   Mind Over Malady • 31
   Avoiding Hearing Loss • 34
   Snore No More...Or At Least Less • 37
   Young Fooled by Cool Legal Drugs • 40
   Surprise! Kids Do Follow Adult Examples • 42
   Kids Will Lead The Way to Non-Smoking Health • 45
   Peace-Loving, Non-Violent America • 48
   Positive Thinking: Good Medicine for Seniors • 51
   Appreciate Your Good Health Now • 54

TABLE OF CONTENTS

2 - The Wonderful Body Machine We Live In

Bad Germs...and Good Ones Too • 63
Pain, Real and Imagined • 66
Red-Blooded Health • 69
White Cells: Microscopic Body-Fixers • 71
The Blood Cell Factory Within Your Bones • 73
Fingernails Fully Explained • 76
It's a Right-Handed World • 78
Your Quietly Efficient Lymph System • 80
Breasts Versus Brains • 83
Stuttering • 85
Hernias • 88
Your Skin Has Holes In It (Thank Goodness) • 90
Bravo For Your Bottom • 93
Forgetting to Remember As You Grow Older • 95
How The Nose Knows • 97
Hormone Tour • 101
Your Thyroid Thermostat • 104
Those Amazing Sphincters • 107
The Useless Prostate • 111
Go Ahead, Have a Good Cry • 113

3 - "Not feeling so good..."

It Must Be a Virus • 122
Those Not So Harmless Childhood Diseases • 125
You May Have More Than Just "A Common Cold" • 128
Not Enough Iron • 130
New Ways to Treat Ulcers and Stones • 133
Gout, No Longer "Rich Man's Disease" • 136
Gas Is No Laughing Matter • 139
Liposuction: A Costly Way To Improve Your Looks • 142
Diabetes: A Serious But Controllable Condition • 144
Amazing New Aids for the Hard of Hearing • 148

TABLE OF CONTENTS

Unhappy Facial Maladies • 150
Hyper/Hypo, Too Much/Too Little • 152
Maybe You Have Lupus; Most Likely You Don't • 155
Lou Gehrig's Disease • 158
Anxiety, Fear and Panic Attacks • 161
Arthritis: Painful, Usually Treatable • 164
"My hand keeps going to sleep..." • 168
A Successful Fix for Dupuytren's Contracture • 169
Vertigo • 172
Depression: It's Not Just "All in Your Head" • 174
To Sleep, Perchance to Dream • 178

4 - "After A Long Illness..."

Smile...It's Only Cancer! • 187
Good News About Cancer in Women • 190
Cancer in the Entertainment Business • 192
Who Needs Those Pap Tests and Mammograms? • 195
Hope for a Leukemia Cure • 197
Three Mothers and Their Cancer Kids • 200
Doctor Parkinson and the Shaking Palsy • 203
Skin Cancer Caused by Child Abuse? • 205
Heart Attack, Hot Brash or Hiatal Hernia? • 209
When is a Heart Attack Not a Heart Attack? • 212
How a Black Egg Helped Me Kick the Cigarette Habit • 215
Love and Disinterest in Nursing Homes • 218

5 - Pills and Other Cures For What Ails You

A Cow, A Milkmaid and Your Good Health • 226
The A-B-C's of Popping Vitamins • 229
Pill and More Pills for High Blood Pressure • 231
Peg-Leg Pete and Chuck the Hook • 235
When Scratching That Itch Isn't Enough • 237
Steroids, Good and Bad • 240

TABLE OF CONTENTS

The Bald Truth About Hair Restorers • 243
How To Avoid Clogged Arteries • 245
Prozac — Good News or Bad? • 248
Medications to Change Behavior • 251
Generic Drugs — Good or Bad? • 255
Laughter Is The Best Medicine
  — No Kidding! • 257

6 - Sex, Babies, And All That Stuff

Can Kissing Be Dangerous to Your Health? • 267
Birth Control, Today and Yesterday • 269
Condoms, STDs and Morality • 273
Newer, Safer Intrauterine Device • 275
Norplant: The Ultimate Contraceptive? • 277
Virginity: New Teen Lifestyle? • 280
The Incredible Egg of Life • 282
Tough Abortion Choices for Lawmakers • 286
Just Call Womb Service • 289
Having Babies, Naturally and the High-Tech Way • 292
Cesarean Sections: A Better Alternative Today • 296
Twins! • 300
Circumspect Circumcision • 303
Dramatic Changes In Adoption • 306
Happy Ending to Teen Pregnancy • 309
Women Are More Than Equal Already • 312
When You're Having Trouble Having Children • 314
PMS Blues...And Worse • 316
Hysterectomies: Too Many? Unnecessary? • 321
Three Paths to Menopausal Happiness • 323
Androgen vs. Estrogen: Man/Woman Stuff • 328
The Myth of Male Menopause • 330
Widows and Widowers Aren't Fourth Class Citizens • 333
The Quest For An Aphrodisiac • 335

TABLE OF CONTENTS

7 - Good and Bad, Right and Wrong

Ethical Preparation By The Next Generation • 343
Doing What Was Right Seemed Much Easier Then • 345
"Above All, Do No Harm" • 349
A Case of Life or Death • 353
Is the Genetic Genie Out of the Bottle? • 355
Research Using Fetal Tissue Can Be Very Pro-Life • 358
It's Getting Difficult to Die With Dignity • 359
Suicide • 361
Pulling the Plug • 364
Living Wills • 368

8 - Doctoring

Diminished Image of The Doctor • 379
Men Medics/Hen Medics • 382
Angels of Mercy • 384
Robot Nurses of the Future • 386
Better Names for Aches and Pains • 389
Healthful Alternatives to Traditional Medicine • 392
Radiation Can Be Vital • 395
Treat Computers With Healthy Respect
 — And Wariness • 397
He Needs His Head Examined • 399
When A Death Can Give The Gift of Life • 402
New Hinges For Your Joints • 405
The Stress of Stress Tests • 408
Doctors Don't Know Everything • 411
Medications Are To Help Your Body Heal Itself • 414
Analgesia, Amnesia, Anesthesia • 417
Pain and Suffering • 419
Medicines Created From the Earth • 423

The Family Doctor, Today and Tomorrow

· FORWARD ·

Forward

Today, as never before in the history of this country, the practice of medicine is undergoing dramatic changes. With rising health care costs, uneven quality of care, and as many as 37 million people without complete access to reasonable care, the political climate is ripe for a major overhaul in our health care system.

In the midst of this maelstrom of reform debate, policy makers have discovered something that medical educators and practicing physicians have known for two or three decades: the United States of America has a shortage of primary care physicians, and the primary physicians we do have are not equally distributed across all areas of need. In short, we have a geographic and specialty maldistribution.

We heard the same conclusions in the late 1960s, but student interest in "general medicine" continued to wane. Primary care academic units in medical schools — including family medicine, general internal medicine, and general pediatrics — have remained anemic at best. Proper role models for the "general docs" have been few and far between.

At the same time, the allure of high-tech medicine, with its comparatively larger incomes, has beguiled far too many formerly altruistic medical students. Along the way many MDs have lost track of the real reason the profession exists, and the only lasting source of professional satisfaction:

• FORWARD •

grateful patients.

The book you are about to read should be devoured by every medical student. It shapes, in human words, a lifetime of service, devotion and hard work of a "general doc." In simple terms which are understandable by all, it paints on unblemished fabric the joy and sense of well being that comes from caring for others. It is too bad a revolution in health care is necessary to bring this simple, unchangeable truth into sharp and undeniable focus.

Listen to the music of the words — they are singing the song of being a physician.

M. Roy Schwarz, M.D.
Senior Vice President, Medical Education and Science
American Medical Association

Introduction

IDA ADDINGTON IS 102. When she came into the office last week for her annual checkup, she told everyone in the waiting room that "Doctor Fox kept me going this long." She's been announcing this for the past fifteen years or so, and of course I thank her each time for her testimonial, but as a physician I know better. Good genes, a good immune system, a good life style and a positive attitude have combined to allow Ida to celebrate her 102nd birthday.

Ida and all the other patients who over the years have passed through my waiting room door have been my daily reminder of the wonders of the human body. Over a lifetime of medical practice, these people have left me with a deep and increasing humility, and an awareness of the magnificence of the human spirit.

Today more and more people cherish good health and are willing to work at it, walking, jogging, biking, aerobic dancing. We are (though sometime grudgingly) accepting the dietetic teaching that steers us away from sugar, fats and cholesterol, munching instead on carrots and broccoli.

Aside from yearning for a brimming, zestful physical life, we seem now to be searching for a better understanding of the mental and spiritual function of the human being, either in a personal quest in our reading and writing, or in a turn toward religion.

• INTRODUCTION •

Today my patients have a healthy hunger for more scientific information about mind and body. We physicians are supposed to be teachers as well as healers, and recognize that we have an obligation to dispense accurate information as well as antibiotics. This attitude is a far cry from the days when we wrote prescriptions in Latin, and let our patients know that we expected them to obediently follow instructions and not ask questions.

If there were a need for further confirmation of the wonders of the human body, reflect upon the fact that Ida's lungs have been pumping oxygen 20 times a minute for more than a hundred years, which means she's taken more than a billion breaths. Her heart has been pulsing life-giving blood through her body at around 70 beats a minute, adding up to about 3.7 billion heartbeats! And Ida's heart and lungs keep right on working, 24 hours a day and night, without any conscious help from her. The world's most complex computer, the human brain, takes care of making that happen, while simultaneously handling sensory information ("Mmm, this is good jam!") and independent thought ("Tomorrow's Tuesday — I'm supposed to go in for my annual physical.")

As we gain more knowledge about our bodies, and as we look forward to more quality years of life, we more willingly accept the principles of preventative medicine. In the final decade of the twentieth century we can look back to the early 1900s, when life expectancy was around 50 years. Now 80-year-old men and women keep right on using their minds and bodies, and century-old Ida's are no longer a rarity.

As I listen to my patients, I continue to learn from them. For making that possible, I owe a vote of thanks to my wife Ellen, a nurse who stood beside me for half a century, steadfastly forgiving me for broken social engagements and re-heated dinners.

• INTRODUCTION •

Thanks also to my sons, John and David, for providing challenging intellectual stimulus, and for encouraging me to collect these essays. Recognition and thanks go to The Coeur d'Alene Press, my hometown north Idaho newspaper where most of them first appeared, as well as to the Western Journal of Medicine, the Journal of the American Medical Association, and the Houston Medical Journal. A special thanks to Malcom S.M. Watts, Editor Emeritus of the Western Journal, who gently prodded me to use what he graciously called "a fertile brain."

And finally my sincere thanks to the many patients who, over the past 57 years, have shared with me their cares and their cures, their births and even their deaths. From these experiences came the fertilizer and the soil from which these earthy essays could spring to life on the printed page. In sickness and in health, people have been my inspiration.

Coeur d'Alene, Idaho
May, 1993

*Toward
A More
Healthy
Life*

Introduction

Too soon we grow old — Too late we get smart

NOW THAT I HAVE ATTAINED what the AARP calls "modern maturity," I've come to the conclusion that Mother was a Health Nut. A wise and sensible wellness enthusiast, expert in the care of her five kids through her motherly intuition.

Long before we had the benefit of good public education in regard to a healthy life style, Mom taught us preventive medicine with her succinct maxims.

"Eat your roughage — it's good for what ails you."

"Don't just sit around — get out of this house and run off some of your energy."

"A little water — inside or out — never hurt anybody."

"Cigarettes are tools of the Devil."

"Sunshine is good for you — but don't let it blister you."

"Wash your hands before you eat — there are a lot of nasty bugs out there."

"You've got a cold — so don't pass it around. Cover your face when you cough or sneeze."

"Think clean — Have a healthy mind in a healthy body."

Today we are discovering the scientific reasons for some of Mom's aphorisms. Now I've learned that Mother was a very smart Health Nut. I think she would have given her approval to the physician's thoughts on the following pages.

1 No Pain, No Gain — Why Hurting Can Make You Feel Good

"No pain, no gain" is a motto favored by coaches and fitness enthusiasts. Is there any truth in it?

Certainly the joggers running by my house seem to be in pain, their brows furrowed, their faces red and contorted. When I asked fellow physician and super runner Dick Caldwell why they put up with this hurt, his answer was brief and direct: "It gives you a high."

On the flip side of the coin, Harvey, my friendly couch potato patient, whose most vigorous exercise is changing TV channels or popping open another can of beer, scoffs and says, "Hey, man, that's all in their head!"

Now it just might be that both Dick and Harvey are right.

Recently researchers have been working hard to learn more about how pain works, and its good and bad effects. Doctors have a good opportunity to observe patients undergoing pain, among other things noting how differently different people react to being hurt.

During my delivery of more than four thousand babies, I repeatedly marvelled at how many women in labor seem almost oblivious to the deep-down searing ache they must feel as an infant weighing eight pounds or more squeezes through their birth canal. Then a moment later I would see these mothers radiant, wearing a jubilant smile, as if to say "Oh, what a beautiful feeling!"

On several occasions, when a baby had to be delivered in great haste, to widen the vaginal outlet I'd quickly make a cut, an episiotomy, without anesthesia. How could I do this without a peep from the mother? Simply to say this patient has a "high threshold of pain" isn't enough of an answer.

At the other extreme, my dentist informs me there are folks who need a shot of Novacaine just to have their teeth cleaned!

What accounts for this variety in reaction to pain? Are some of us simply stoics, others wimps? Do some people actually derive a gain — a high — from their pain? Or is it, as Harvey insists, all in their head?

Dr. Choh Hao Li, Director of the Hormone Research Laboratory in San Francisco, believes that, yes, there can be an actual gain from pain. That its benefits are not imagined.

Dr. Li postulates that the sensation of pain passes with literally lightning speed through the sensory nerves to the spinal cord, up to the base of the brain. There the pain impulse zaps the tiny pituitary gland into action, stimulating the production of a hormone called beta-endorphin, our body's own "natural" morphine.

Presumably this pain killer, endorphin, is then fired back through the spinal column to the nerve endings in the cut finger or the stubbed toe, producing a temporary relief of the pain — the initial numbing effect.

There are other wide-ranging implications in this beta-endorphin story. There may be some surprises ahead.

Doctor Terrence Murphy, of the Department of Anesthesia of the University of Washington School of Medicine, conjectures that these endorphin substances could explain why acupuncture is occasionally successful in relieving pain. The needle manipulation could send an electric impulse to the brain, stimulating the production of this pain-preventing beta-endorphin hormone.

If we accept the theory that it is the trauma to the tissues that results in the relief of pain, then we can understand why the new mother would wear that beatific smile. And why there continues to be strong support for "natural childbirth."

Women who are afflicted with the curse of a monthly bout of PMS — Pre-Menstrual Stress — have found that vigorous exercise can offset the mental and physical discomfort they so often experience just prior to the menses. Apparently a brisk walk, a jog around a half dozen blocks, or ten or fifteen laps in the pool can stimulate the production of enough endorphin to relieve the stress of PMS.

Dr. Li's experiments with endorphin suggest that this mysterious substance could be labeled "The Happiness Hormone." He injected a feisty laboratory tom-cat with endorphin, then put him in a cage with a troop of white mice. The hormone had turned Old Tom into a mellow fellow: he and the laboratory mice cavorted about in peaceful harmony.

The tom-cat/mouse experiment made a point. But now Dr. Li may be onto something of even greater significance.

Other experiments have determined that beta-endorphin has an opiate-like activity many times stronger than morphine. On a hunch, Dr. Li and his co-workers injected synthetic endorphin into morphine addicts and methadone abusers, achieving surprising results. After one, or at most two, injections of the chemical, every person in both groups lost the desire or the need for any more narcotics. And, amazingly, the treatment appeared to have lasting effectiveness.

Just why this is so remains unexplained. Dr. Li suggests that the hormone endorphin acts on the central nervous system, somehow blocking out the awful urge the addict has, dulling the driving need for additional narcotic injections. If further study bears out that contention, what a great benefit for society this will be!

This fascinating substance, beta-endorphin, now takes its place in a family of hormones, both male and female: estrogen, progesterone, testosterone, prolactin, adrenalin. Mysterious chemicals that each day do their silent work within our minds and bodies.

Our ancestral physicians must have known that something of this nature was going on within us. They wrote about the importance of body "humours" in sickness and in health. They contended that the fluctuations in these humours determined whether our minds and bodies would have radiant health or be afflicted with disease; whether we would be depressed or euphoric; whether we would be stoics or pain-prone weaklings.

If we substitute "hormones" for "humours" it becomes obvious that our medical forefathers were intuitively on the right track. They already knew what our research scientists are only now revealing to us. That pain control is "all in our heads."

2 Diet Fads and Frauds: How to Keep Pounds Off Forever

ATTEMPTS AT WEIGHT LOSS through dieting long have been favorite topics of conversation. Diets have come and gone. Successes have been few, but the public remains fascinated with new ways to lose weight easily. Weight loss pills and liquid diets are the two most recent methods extolled in the mass media.

"Doctors Invent 'Lazy Way to Lose Weight'" reads the irresistible headline in a newspaper advertisement, promoting "US Government Approved" diet pills that are sweeping the country. Their maker promises that these "fat-magnet" pills will flush excess pounds right out of your body.

At last, the answer to a fat person's prayer. A simple, painless, lazy way to lose weight. You don't even need to diet. Just take twenty dollars worth of pills. Apparently, some people fall for such claims and promises.

Meanwhile, happy, talented and formerly chubby talk show host Oprah Winfrey proudly shows off her new slim figure, 67 pounds lighter, all thanks to a liquid diet. For four months she consumed no solid food — except one lone cheeseburger, the only moment when she lost her willpower.

Judging from these reports, it might seem the only decision facing obese Americans is whether to swallow a "fat magnet" pill or to drink a high protein liquid.

Every physician who works with patients who are (or who believe they are) obese wishes it could be that easy to help them lose weight. But it's not. Let's take a closer look at "The Lazy Way to Lose Weight" pills, and Oprah's more difficult liquid way to attain a slim and svelte figure.

The one basic premise that physicians accept is that obesity can be treated but not cured. As in the treatment of any chronic disease, such as high blood pressure or diabetes, at best the patient hopes to get the condition under control.

Two nutrition specialists doing research in a weight control clinic at the University of Southern California School of Medicine arrived at several conclusions that could be most helpful for people who are trying to control their weight.

One of the most surprising findings was that, yes, low calorie diets, along with exercise, are the cornerstones of any weight reduction program. But these two researchers contend that, unless the weight control program is accompanied by a deep desire to lose weight, and by a willingness to use continuous and persistent "behavior modification," the effort is doomed to ultimate failure. There you have the two keys to a lifetime of slenderness: motivation and behavior modification.

Diet pills for long-term use were dismissed out-of-hand by these two doctors. They list a dozen medications that are available for appetite control, and conclude that these can be of limited usefulness, but only on a short-term basis.

Their findings should dismiss the "lazy way to lose" by taking pills. Any sensible person who has fought the battle of obesity must know that twenty dollars worth of pills is just not going to solve the weight control dilemma.

On the other hand there is slim and vivacious Oprah, a living, breathing testimony to a person's ability to lose weight by dieting. She made those cans of magic liquid food into hot items.

When Oprah's star began streaking across the electronic sky, her weight also began rocketing up, to a peak of 217 pounds. At this point she suddenly realized that, because of her obesity, not only was her health at risk but so also was her continued success as a TV personality. She became determined not to let that happen.

When she made that decision she took firmly in hand one of the two keys to a successful weight control program — motivation. This intelligent, gutsy lady was already outshining several other well established talk show hosts, and no way was she going to let her plumpness plunge her ratings star back to earth.

To accomplish her goal she knew she would need to make a drastic revision in her life style, a change in her eating habits by way of "behavior modification."

Behavioral treatment of obesity can be broken down into three self-disciplines:

(1) Self Monitoring: The patient must carefully observe

and record his or her eating habits. Where, when, why and what foods are eaten.

(2) Stimulus Control: This means taking the fun out of eating. Chewing each bit of food 20 times before swallowing, sipping water between bites, and avoiding the pleasant events that trigger eating.

(3) Self Reward: Promising a prize for being "good." That new dress, that piece of jewelry, a trip, or simply that satisfaction that comes with increased self assertiveness and self image.

Oprah employed all these disciplines. She had a gimmick, liquid food, which took the fun out eating. She had an intense motivation to stay beautiful. And she rewarded herself by becoming more attractive and more admired by her TV audience.

Of course, she wasn't the first one to discover liquid diets. They've been around for quite a while. We know they can be dangerous and should not be used indiscriminately. Over the years people have died using these liquid diet weight loss "systems."

Oprah surely knew this. She had the time and the financial resources to obtain careful supervision. Every Thursday she would visit her doctor, have heart tracings and blood tests, coupled with counseling. All this added to her motivation and her behavior modification. And she maintained a regular exercise program.

Anyone can do what Oprah did, even without the liquid diet gimmick. All you need is deep motivation, persistence in behavior modification, and then — and this is a biggy — sincere determination.

The Weightwatchers program, with its excellent diet, has proven its worth. Self-help groups can work for the person who can benefit from group support in maintaining behavior modification. And diet clinics work for the person who needs more careful — and more costly — supervision.

Just one word about the more exotic means of weight reduction such as stomach stapling, stomach by-pass, gastric bubbles, jaw wiring. These are invasive procedures which carry a risk. They are to be considered only in the patient who is grossly overweight, who has what's called "morbid obesity."

Then finally we come to that all important "self-determination." Why so many programs fail is because the person's determination to lose weight is dependent on external help, from a doctor, a weight loss group or a diet clinic. When this support is withdrawn the pounds go right back on. At this point the ultimate success hinges upon that person's willingness and courage to stay with the program.

At this crossroad the dieter must say to himself, "Now that I have lost my ten pounds (or 20 or 67), and now that I am no longer part of a support group, now I will have to call on my courage and determination to stick with my own behavior modification program."

This will be the turning point for you. Oprah, because she is a public figure, had plenty of motivation to embark on, and persist in her quest to return to a slender size 12. The ordinary, non-celebrity Jill or Joe deserves all the more credit when they summon up the courage and willpower to undertake and continue their personal program of diet, exercise and, most important of all, behavior modification.

And then to stay with it — forever.

3 Slim and Thin Isn't "Normal" If You're Starving

ATTENTION ALL YOU curvaceous, full-figured ladies. Rejoice! Twiggie is out, Fergie is in. Those gaunt and bony females in the pages of Harper's Bazaar are giving way to the more shapely, size-16 women in, believe it or not, the annual swimsuit section of Sports Illustrated.

Physicians welcome this change. We know that the well-rounded thigh and bosom actually can be a sign of good health. And we also are aware that during the 1960s and 1970s women were seduced into an unhealthy worship of slimness. The resulting starvation craze forced the medical profession to take a closer look at two diseases linked to weight loss, bulimia and anorexia nervosa.

Some medical practitioners blame the designers of women's fashions for propelling women to seek an unwholesome and emaciated thinness. When we see photos of models parading down the runways in the fashion shows, we can't miss their sunken cheeks and their protruding hip bones. We just know they must be bulimic, or even anorectic. (Incidentally, have you ever seen one of them smile?)

The attainment of slimness is the motivating force behind both bulimia and anorexia, but there are important differences between the two. Bulimia, simply stated, is "uncontrolled episodic binge eating of large quantities of food over a short period of time." Then, to compensate for her excesses, a woman will induce vomiting, or take laxatives, or try to lose pounds by taking a diuretic. Bulimia is an on-again-off-again thing, usually self-limited.

Anorexia nervosa, on the other hand, can be a chronic disorder of a much more serious nature. It is characterized by continuous, pathologic starvation, which can lead to dangerous physical damage, even death.

Bulimic women are usually of low normal weight, and are hungry all the time. Anorectic patients are not consciously hungry, and are usually abnormally thin, a pathetic picture of "skin and bones."

Both the bulimic and anorectic patients have some characteristics in common: nine out of ten are young and female, coming from middle- or upper-class families. They are intelligent overachievers, trying desperately to overcome the presumed deficiencies of their self-image. They fear rejection by their families or their peers. Their lives are punctuated by one crisis after another, often involving the loss of a friend, or perhaps a divorce or a death in the family.

We can agree that the women's fashion industry must shoulder some of the blame for the spread of these two eating disorders, along with the news media, women's magazines and television. They all project an image of the "ideal" woman's figure as being extremely thin. Even certain cigarette ads show an extremely slim but beautiful lady holding a long and very slim cigarette — skillful but sneaky subliminal suggestion!

Advertisements promoting weight loss clinics and health spas also send a message about the ideal of slimness, but they are targeting obesity. Their commendable objective is to achieve a careful weight reduction program for the overweight person who wants to take off pounds. These establishments, along with various self-help support groups and Weight-watchers clubs, use carefully supervised diet control in conjunction with behavior modification, teaching us how to change our ways of living and eating.

Weight loss enthusiasts are in no way pushing ladies toward attainment of a Twiggie figure. Normalcy is their goal. They will concede that Fergie's curves can be both attractive and healthy.

So it would seem that the cult of thinness that has lasted through the 60s and 70s is now giving way to the more sensible teachings of the 80s and 90s. Indeed, the tables of "normal" weight-for-height ranges published by the Metropolitan Life Insurance company were revised upward in 1987. An article in the Journal of the American Dietetic Association noted that "the latest figures indicated that today's adults can weigh more than their 1959 counterparts and still anticipate favorable longevity."

This doesn't mean that what you weigh no longer matters, just that your "healthy" weight now is figured to be a little higher than before. It also means that the fashion industry is taking a more sensible approach in their design of women's clothes, including providing style for "plus-size" women. The end result is more women feeling good about themselves, and feeling better because they're healthier.

Of course, bulimia and anorexia nervosa won't disappear over night. There will always be hyper-active, over-achieving young women who still starve or binge in reaction to their life stresses. But there surely will be much less pressure to be thin. And now those curvaceous, full-figured ladies will once again proudly make their way to the beach!

3 Cholesterol Facts, Including a Few Good Yokes

"Look, Ma, double yolks!" When I was a boy that was always a thrilling discovery, as my mother cracked our morning eggs into the big black frying pan. It made us think we were getting more for our money. But today that's all reversed. Egg yolks are a no-no, because they contain cholesterol, and cholesterol is today's negative buzzword.

In our better-health-oriented culture we physicians are spending more time than ever practicing preventive medicine — educating our patients and the general public on how to live longer and healthier lives. This is all to the good — if we don't overdo it.

Along with trying to raise our patients' cardiac consciousness and their cancer consciousness, we've also talked a great deal about cholesterol consciousness. We warn against these double egg yolks, cheeseburgers with fries, creamy desserts, well-marbled beef and animal flesh of all kinds.

Sometimes it seems a person doesn't know what to believe — or what to eat. At one time high-protein foods such as these were lauded as muscle-builders for athletes, and waist-line slimmers for chubbies.

Now the pendulum has swung away from the practice of eating a steak before the game, and over to carbohydrate-loading for the marathon runners. Currently "fat" continues to be a dirty word, and physicians counsel against all rich and oily foods.

And then along comes fatty fish oil, omega-3, supposedly so very good for you that they've put it into capsules. At the same time government and university researchers inform us that soybean, linseed and rapeseed oils, (such as the new canola oil) are good for us because they are high in "unsaturates." It gets a little confusing, doesn't it?

One fact stands out above the confusion: a high level of cholesterol in your blood can increase the "rust" in your pipes. Over time arteries become narrowed by this buildup, reducing blood flow to various organs, such as the heart and the brain. This can lead to heart disease and strokes.

The good news is that, even though animal fats do raise a person's cholesterol level, this condition can be reversed. And furthermore, eggs may not be that sinful. A study by physicians in Oxford, England found that patients who ate an egg every day experienced no more change in cholesterol counts than those who ate only two eggs a week.

Cholesterol tolerance apparently varies from person to person, inherited in our genes. If your mom or dad or your grandparents possessed the cholesterol tolerant genes, there's a good chance they passed them on to you.

You can't do much about your genetic inheritance, but you can control your lifestyle, to control your cholesterol levels. Keeping your weight down is certainly important. And we know that cholesterol levels are markedly elevated in cigarette smokers. Losing weight and quitting smoking (admittedly tough to do at the same time) will lower your cholesterol levels, thereby reducing your risk of heart attack and stroke.

Incidentally, before I hear you complain that "doctors are trying to take all the fun out of life," let me comment that some heart specialists contend that a drink or two a day may have a beneficial effect on the coronary blood vessels.

If you're in your forties or older you should know your cholesterol level. This information is routinely and easily obtained from a blood test. Many factors enter into the evaluation of this analysis, and there is no precise magic "good" number for everyone, although 200 to 220 is accepted as the upper range of normal. But a healthy 20 year-old will have a lower reading than a 50 year-old, and women generally have a lower reading than men.

When your doctor talks to you about cholesterol, he or she will refer to two additional terms, the low density lipids, LDLs, and the high density lipids, HDLs. The HDLs are thought of as the "good lipids." If your HDL level is high you presumably have a lower risk of developing heart disease.

Why do women not only suffer fewer heart attacks, but also live longer? One reason probably is because the female hormone, estrogen, raises the HDL level, while the male hormone, testosterone, lowers it. Sorry, men, that's just the way nature works.

A variety of medications have been created in an effort to lower cholesterol counts and raise the HDL level. Among the brand names: Lopid, Lorelco, Questran, Niacin, Colestid. They all have side effects such as upset stomach, constipation, nausea, muscle and joint aches, and so are used only after all other efforts have failed. Diet, weight loss and exercise comprise the first line of attack.

Research continues on new prescription drugs to lower cholesterol levels. A few years ago a new generation of "wonder drugs" such as Lovastatin were developed and tested. But like so many "wonder drugs," Lovastatin had one very serious side effect, not on the stomach but on the pocket-book: initially it cost $500 a month!

And so we come back to the basic question, "What shall we do when we find out we have a high cholesterol count?" Here are a half dozen simple answers: 1. Select a low cholesterol diet and choose the foods you can cut down on. Stick to low fat dairy products. 2. Cut total calories and lose weight. (And eat your oatmeal!) 3. Exercise — ride your bike, swim, walk. 4. Quit those coffin nails — cigarettes. 5. If you use alcohol, do so in moderation. 6. Finally, thank the Lord for parents who were long-livers!

5 Mellow Out To Save Your Life

IN THE MID-NINETEEN-FIFTIES two heart specialists in San Francisco, Meyer Friedman and Ray Reinemann, observed that most of their patients who had suffered heart attacks had similar personalities: they tended to be antagonistic, anxious, aggressive and antsy — people in a rush to get things done. The doctors concluded that people in this group had a high risk of succumbing to heart attacks, then as now our nation's leading killer. They designated them as having "Type A" personalities.

On the other end of the human spectrum they found the "Type B" persons. Type A people lived a life of constant frustration, always ready to find fault, always ready to strike out in anger and hostility. The Type B person, on the other hand, was more laid back, more level-headed, more willing to see both sides of the question.

Their theory of heart disease being linked to personality type later was put to more careful statistical analysis by Doctor Redford Williams at Duke University. He felt that Friedman and Rosenmann were at least partly right, but that they failed to differentiate between two distinct parts of the Type A personality. One they called the Urgency Factor, that antsy/anxious tendency of some people to be impatient to get things done right now. The other, much more harmful character trait they called the Hostility Factor, the general attitude of anger and the aggressiveness, which was especially linked to increased risk of heart attacks.

To test the importance of these two traits, Williams and his co-workers gave the Cook-Medley Hostility Test to thousands of students, blue- and white-collar workers and executives. Results from over thirty years of testing showed those who scored high on the hostility scale had a statistically greater incidence of heart disease. Dr. Williams and his colleagues concluded that anger and aggressiveness ranked right alongside hypertension, lack of exercise, smoking and diet as behavior increasing a person's risk of developing heart problems. They noted, also, that the chronically angry person got angry more frequently, and that they stayed angry longer.

In an effort to find reasons for all this Doctor Larry Scherwitz, a psychologist at the University of California at San Francisco, conjectured that "Hostility is not just an inner trait. It's related to a range of things that affect us — interpersonal relationships, behavior, and habits." People with high hostility scores smoked twice as much as those having lower scores, consumed twice as much alcohol, and ate an average of 600 more calories each day.

Is there a scientific explanation explanation for why the hostile person is more likely to have crackling coronaries?

How can emotion cause physical harm? The physiological theory is that, under the stress of anger or fighting, the hypothalamus gland in the base of the brain sends out danger signals to the adrenal glands, and secondarily to the liver.

As a result, adrenalin is pumped out into the system, causing the heart to thrash harder and the peripheral blood vessels to go into spasm. Simultaneously, the liver is stimulated to produce more cholesterol, the stuff that over time clogs blood vessels.

All of this is under the control of your autonomic (automatic) nervous system, which manages all of your internal operations, through two sub-systems, the sympathetic and the para-sympathetic nerve hook-ups. How these sub-systems function will determine your "fight or flight" reaction — whether you strike out to make war, or you retreat to embrace peace.

The sympathetic system takes over in periods of stress — it controls anger and hostility. This is the Adrenalin System, useful when used properly and not allowed to get out of hand. The para-sympathetic is the peace-making system, as it lowers the blood pressure, slows the heartbeat, and improves circulation. It combats stress as it evokes good emotions, such as love and affection.

What, then, is the prescription for avoiding hostility-induced coronary heart attacks? It's simple and it's cheap:

Being good is good for you

Make love (peace) not war (anger)

Don't fight, take flight

Mellow out, man

Don't worry, be happy!

Compared to the high prices for heart medications, this prescription is a fantastic bargain. Try it. You'll like it.

6 Naturally Regular

MOTHER WAS RIGHT, of course, when she told us kids, "Now you eat that, it's good for what ails you." She meant that eating our veggies would keep us "regular."

Being regular, avoiding constipation, was in her opinion the way to stay healthy. So Mom fed us plenty of "roughage" — bran muffins and garden produce were always on the menu.

If anyone in the family had even a hint of irregularity, she would prescribe natural medicines such as stewed prunes, prune whip and rhubarb sauce. Mom would even cook up a pot of "psyllium soup" — psyllium seeds steeped in boiling water. We would be given a tablespoon of that glary goo at bedtime, to make sure that all that poisonous excrement would be flushed out of our systems the next morning.

With such a "regular" background, kids of my generation naturally carried to our adulthood the belief that a bowel movement every day is essential for a strong body and a clean and healthy mind.

The next generation used the term "bulk" rather than "roughage," and glorified "cellulose" as the food element that would contribute to alimentary regularity, to keep us healthy and happy.

Cellulose got extra points, especially from dieters, because it has few calories. And if we couldn't consume enough veggies to supply our daily quota of bowel bulk, we no longer needed that yucky psyllium soup. Instead we could purchase a wide variety of over-the-counter bulk producing products.

Metamucil is one of them, and actually is made from finely ground psyllium seed, with sugar and flavoring added. The instructions say to stir a teaspoonful of the powder into a glass of liquid and then drink promptly. Very promptly. We soon learned that if we hesitated before gulping it down, the stuff would gel into a mucillaginous mess.

Nutritional trends never stand still. Yesterday's stress on "bulk" was soon flushed away, to be replaced by "fiber." Today supermarket cereal aisles display a dazzling selection of high-fiber foods; TV commercials brag that you'd need to eat twice as many bowls of rival cereal B, to get the amount of fiber contained in just one bowl of superior product A.

Mother was really onto something several decades ago. She didn't understand the anatomy and physiology of the gastro-intestinal tract, but she certainly was well aware of its basic functions.

How many of us really give a second thought to our GI tract, unless something gets out of kilter? Three times a day we put food and drink in at the top. Then, paying little attention to the intervening alimentary process, we expect that at least once a day there will be an excremental ablution at the other end.

And most of us will admit to experiencing a certain amount of pleasure at both ends of the digestive process. From infancy on we enjoy chewing, tasting, swallowing. Then, in later years, after some of the other pleasures of the flesh have dulled a bit, the satisfaction of regular elimination may represent one of the high points of the day.

What is your gastrointestinal tract all about? Put simply, your "GI tract" is an open tube, approximately 30 feet in length, with valves located at various strategic levels, to regulate the ebb and flow of the bowel contents.

At the upper end an ingenious valve mechanism allows food to pass down your esophagus — the swallowing tube — into your stomach. But it keeps everything you've chewed and swallowed from getting into your trachea — the breathing tube — or into your lungs. We take this for granted — until some of the food inadvertently gets into our "Sunday throat," making us choke and spew and cough our heads off.

At the other end of our food tube there is another set of valves ingeniously designed to retain or release gas or feces. We pay attention to these valves only when we are angered or embarrassed by an accidental passage of stool or gaseous effluvium.

Between the top and the bottom of this hollow viscus are the intestinal organs, the small and the large bowel. They writhe and squirm as they digest nutrients, advancing the food and fluid down the pipeline by a process known as peristalsis. Only when the writhing and squirming becomes too vigorous are we aware of this bowel function. Then we complain of gas pains and colic — a bellyache.

As intestinal contents pass on through the small bowel, nutrients are extracted from the food. In the large bowel, the colon, water is absorbed, and the fecal content begins to assume a semi-solid consistency. It is here that a misfunction could result in constipation, the ailment that all our mothers fretted about.

Although constipation is not ordinarily considered a serious health problem, recent scientific studies indicate that sluggish movement of the fecal mass through the colon may contribute to the development of weak spots in the bowel, little pockets called diverticula. When these pockets become inflamed, the condition is called diverticulitis.

Sluggish bowel function may also contribute to heart disease, diabetes, even colon cancer. How could this be? These studies also suggest that the slow movement of the BM material through the colon — the technical term for that is "decreased fecal transit time" — allows the absorption of chemicals or carcinogens that could lead to such pathologic conditions.

Unusual as this may seem, there just may be some truth in these theories. I well remember when I first began to become a believer. It was back in 1970 at a meeting of the American College of Surgeons — a breakfast seminar, in fact — where a Dr. Denis Burkitt, an English research scientist, described his investigative work that led him to believe that eliminating constipation by increasing the fiber in the diet could reduce the incidence of diabetes, heart disease, and cancer.

He arrived at this theory by a circuitous route. He had learned that in Africa people had a far lower incidence of these three maladies than did his fellow Londoners. As a true scientist he asked "Why?" In searching for an answer he concluded that diet must be a determining factor.

The obvious differences between the African and British diet was fiber. African natives consumed large quantities of corn, millet, potatoes (skin and all), and leafy fruits and vegetables. In contrast, British food was soft-cooked and bland.

But here was the problem: How could cause and effect be proven? The good doctor reasoned that even though he couldn't measure the food that went into the native he could at least attempt to measure the residue that came out.

So at this breakfast meeting the professor told us — with vivid slides to prove it — how with true scientific zeal he went about gathering up stool specimens, carefully measuring, weighing and recording them. Can't we just picture this British doctor tip-toeing through the jungle, pooper-scooper in one hand, a scale in the other, retrieving and weighing these fresh fecal donations?

When Doctor Burkitt had accumulated enough African data, he returned to London and repeated the experiment on a similar number of stool specimens gathered in the large hospital in which he worked.

He found, to his scientific satisfaction, that the large average African specimen out-weighed the British output two to one. The logical conclusion then had to be that a high intake of fiber increased the bulk which thereby hastened the transit time. Carrying the reasoning one step farther, fiber just had to be the reason for the lower rates of heart disease, cancer of the colon and diabetes among the Africans.

Similar studies have now given us additional convincing evidence that a high fiber diet reduces serum cholesterol, secondarily lowering the incidence of heart disease and hardening of the arteries. Bran, especially oat bran, has had an upswing in popularity.

There is more good news. When fiber hits the GI tract it swells, making you feel full. If you're dieting, low calorie fiber may fill you up as it slims you down.

Yes, Mom surely possessed the wisdom of the ages. Even though she didn't know why, she knew what was good for what ailed us.

At your dinner hour you may have seen a kindly face peer out at your from the TV screen advising you that, "MOM knows just what you need. Nobody treats you better than MOM."

Be not mislead. The stuff that man's talking about is magnesia, a laxative. Mother would have favored fiber.

7 *Ironing Wrinkled Skin*

MY TELEPHONE IS RINGING OFF THE HOOK. Everyone wants a prescription for Retin-A, the new wonder drug that promises to wipe away all your ugly wrinkles.

An article in the Journal of the American Medical Association, "Topical Tretinoin Improves Photo-aged Skin," was the start of all the fuss. The mass media latched on to the findings that wrinkles caused by an overdose of sunshine might show some improvement, at least temporarily, by an extended period of treatment with Retin-A.

The folks in the media rushed this exciting human interest story into newsprint and on the air. I have to wonder if any of these reporters took the trouble to trudge through the original, scientific article.

Here, in a nutshell, is what the researchers concluded:

(1) After 16 weeks of application of Retin-A to the faces and forearms of 30 volunteers, there were varying degrees of reduction in wrinkling in those patients who stayed with the treatment for the entire four months.

(2) 92% of the patients experienced a fairly nasty skin irritation, characterized by burning, tingling, itching, and scaling, severe enough to require treatment with cortisone cream. For some patients this dermatitis lasted as long as three months.

(3) Forearm skin showed more improvement than the skin of the face.

(4) This report was only of a preliminary study on a small group of volunteers, and, to quote the article, "Other studies will be required to determine whether changes induced by tretinoin will persist after therapy is stopped."

There you have it. This preliminary report was probably given more credence than it deserved, raising our hopes too quickly. And, as so often happens with such "medical breakthroughs," after the initial excitement has evaporated we learn the use of the medication carries with it adverse reactions, even failures.

On the plus side, this intense focus on wrinkles brought to the public a better understanding of what causes wrinkles in your skin, and what you can do to prevent them.

The study which got my phone ringing involved 30 people in the 50-year-old age group, assuming, I suppose, that there wasn't much hope for improvement in the faces or forearms of older, "mature Americans." Therefore, this sermonette on preventive medicine will be aimed at the younger group who still may be able to prevent the skin damage that produces wrinkles.

Will they listen to sage advice from their elders? It's worth a try.

The two most important causes of wrinkling are smoking and sun exposure. Because more and more people are giving up — or not starting — smoking, this trend alone happily portends a marked improvement in the collective skin of the next generation. So I'll speak here only about sunshine, and how and why it can cause skin damage, wrinkles, even skin cancer.

We love the sun's power to chase away our wintry aches and chills, but sunshine contains ultraviolet light (UVL), the portion of sunlight's spectrum that causes our worries about wrinkles.

There are three kinds of ultraviolet light, types A, B, and C, each with its own special characteristics.

Ultraviolet "C" (UVC) contains the most damaging rays, and is valuable only for use in germicidal lamps. So far we're protected by the ozone layer in the atmosphere that effectively shields us from UVC.

UVB is the sunburn portion of sunlight. It's what gives us our "tan," but also our wrinkles and skin cancer.

UVA is the so-called "safe" ultraviolet, touted by the tanning parlors. Used in moderation it tans without burning, but it will wrinkle and leatherize the skin when received in high doses.

How to avoid the bad long-term effects of the sun? Here are a few tips.

We know that the maximum strength of sunburn producing ultraviolet UVB occurs when the sun is high in the sky. As spring approaches we are working toward the longest and sunniest day of the year, June 20th or 21st. Around the third week in June, 60% of the UVB rays will strike the earth's surface between 10:00 AM and 2:00 PM. That's the time to avoid long exposure.

And whether or not you're going out in the sun in mid-day, use sun screen that matches your particular skin sensitivity. If you're fair-haired or a red-head, you should apply a sun screen with a Sun Protective Factor (SPF) rated 15 or better.

If you insist in not using high-rated sun screen, and insist on hitting the beach between ten and two, please allow your self no more than 15 or 20 minutes of unprotected exposure to old UVB, especially if this is your first time out. After that first exposure, gob on the SPF and even slip into a shirt and put on a hat. You'll sleep better that night, and you'll get a better tan, instead of a blistering burn.

The same advice applies if you're heading for the slopes. Remember that every 1000 feet of increase in altitude increases the power of UVB rays by 5%. Moreover, whether skiing or swimming, snow and water reflect the rays right back up and at you, doubling your chance for a bad burn.

If you are taking children along on your sunny excursions, even just to an open-air mall or to the zoo, be sure to apply adequate sun protection, because young skin is extremely sensitive to the sun. Leaving little ones to swelter in a stroller is a form of child abuse.

Here are four additional points about getting the best — and avoiding the worst — from the sun. First, gobbing "suntan" or any other kind of oil on the skin will increase the likelihood of a bad burn, because oil enhances the ultraviolet penetration.

Second, wearing a wet T-shirt not only doesn't protect you from the sun, it actually increases the chance of a burn.

Third, a person on certain medications may be surprised

by a quick and painful sunburn, even on short exposure. Tetracycline, sulfa, arthritis medicines, and water retention pills are examples of drugs which can greatly increase photo-sensitivity.

Finally, while talking about the sun and our bodies, here's one more piece of important advice. Everyone knows that sunlight can blister bald heads and tender insteps, but not much has been said about the damage these rays can inflict upon our eyeballs. Medical researchers now have reason to believe that ultraviolet sunlight plays a major role in the formation of cataracts.

Eye-glass manufacturers are paying attention. Lenses that filter out harmful ultraviolet rays are now available. Your glasses or sunglasses already may be so equipped. To find out, check the bow or the temple piece for a statement that they are. If they are not, you might investigate obtaining sunglasses with this additional sunscreen for your eyes.

As for wrinkles, instead of trying to erase those handsome laugh lines, I suggest you take steps to avoid creating any more:

(1) If you smoke, quit. If you don't smoke, don't start.

(2) Tan your hide if you must, but do it wisely and in moderation.

And, for your good sight's sake, don't cook your corneas!

8 *More Advice for Sun-Worshippers*

MOST AMERICANS ARE heliophiles, sun-lovers, sun-bathers, sun-worshippers. We bask in the sunshine for its warmth, and with the hope of acquiring a "healthy tan."

But now there is mounting evidence that, rather than being a loyal friend, Old Sol can turn against us if we let down our guard. We know that over exposure to his rays can give us thick, wrinkled, elephantine skin as well as skin cancer and malignant melanoma. Two of the most common causes of blindness, cataracts and macular degeneration, also may be due to over-exposure to ultraviolet rays.

Dermatologists tell us that there are wide variations in people's susceptibility to damage from exposure to sunshine. They rank us into six classes of genetic skin types, the most susceptible being Type One, the freckled red-head who invariably burns, and Type Two, pale-skinned blondes. The range continues through the brunettes, Asians and Blacks who rarely burn. Of course, the people who burn and tan most easily are the ones who are in the greatest danger of developing skin cancer and malignant melanoma.

This awareness has prompted us to try to learn more about sunlight, and what this golden ball in the sky does for us — and to us. The most obvious beneficial effect of sunlight is to warm Planet Earth. The ultra-violet rays in sun shine act upon our skin to produce essential Vitamin D. The ultra-violet rays also produce life-sustaining chlorophyll, the green substance in the leaves of plants, trees and in blades of grass.

Physicians use ultra-violet rays to treat certain skin diseases such as psoriasis, and the patchy white skin of vitligo. If you pass by the nursery at the hospital you may see a baby lying beneath a blue light for the treatment of newborn jaundice. It works.

We take the favorable aspects of sunlight for granted. Yet, as we lie on the beach, sit in our boat, or ski down the slopes we give little thought to what the rays of UVA, UVB and UVC may actually be doing to us. And even though it is a "wellness" consideration, many of us are reluctant to take even the simplest of precautions.

Suncreens are available with "sun protective factors" (SPF) up to 50, but none of them give perfect protection.

Some may protect against UVA but not UVB, or vice versa. And, because most sunscreens are water-soluble, you need to re-apply them after swimming.

For example, improved products such as Photoplex, Shade 45 and Filteray protect against both UBA and UBV, but are not waterproof. For those people who resist using a sunscreen but would use a "moisturizer" there is a product called Neutrogena Moisture 15. Research continues on the feasibility of combining various chemicals (even Vitamin C) with creams or ointments, in the hope of finding a superior protective skin coating.

The most sensible protection is, of course, to avoid over-exposure in the first place. That means exercising greater care during the midday hours, from 10:00 AM to 2:00 PM, when the radiation levels are the highest. Suncreens do help. For additional eye protection there are several specially designed goggles, such as "Super-Visor," now available.

Use good sense when you worship the sun. Stay on good terms with Old Sol.

9 *Chemicals in Our Lives*

PITY THE POOR APPLE. It's been maligned and derided, it's been poisoned and it's been shot at. But, praise be, it always bounces back.

The apple's bad name began way back in the Garden of Eden. You may have your own ideas about what went on between Adam and Eve when they first sampled the apple and learned about "sin." Though the First Couple, a couple of innocents, were banished from the Garden for partaking of the forbidden fruit, the apple survived and had its good name restored.

However, the apple's reputation through the ages has been decidedly mixed. First there was Snow White who drifted out into an eternal dreamland after biting into a poisoned apple. Luckily Prince Charming dropped by and revived her with a kiss.

Then there was the fellow by the name of William Tell, who went around splattering his arrows into apples perched on his son's head. Why couldn't old Bill just as well have used a melon, or better yet, a cabbage, instead of desecrating the apple?

In spite of these setbacks the apple rebounded, constantly gaining in popularity. "An apple a day keeps the doctor away."

With a little help from Johnny Appleseed, apple trees sprouted across America, and the apple became the favorite fruit of our children and our grandchildren. When baked in a pie crust, we proudly lavish the apple with superlatives. "As American as Motherhood and apple pie."

That is until a movie star, after watching "60 Minutes," was panic-stricken to learn how sinful apples treated with alar really are. She promptly marched before a Congressional Committee to air her complaints. (Wouldn't it be nice if we all could do that?) Her testimony stirred up a whirlwind of worries in the minds and hearts of mothers all across America. "Don't let them use chemicals that will give my children cancer!" was the cry that went out over the airwaves.

It mattered little that these reports were quickly discredited by the Food and Drug Administration, the Environmental Protection Agency, and the U.S. Department of Agriculture. The damage was done. One movie star and one report on one TV show threw our country into a panic. And the apple industry lost millions.

A little later the American public and our federal government flew into similar hysterical tizzies over two Chilean grapes that may or may not have been injected with a little drop of cyanide.

Now even the lowly potato is suspect. A hard-working reporter discovered that a chemical called aldicarb has been used to stimulate the growth of larger and healthier Idaho bakers. It has been rumored that chickens often may harbor salmonella, and some time ago we were warned that fish may be loaded with mercury.

So our lives are filled with fear, not only the fear of cancer — cancerophobia — but also the fear of chemicals — chemophobia.

To make matters worse, now we're told that some organic foods might be bad for us. As wheat, corn and peanuts grow out in the field they may acquire tiny amounts of a poison called aflatoxin. Fortunately, that's not going to stop you or me from having our peanut butter and jelly sandwich.

There are other chemicals out there lurking in the shadows that probably should be given a little more attention. We now know that beer contains one part per billion of formaldehyde, and scotch whiskey has a squinch of fusel oil in it. The nicotine and hydrocarbons in tobacco kill 339,000 Americans each year. (Ironically, the government subsidizes tobacco growers and in some states runs liquor stores.)

The irrationality of all this carries over into the practice of medicine. For many years we doctors used a pill called Bendectin to control morning sickness in early pregnancy. It worked.

But then a few of the women who had used the drug gave birth to babies with minor defects. In this litigious climate they naturally sued the drug company. After many lengthy and expensive law suits the courts finally found that Bendectin was harmless. But now no drug company will risk bringing Bendectin back on the market.

Immunization of infants with DPT has long been recognized as a life-saving procedure. However a few isolated reactions from the shots caused a public panic and more lawsuits. As a result many pharmaceutical companies withdrew from this category, so we now have a limited supply of the immunization material. And, of course, the cost of the shots has risen from pennies to dollars.

Thalidomide was perhaps the first drug to produce nationwide fear, and it certainly was the drug that put the Food and Drug Administration into business. Now, through another twist of fate, thalidomide is being heaped with praise as the magic potion that assists doctors in succeeding with bone marrow transplants.

Faced by all these poisons, all these carcinogens in what we eat, drink or breathe, you have to wonder how we so far have survived them all. We are being reminded each day that life itself is carcinogenic.

How did we manage to raise our life expectancy from 48 at the turn of this century to 78 today? We must be doing something right.

We realize now that we shouldn't have been panicked by the alar apples and the Chilean grapes. We've learned that aldicarb and aflatoxin are not life-threatening. But next time will we remember to keep our cool?

Today we can once more let our kids bite into a crisp apple, and we can pour another cup of apple juice for the little ones. And for dessert tonight let's cut ourselves a slice of apple pie, the kind that Mother used to bake.

10 Mind Over Malady

THE "PLACEBO EFFECT" IS REAL, the placebo itself is a fake. Placebo, in its Latin derivation, means "I shall please." Placebos used by physicians are inert substances that we give to patients, implicitly asking them to believe that they will prove to be "pleasingly beneficial."

But isn't it wrong for physicians to use placebos? I've often felt guilty when I've prescribed a medication that could be considered a placebo, feeling vaguely dishonest or even unethical. Yet I know that when I offer this pill to my patient, just as when I prescribe a powerful and specific drug, I give each with a full measure of my confidence, a strong component of the "placebo effect."

When the Food and Drug Administration tests a drug, placebos are used in "double blind" studies. If one hundred volunteers agree to try a new drug, fifty of them will be given the medication being tested, fifty a placebo which appears exactly the same to the volunteers (same size, color, etc.) but which contains no active ingredients.

In this trial, fifty percent or sixty percent of the people taking the new drug may show improvement. But ten percent or more of those taking the placebo may also report improvement, illustrating how the power of suggestion can have a very real therapeutic effect.

This control of the mind over the body through the power of suggestion has been used for centuries in various forms of meditation, in the silent repetition of a mantra, even in hypnotism. And there is plenty of scientific support for the concept that the mind can help or hinder the body in times of illness or stress.

Dr. Jan Fawcett, chairman of psychiatry at the Rush/Presbyterian Medical Center in Chicago, believes that mental outlook has a direct effect on physical health or mental illness. Fawcett refers to research that documents how "an optimistic attitude can affect the immune system to protect against illness and increase the numbers of 'killer cells' — the white blood cells that attack malignant tumors." And the reverse can be true: "Depression can lower the immune system's activity and possibly invite physical illness."

In a 1984 study at Stanford University Medical School,

Dr. David Spiegel evaluated the effect of emotional support on the prognosis of 84 women with advanced breast cancer. All were given the same standard cancer therapy, but 50 of these women, randomly selected, also were assigned to weekly discussion groups in which they were encouraged to air their complaints.

After a year Spiegel found the women in the emotional support group were experiencing less depression and less pain, and had a more positive outlook, compared to the women receiving only physical treatment for their cancer. More surprisingly, the women who received only conventional treatment survived an average of 19 months, while the women in the support group lived an average of 37 months.

Dr. Erich E. Brueschke, head of the department of family practice at the University of Illinois Medical School, believes that "physical symptoms can occur in response to life stresses in the environment, leading to gastro-intestinal problems, chest pains, palpitations, abdominal pains, muscular aches and pains."

It has been conjectured that 80% of the complaints patients bring to the physician's office have no identifiable organic dysfunction: the mind can make the body sick. The wise physician will accept this and may, with a clear conscience, resort to the use of a placebo to make the body well by treating the mind.

Nonetheless, many physicians consider the use of placebos unscientific, and the use of "sugar pills" deceptive. But Dr. Howard Brody, writing in the Annals of Internal Medicine, complains that "instead of listening to what the patient has to say, physicians may tend to look at monitors, lab reports and diagnostic images." Brody contends that treating the patient's symptoms is an acceptable first step before ordering a battery of lab tests and procedures.

Furthermore, any physician must admit he or she unintentionally — and unavoidably — utilizes the placebo effect by simply sitting back and listening, allowing the patient to "talk it out." No wonder patients often say, as they leave the doctor's office, "I always feel better after talking with you!"

Mind over malady? Placebo effect? Don't knock it — it works!

11 Avoiding Hearing Loss

IN THE "GOOD OLD DAYS" a gold watch was the traditional retirement gift for the sawmill worker. Perhaps the watch was to help tick away the hours, days and years of his retirement

A hearing aid would have been more appropriate. Practicing medicine in a north Idaho town for more than fifty years, I've observed the majority of the long-time mill workers retiring with a severe hearing loss. The screeching and snarling of the saws and planers almost always inflicted irreparable deafness on these men .

Today the Occupational Safety and Health Administration (OSHA) requires that any worker exposed to loud sounds in the workplace be provided with a hearing protection device. And not only do factory workers and airport ramp attendants gladly don such protection, some rock musicians damp their own artistic noise with ear plugs.

Most companies take the threat of hearing loss quite seriously. Many require pre-employment hearing examinations, and hand out fresh ear protection each day. Like hard hats and steel-toe shoes, ear plugs are now a normal part of the working man's attire.

Occupational hearing loss is not limited to the mill or the factory. If you've ever attended a disco or a rock concert, you might have concluded that the noise is literally deafening. You know why the rockers have that pained expression on their faces as they belt out their lyrics: Their ears hurt.

A recent article in The Hearing Journal lamented "the degree of ignorance that exists in our society when it comes to the workings and the vulnerability of our hearing system." The writer deplored the use of head sets, walk-men, "boom boxes" and car "superstereos" turned to a "full high." The "sound bashes," the "quake shakes," the "thunder on wheels."

Many teenagers are sublimely unaware that young people can go deaf. Or they rebelliously choose to ignore the facts. One 22-year old stereo buff boasted, "Sure I'm going partially deaf, but I blast mine as loud as I can wherever I go."

School administrators are aware that hearing disability can cause learning disability. Often, when a student begins failing in his studies, a hearing test may reveal partial deafness.

Kristi Reed, our local audiologist, agrees that high decibel noise can be damaging to youthful ears. She relates the unhappy story of an 18-year-old who had his heart set on joining the military, only to be turned down because of an acquired hearing loss.

Some years ago I visited Iran on a medical study mission. As we moved about in the beautiful city of Teheran I was impressed by the absolute quiet — no horns or car radios blasting in the air, no street music. Why, I asked?

"Ah yes," our guide explained. "Here in Iran the Ayatollah Khomeini has banned all music. He believes it to be the opiate of the masses." I thought — "What a pity, what a loss!"

This incident came back to me last week as our local high school band performed in concert. Far from being an opiate, the music these young people produced was inspiring, enlivening. How lucky these students are to be acquiring a love and understanding of the good sounds of music, and an abhorrence of the harsh, high decibel noises that can induce senseless hearing loss.

The Ayatollah's elimination of all music by dictatorial fiat solved the problem for Iran. But that won't work in our democratic society, though limits can be set. Our local government limits noise emissions to 92 decibels daytime, and to 70 decibels at night, far below the damaging limits.

This is a good start, but we need more than city ordinances. Being young means that you have the right to reject the advice and admonitions of the Establishment — parents, educators, governmental authorities. We need only to reflect upon our lack of success in discouraging smoking among young people.

But here are a few ideas that might work:

✦ Even though our youngsters won't willingly accept our advice, they very often imitate us, perhaps unconsciously. If we make a practice of using ear protective devices, they may follow suit. Also, we can point out that machine operators, airport workers, and chainsaw users all use ear muffs or ear plugs. These guys are not sissies.

✦ In some school systems rock stars who have suffered a hearing loss are willing to come before the school assemblies to tell of their personal unhappy experience. Students will listen to their peers.

✦ Kids hate to think about growing old. Somehow they must be reminded that exposing their ears to repetitive loud noises induces hearing loss and accelerates the aging process. That's called "presbycusis." Just the fear of catching it might discourage them.

12 Snore No More...Or At Least Less

TALK TO A LOT of people about snoring and you'll soon be swapping funny stories. There'll be good-natured tales of how friend husband's snoring will send the lamp shades swaying and the windows rattling. His snoring is variously described as raucous or rhythmical, lyrical or laughable.

However, many wives speak of their husband's snoring with far less flattering words. And they admit that their patience is wearing thin. "Joe's snores are driving me up the wall. I'm losing sleep while he lies there sawing logs. Doc, either we find a way to stop this noise, or he and I are splitting!"

Such murderous thoughts have been expressed to me by more than a few of these tormented ladies. One wife complained that her husband snored so loudly that the people in the next apartment complained. "Isn't there something you can do to quiet him down?" they asked. "Yes," she replied, "but it's against the law."

Just what is a snore? In medical terms it's the raspy, snorting sound created by the flapping of the soft palate in the back of the throat, as air is sucked in and forced out. The narrowing of the air passage back there makes the stream of air more forceful.

Numerous explanations are given for this phenomenon. Because snoring occurs most frequently in "back sleepers," in this position the tongue may be dropping back on the throat, causing air-way obstruction. Malformation of the jaw, muscle relaxation, nasal obstruction, polyps, allergies, sinusitis — all these have been blamed, without any one of them being singled out as the most probable cause.

Certain traits and physical characteristics are known to play a part. Obesity is invariably a factor. Thyroid insufficiency, "glandular problems," have been indicted. Overindulgence in alcohol and cigarettes share the blame. Emotional tension and the lack of exercise also are mentioned by researchers. Typically, these people are the "day-time sleepers," who can nod off the moment they drop into a chair.

Middle-aged men are the group most often accused by the wives who are the sleepless victims of this "listener's disease." But a good many women are hefty snorers as well. It just may be that (1) ladies snore more gently, or (2) men sleep more soundly, or (3) husbands are more forgiving. It's difficult to get an unbiased opinion.

Obviously, it's the spouse of a snorer who usually seeks a cure. A wide variety of remedies have been tried. Sewing a couple of ping-pong balls into the back of the pajama top has met with some success. The idea is, of course, to prevent the fellow from sleeping on his back. But what if he insists on sleeping in his birthday suit?

Chin straps, mouth pieces, taped lips, double-chin beauty caps have all been tried. Sedatives and ear plugs have been suggested for exasperated, wakeful victims. But what if the children should cry out during the night, or the telephone should ring? And sleeping in separate bedrooms is hardly conducive to marital bliss. It has been said that the best way to cope with a snorer is to fall asleep before he does. But that puts limits on love-making.

Our tendency as physicians has been to look upon snoring as a harmless but aggravating problem. But recently we've learned that snoring can have a dark and dangerous side. It may, indeed, be a pathologic sleep disorder. In its severe form it may result in "sleep apnea," which in rare instances could be fatal.

Sleep apnea occurs when — as the wife describes it — her husband has been snoring raucously, will suddenly let out an especially loud snort, then stop breathing completely. Then, after a lengthy and disturbing pause he'll resume his labored breathing and snoring. This sequence may recur again and again through the night.

During these brief bouts of sleep apnea the snorer goes into a period of what doctors call "hypoxia" or "oxygen desaturation." This simply means that, because the sleeper's breathing has stopped, there is not enough oxygen being pumped back into the blood stream. The respiratory center in the brain that regulates breathing temporarily fails to respond. Researchers feel that repeated episodes of hypoxia eventually can lead to brain damage.

There have been instances of sudden death resulting from sleep apnea. This has been likened to SIDS — sudden infant death) syndrome — because both of these catastrophic events result from an unexplained failure of this regulatory center in the brain.

There may be as many as 35 million snorers in America. Certainly very few are victims of sleep apnea serious enough to lead to dangerous oxygen deprivation. But any spouse who is concerned about the partner's snoring habits should obtain further information.

What must the apneic snorer do? First and most important, lose weight. Then, quit smoking and kick the night-cap habit. Obviously, any nasal or throat obstruction should be attended to. A physical check-up is in order, to rule out any significant physical ailment.

It's not surprising that these sleeping disorders have led to the establishment of "sleep labs," scientific laboratories where our sleeping habits can be carefully traced and documented. Tests in these labs can determine whether the snores and snorts could be the kind that could eventually lead to a dangerous sleep apnea.

Formerly the only relief for the severely apneic patient was a tracheostomy — a tube inserted into the front of the neck to allow air to pass by the obstruction in the back of the throat. That's pretty radical, but it could be life-saving.

Medications such as progesterone and protriptyline have been tried, but with little success. The use of intranasal oxygen has some serious drawbacks. Up until now medical management has not given us a solution to the problem.

Now we find there is new hope for these snorters and snorers, who have a serious degree of hypoxia. It's called "Continuous Positive Air Pressure" — C-PAP (pronounced "see-pap"), and in some cases this shows great promise. A special device is required, and it is used under the direction of a pulmonary specialist.

Snoring can be laughable, but in rare instances it can be serious, even life threatening. And so before a maddened wife whips out her Saturday Night Special, to silence the bedroom bedlam, let's remind her that, hallelujah, there now is medical help for this horrible human ailment.

13 *Young Fooled by Cool, Legal Drugs*

THE STAGE SETTING was simple, a microphone and two stools. One tall stool just behind the mike, another six feet back on the stage, on which an attendant had placed an ashtray and two large plastic cups. As the theater lights dimmed a middle-aged man with a boyish smile walked into center stage, puffing away on his cigarette.

Here was John Prine, popular folk and country singer, song writer, humorist, philosopher. Slightly pudgy, with a dimpled cheek, and a charming stage presence.

After thanking his audience for a tumultuous welcome, he rested his cigarette in the ashtray, then strummed and sang his way into the hearts and minds of his youthful listeners. He was at times happy, then sad, then angry. He railed at an uncaring society.

Each time he finished a song he would turn and walk back to the other stool, where he would sip liquid from the two plastic cups, then re-light his cigarette, drag deeply from it, and blast out a great billow of smoke to float over the audience.

Throughout the program, following the enthusiastic applause after each song, Mr. Prine would sip his drinks, inhale his smoke, and return to the mike. The crowd loved him, and at the end gave him a standing ovation.

As I walked out of our local college auditorium into the brisk autumn evening, I struggled with my mixed emotions toward this performer. John Prine is a skilled musician, who has written songs with social significance, many carrying an important message to his listeners.

Yet it troubled me to see him smoke and drink between each rendition. For all his call for social change, what was the subliminal message these young people would take away with them? Was Prine telling them, "Hey, man, what I'm doing is cool?" Would his listeners presume that puffing and sipping would somehow improve their wits, or increase productivity?

Reaching home I clicked on the TV, and by coincidence was tuned to the "old film classics" channel, where Clark Gable and Bette Davis were lighting one cigarette after another. I was struck by how different that was from what we see on film today.

As I listened to John Prine that evening in his hoarse, husky voice, the physician in me naturally attempted a clinical analysis. Taking a look down his throat with a laryngoscope mirror, what would his vocal cords look like? Would they be stubbed with "singer's nodes" or inflamed by cigarette smoke? Would inspecting Prine's lungs with a bronchoscope reveal gray and black smirches of soot?

I recently was reminded of just how much our attitudes toward smoking have changed, when two of my emphysema patients, Eileen and Arthur, came into the office for check-ups. They weren't alone; as they slowly walked into the waiting room they trailed behind them their constant two-wheeled companions — oxygen tanks.

They grew up in the Clark Gable/Bette Davis era in which smoking was still considered chic, smart, fashionable. Before we learned the grim lesson that smoking causes emphysema, throat and lung cancer, and heart disease.

As a callow youth I smoked. I thought it made me look mature, sophisticated. Luckily, I gave it up, saying goodbye to that very addictive drug, nicotine. But, sadly, John Prine is hooked. He was obviously totally dependent, needing that help to get through his concert. We can only hope that through some miracle he dumps this addiction, before his voice becomes even more husky, and we are forever robbed of his remarkable talents.

I am confident the young people who whooped and whistled were applauding his songs and lyrics, not his between-song use of recreational chemicals. The wise members of the Now generation will not be bamboozled into believing that any drug, whether smoked or sipped, is chic, smart, or fashionable. Or cool. Or necessary for high performance.

14 Surprise! Kids Do Follow Adult Examples

IT'S THE OLD STORY of "nature" over "nurture." Are we human beings more the product of the genes we inherit, or of the environment in which we grow up?

A few years ago psychiatrist Herbert Leiderman of

Stanford University argued that the pendulum is definitely swinging toward "nature," away from "nurture." He contended that how people think and act — their very personality — is determined more by the DNA in their body cells than by the influences of home or society.

Following this contention to its logical conclusion would predict that whether we will be rich or poor, smart or stupid, aggressive or timid, law-abiding or criminal will be a result of the genetic traits passed down from grandparents to parents to children.

That's a rather convenient cop-out, isn't it? Our life's mold is set at the moment of conception, and there's just nothing we can do about it. This would lift a heavy load off the shoulders of parents, teachers, the clergy, the courts, the social agencies.

Most of us won't buy that. We are quite willing to accept the responsibility for guiding and shaping our children's character and personality. We also want to have some of the credit for turning out good kids.

A remark made in passing by my anesthetist colleague Jim Brinton brought this home to me in a down-to-earth manner. Each day Jim gently lulls patients to sleep at our hospital, but he really shook me awake when he pleaded, as we were chatting during a surgical operation, "Why doesn't somebody do something about those kids in the junior baseball league who chew tobacco?"

I was surprised and responded with something like "Come on, Jim, that can't be true." But several of the nurses in the operating room, mothers of such youthful baseball players, chimed in "You bet it's true — a lot of them think it's the thing to do."

Well, if it's true we must ask "why do they do it?" Obviously these youngsters were not programmed in utero to be tobacco chewers, like addicted crack babies.

Someone or something in their environment must have encouraged them to start to chew. I can't believe they were copying their parents or their coaches.

They were, of course, simply copying what they've seen their baseball heroes do on TV. The stars stand at home plate or on the pitcher's mound, their checks bulging with a huge cud. Then, like as not, these youths will see their role models hitch up their pants at the crotch, then nonchalantly spit out a big brown blob.

No wonder our youngsters on the local baseball diamonds indulge in "Chawin' tobaccer." Only now it's lumberjack "snoose," the round can stuff, so visibly displayed in the hip pocket. Advertisements suggest that it's harmless because it's "smokeless."

At a recent board meeting of the local cancer society, president Nancy Flagan commented that the American Cancer Society is undertaking a nation-wide campaign against the use of this "smokeless tobacco." The inherent dangers, so far not too well-publicized, are the development of cancer of the lips, tongue and throat. A lot more help is needed from the parents, the teachers, the public.

Unfortunately, kids have an abiding faith in their own immortality. If they give it any thought at all, they perceive cancer as something that happens only to other people, mainly to older folks.

In many communities, concerned parents and health care workers are advancing eduction programs about the dangers of using tobacco in any form, including "smokeless tobacco." But they can't do it alone. And, though on the surface kids are hard to persuade, and even though our children so often outwardly rebel at us, we should remember that parents, teachers, in fact all adults, are their role models. Ultimately, whether they want to admit it or not, they will copy what we do and say, good or bad.

Many years ago a Russian scientist named Ivan Pavlov

demonstrated that all our actions and reactions are the result of what he called "conditioned responses." The experiences we have, what we see, what we hear or feel, all combine to shape our future reflex responses. Impressionable youngsters, when they see their favorite big league TV star chew and spit, will follow that example. At the same time more mature adults, who have been differently conditioned, will find that in poor taste, even disgusting.

Those who argue that it's "nature," not "nurture" that has the strongest effect on the development of young people will have to accept some middle-ground compromise. It's true, our genetic inheritance is all-important to get us off to a good start in life. But once out of the womb, our character traits, our personalities, our conditioned reflexes are, without question, largely the result of our environment.

We parents and teachers, we are the somebodies who have the great responsibility of providing the very best "nurture" possible for the next generation.

15 Kids Will Lead The Way To Non-Smoking Health

THE PROPHET SAID, "And a child shall lead them." From what I've seen in our elementary schools, I might amplify the proverb to say that our children will lead us toward a healthy, smoke-free environment in the future.

Isn't it ironic to observe that our youngsters, even the first-graders, might be able to accomplish what we adults haven't been able to able to bring about during the past two decades?

They're not doing it on their own. A few years ago the

American Cancer Society, the American Heart Association and the American Lung Association cooperated in an effort to enlist the help of children in an educational program dealing with substance abuse — particularly smoking. The hope is the little ones will be able to influence older brothers and sisters, while learning an important lesson. Included were packets of information to teach "how smoking affects the lungs and how the environment affects health."

All this is happening with the enthusiastic involvement of teachers, who teach lessons of a healthy lifestyle, and bring the youngsters an awareness that will stay with them forever.

The importance of youthful learning came back to me as I re-read that delightful best-seller of a few years back, "All I Really Need To Know I Learned in Kindergarten." In that light-hearted book author Robert Fulghum gives us some important life-guiding commandments that, as he says, he learned while playing in the sand box. Here they are:

- Share everything — play fair.
- Don't hit people.
- Clean up your own mess. Flush.
- Don't take things that aren't yours.
- Say you are sorry when you hurt someone.
- Wash your hands before your eat.
- Warm cookies and cold milk are good for you.
- Be aware of wonder — remember to look.
- When you go out into the world watch out for traffic, hold hands, and stick together.

Fulghum insists, "Everything you need to know is in there somewhere. The Golden Rule and love and basic sanitation and sane living." If we extrapolate these simple concepts into terms we use regarding cigarette smoking and drug abuse, we see how aptly they fit.

We can hope this nationwide approach in our elementary

schools will succeed where our previous efforts were slow in achieving results. Because we learn from our failures, it's worthwhile to evaluate previous programs and reflect upon their lack of quick success.

To do this, I go back more than ten years, to when our Idaho Medical Association and the American Cancer Society cooperated in an effort to discourage smoking, especially among teen-agers.

Cancer Society volunteers went to high schools to put on programs and hand out brochures. A resolution was passed by the medical association condemning cigarette advertising, and urging use of a more effective warning on cigarette packages.

Though the public remained apathetic, these efforts continued. At the same time, the scientific community presented more information about damage to the heart and lungs by inhaled smoke, not only to the smoker, but to those within breathing distance.

Restaurants began to segregate smokers and non-smokers, and at airport check-in counters you were asked, "Smoking or non-smoking?" But the warning on the cigarette pack continued to say only, "Smoking may be harmful to your health" — not a very powerful or convincing deterrent. And cigarette advertising continued to glamorize smoking, especially for young women.

Early efforts began to show effect. The surgeon general's warning on the cigarette pack now states: "Smoking Causes Lung Cancer, Heart Disease, Emphysema, and May Complicate Pregnancy." Magazine ads are becoming less seductive, with fewer pictures of those slim, svelte, emaciated models, gracefully holding those long, slender cigarettes.

But girls and young women still constitute the only segment of our society showing an increase in cigarette smoking, and fewer boys are taking up the tough-to-break habit. Women seem to find it harder to quit smoking once they've acquired the habit and become addicted more easily than men.

Perhaps they wouldn't have begun if they'd learned about the bad effects of smoking when they were very young. Which is why educational programs in elementary schools are so exciting, and so promising.

16 *Peace-Loving, Non-Violent America*

NEWS RELEASE...On May 23, during Game 3 of the National Baseball Association's Eastern Conference Finals, Detroit center Bill Laimbeer seized Boston's Larry Bird — who wasn't so much as looking at him — by the throat and flung him to the floor. The next day, during Game Four of the National Hockey League's Stanley Cup finals, Philadelphia goaltender Ron Hextall nearly ended the career of Edmonton's Kent Nilsson by knocking Nilsson — who was blithely skating past Hextall — to the ice with a two-handed baseball swing of his massive goalie stick. Two days later, during Game Five of the NBA's Eastern finals, Boston's Robert Parish punched out Laimbeer, who was looking the other way.

By fortunate chance we were born into a highly civilized society here in the United States. We live in the company of peace-loving people, people who abhor violence. As American Citizens, you and I are rewarded with health, security, long life. Society protects us from harm in every possible way.

As infants we were immunized against illness, and as we grew through childhood into adulthood we were alerted to the evils of alcohol, nicotine and adulterated foods. We were warned about the dangers of highway travel and of drinking while driving.

In our culture we try to protect our children from physical or emotional abuse. The law deals harshly with adults who batter their offspring or their spouses. Teachers have learned that they had better not wallop their miscreant students, or the courts may descend upon them.

We show deep concern for our household animals. Owners who starve or mistreat their pets are publicly chastised. We have laws to prevent cockfights, and at least some of us are horrified at the torture animals are subjected to in the bull ring.

Out here in Idaho even the lowly (and prolific) jack rabbit gets sympathy and protection. Some time ago, when hordes of these bunnies chewed away at the field crops, the farmers got a little angry and took after them with baseball bats. Then the public was outraged and protested loudly at this inhumane treatment of jack rabbits.

Further evidence of our society's cultural progress is shown by our concern for the human participants in various sporting events. In the game of baseball, for example, the batter wears a solid plastic helmet with a flap down over his ear. This is designed to guard the integrity of the player's cerebral cortex should a 90-mile an hour "bean ball" inadvertently strike that area.

All the players are equipped with the most modern paraphernalia. They have spikes on their shoes to afford better traction. These spikes also help clear the way whenever a player is sliding, feet first, into second base. Managers give preference to second basemen who are agile and who can leap high to avoid the advancing spikes. Managers want to keep their players healthy.

In football the players are all well protected. They are equipped with firm padding for their loins and groins, and other vulnerable areas. And there are rock-hard helmets atop the heads of the 22 players in this war-like game. The use of these helmets to ram into an unsuspecting opponent's midriff (it's called "spearing") is officially looked upon as a naughty, unsportsmanlike activity. But it is acknowledged that this maneuver does discourage an opponent from being too aggressive. The well-meaning, health-oriented owners do make certain to have orthopedic surgeons and superbly-equipped ambulances at the ready to care for any broken bones, torn ligaments or brain concussions.

Another cultural activity in the sporting world is called "boxing." This game is played by only two participants. They dance lightly around the ring (actually it's square), jabbing at each other with soft, padded gloves. So far as I can ascertain, the sport is called "boxing" because one player tries to box the other into a corner of the "ring," where he can practice his gentle jabbing more effectively.

Here too, every consideration is given to the health and welfare of the players. They are put through a long and strenuous period of training in a "camp" (as in "boot camp"), where they strengthen their muscles, sweat a lot, and toughen up their fists by banging them against other human beings called "sparring partners." These friendly partners are paid well for taking their lumps and bruises and bloody noses.

Once in the ring at the final event the promoters are again most solicitous of the comfort and well being of the participants. The atmosphere is warm and cozy, tinged with the heady fragrance of cigar and cigarette smoke, with a touch of ethanol. The genteel sports enthusiasts who sit at ringside are privileged to yell such words of encouragement as "Hit the bum harder," or "Kill the s.o.b."

We are told this builds character. But we aren't sure whether this character-building is meant to benefit the spectators or the bloodied gladiators, who for 10 or even 15 rounds give and get the lumps that make boxing the "manly sport."

But how lucky we are to be born into a civilized society where violence is abhorred!

17 Positive Thinking: Good Medicine for Seniors

A HAPPY LITTLE DITTY titled "Don't Worry, Be Happy" a few years ago won the top Emmy Award for best song. It's catchy, toe-tapping music, expressing a laid back philosophy of life.

Songwriter Bobby McFerrin sends a simple message: When trials and tribulations beset you, when nothing seems to go right, don't worry, just be happy, soon the sun will once again shine bright. Positive thinking. Just what we need when the skies are overcast, and when we are trying to recover from a severe case of winter blahs.

But down at the office this particular morning, my friend Maggie wasn't buying any of that Pollyanna stuff, let alone any upbeat, soft rock song titles. More fitting for her present mood would have been, "Life is not just a bowl of cherries!"

"I think I'm falling apart, Doc," was Maggie's greeting to me. "Old age is creeping up on me. I have sore knees, a backache, I'm constipated, my stomach's upset, and I've lot all my get-up-and-go."

"How come we older folks have to put up with all these miseries, when we no longer have the gumption to cope with them? Why couldn't the good Lord have figured out a way to let young people have some of these problems, when they've got the vigor and vitality to handle them?"

Letting Maggie air her complaints, getting these troubles off her chest was good therapy — it's called mental catharsis. Moreover, there was truth in what she was saying. The elderly among us do have more than their share of lumps and bumps to carry through later life.

There are the aches and pains that affect the aging body. The osteoporosis that thins the bones, shriveling the spine, and predisposing bodies to broken hips and wrists. As the years roll by the aging blood vessels narrow and become brittle, putting the senior at risk for coronary attacks, strokes and heart failure. There is, in addition, a lessening of the body's immunity, increasing the chances of infections such as pneumonia, influenza, bronchitis, and the nasty viral diseases, such as shingles. Then there is the black cloud of mental depression that may settle down over the older person. All too often the thought comes to him that his productive life is over, that he is only a burden on his family and on society. He wonders if life is worth living.

Probably the worst penalty inflicted by the aging process is the older person's vulnerability to cancer. It seems grossly unfair that cancer picks on the elderly.

Just take a look at the statistics. The American Cancer Society estimates that this year 985,000 Americans will be diagnosed as having cancer. More than half of these will be over age 65. Nine out of ten of the patients diagnosed with colon cancer will be over age 50, and by far the majority of the deaths from breast cancer will be in women over 55. Lung cancer in both men and women is on the increase, and here again the death rates increase sharply after age 55. A man who lives over 65 has a 50/50 chance of developing cancer of the prostate. Don't you hate those kind of statistics?

How can a doctor say to his older patients, "Don't worry, be happy?"

But there must be some good news I can pass on to Maggie. Like telling her, first of all, that she can rejoice at just being alive. It was elder statesman Bernard Baruch who, when he was asked "How does it feel to be alive at 85?" replied, "Just fine, considering the alternative."

Remember, Maggie, that during the 20th Century our life expectancy has increased by leaps and bounds. Some of our grandparents didn't live long enough to get cancer. Many grandmothers didn't even live long enough to experience change of life. Now as we achieve a longer life we learn to accept these adversities as part of the aging process.

Moreover, the future is full of promise. As we learn more about the aging process we are finding new ways of coping with the problems that come with it. We now have a baker's dozen of medications to bring relief to Maggie's aching knees and back. Cancer research is bringing us new and better and gentler anti-cancer chemicals. And, thanks largely to the Cancer Society's excellent educational programs, we are finding cancers earlier, when they can be treated successfully.

Every now and then I will offer this challenge to an older patient: "Let's assume that a new magical serum has been discovered that would, abracadabra, make you 20 years younger. Would you go for that?"

Invariably the emphatic answer is "No!" Our elders, in their accumulated wisdom, accept the fact that life must go on. We can't go back. Way back in 300 B.C. Greek philosopher Heraclitus said it well: "We can never stand twice in the same river."

Moreover, I've found that most seniors are quite content with their lot in life. They remember yesterday with pleasure, they enjoy living today, and they're looking forward to tomorrow. They agree with Francis Bacon who wrote:

"There are four ways aging is better:
- Old wood to burn
- Old authors to read
- Old wine to drink
- Old friends to trust

So, just sing out "Don't worry, be happy!"

18 Appreciate Your Good Health Now

ALL TOO OFTEN we take good health and happiness for granted. Sometimes we need a moment of unhappiness, a period of pain, to bring back those words of wisdom, "He who has health, has happiness."

Isn't it too bad that it takes a painful experience, an illness, a stay in the hospital to teach us how lucky we are to have the God-given gift of mental and physical well-being?

One of my medical school professors reminded us that to become good and compassionate doctors we would first have to suffer a serious illness, or at least a painful bodily disablement. He recommended such a personal experience for each of us. He said we complacently take our good health, our freedom from illness for granted. The members of the younger generation, he said, cannot fully appreciate the bountiful healthiness they now enjoy.

Let's relate that to our present life style. It's true that we have come to believe that we are entitled to constant "wellness." We would like a pill for every ailment. We want to be able to trot to the pharmacy with a prescription for every sore throat, every skin infection. We accept the good news that we can have an appendectomy — or a baby — and be out of the hospital in 48 hours. The good life.

A few of you seniors can remember when a home in which a child was ill with scarlet fever would be quarantined with a red sign "Do Not Enter" placed on the door. Then at the end of the quarantine period the local "health officer" would come by to burn sulfur candles to "fumigate" the house.

Today that sounds pretty silly, especially to my younger colleagues. We now have an almost unlimited repertory of magic medicines to combat nearly every bacterial infection.

Almost every week we physicians read in our medical magazines about yet another antibiotic that's far more efficient than the one we read about last week.

It would sharpen our perspective if we could turn back several decades to the pre-penicillin era, when the son of President Coolidge died of "blood poisoning." The young man had developed a blister on one foot while playing tennis. That simple illness took his life.

A personal incident takes me back to the time when, as an over-worked and exhausted intern back at City and County Hospital in St. Paul, I spent two long weeks as a hospital patient fighting the chills and fever and delirium of lobar pneumonia. As my final doom seemed sealed, the attending physicians decided to risk trying a new experimental drug brought over from England. I survived by the grace of God and this earliest of the antibiotics, Sulfanilamide. Through this experience I took my first big step toward an appreciation of the precious gift of life.

Moreover, looking back to those days gives me a gratefulness for the magnificent progress medicine has made. Here is a flashback to illustrate my point.

Adjoining good old City and County Hospital there was separate building referred to only as "Contagion." We called it the "pest house." It was the isolation area where they put the unlucky patients who had communicable disease.

There we fledgling doctors would see the tuberculous patients who coughed up gobs of bloody pus from holes in their lungs. There we would get to see an elderly man, his body covered with pustules, as he lay dying of small-pox. There we would watch the labored breathing of a teenager, encased in an "iron lung." This was polio-myelitis, the terrifying "infantile paralysis."

Today the white plague of tuberculosis has all but disappeared from our continent. The doctors in training today will never see a case of smallpox, thanks to vaccination.

Tiny drops of vaccine on a sugar cube have wiped away the scourge of polio.

Thanks to childhood vaccination we will hope never again to look into a throat to see that gray membrane of diphtheria with its evil stench. And only rarely will we hear the anguished "hoop" of pertussis.

Now, thanks to antibiotics, we can stop the vicious "strep" bug in its tracks. Scarlet fever and rheumatic fever no longer hold any fear for us. An infected blister need never again take a young life by blood poisoning. The pneumonia patient may never need to spend a four-hundred-dollar day in the hospital, thanks to forty dollars worth of antibiotic pills.

A child born today can look forward to a long and healthy life expectancy. Because of preventive medicine, good living conditions and technological progress, that child need never experience those diseases that crippled or ended young lives just a few generations ago.

The Wonderful Body Machine We Live In

Introduction

WHEN I WAS A FRESHMAN IN MEDICAL SCHOOL, laboriously picking away at my assigned cadaver's embalmed nerves, blood vessels and dried up internal organs, in an anatomy lab that smelled to high heaven of formaldeyhyde, I questioned whether this uninspiring introduction to the practice of medicine should be required at all.

In physiological chemistry, my fellow students and I held our noses when we created ferrous sulfide, with its rotten egg stench. We couldn't help but wonder why we had to suffer such academic indignities, to get that Medical Doctor degree.

After all, we came to this school to become physicians, to be trained to treat the ills of living people. To learn how to listen with wisdom to pumping hearts, to lay our hands on aching abdomens and feel what might be wrong, to care for and to cure human suffering.

Now as I look back over those fifteen years of pre-medical and medical training, with the perspective of more than a half century of medical practice, I realize that medical apprenticeship was meant first to teach me how to care for people, and second to provide me with a basic understanding of the anatomy and physiology of the amazing human body.

My admiration of our bodies and how they function continues to grow with each passing day. And because the Latin root word for doctor is "docere," meaning "to teach or to lead," I gladly accept the physician's obligation to teach his patients about the human body, in sickness and in health. And, at the same time, to share with others a sense of the majesty of the human person.

I hope some of these essays may bring you a greater understanding of that wonderful machine that is your body, as well a renewed appreciation of the human mind, perhaps even of the human soul.

1 Bad Germs ... and Good Ones Too

MAMA HAD ONLY A HIGH SCHOOL education, but she surely knew the basic facts of preventive health care. She would tell us kids, "Now, you be sure to wash your hands, there are a lot of bad germs out there." She also told us about "the five-foot barrage," warning us to keep our distance from any person with a cold or the flu: a cough or a sneeze sends out a shower of droplets heavily laden with "bad germs" that could make us sick.

Mama may not have had much "book learning," but she had womanly intuition and common sense when it came to health matters. She also had an enduring curiosity, and would have been thrilled by the wonders of modern microbiology, the microscopic world of "micro-organisms" — the millions of bacteria, viruses, fungi and other tiny living things that inhabit our bodies, our skin, the soil we walk on, the air we breathe. But she might have been surprised to have learned that all the "germs" she worried about aren't all bad.

The first person to see micro-organisms was surprised to find them at all. In 1674 Anton Van Loeuwenhoec, a Dutch shopkeeper whose hobby was grinding lenses out of hunks of glass, found that by stacking several lenses together he could greatly increase magnification.

Out of sheer curiosity he picked some matter from between his teeth, and put it under his home-made microscope. To his amazement he saw some movement down there. In his journal he wrote, "I saw with great wonder... many very little living animalcules, very prettily a-moving."

It wasn't until 200 years later that Louis Pasteur proved that these little living "animalcules" were the cause of "sores and festers and fevers," and thereby established the germ theory of infectious disease. This knowledge led to the process of heating milk to kill disease-causing microorganisms, "pasteurization," the first step in the elimination of the great white plague, tuberculosis.

Although Mama didn't have access to penicillin or sulfa drugs, and she didn't know about the streptococcus, she did know about rheumatic fever, and that this disease could cause "heart trouble." Consequently, when any of us kids had a sore throat, "quinsy" or swollen glands, she made sure that we got plenty of bed rest, fluids, chicken soup, and tender loving care.

Mama didn't know about that "bad germ," staphylococcus, but she did know about cleanliness, soap and water, hot packs and poultices. And she knew that when the "laudable pus" in pimples or boils was released, the sores would begin to heal.

Had she lived on into the second half of the twentieth century, Mama would have been lost in wonder at the vast array of anti-microbial medications today's physicians have at their command to fight infection. In checking a recent Physician's Desk Reference I counted 457 different antibiotic and anti-bacterial medications available to your physician, to be swallowed, injected or applied locally. And we are getting new ones each week.

Now we doctors have not only the penicillins and the sulfas and the dependable old tetracyclines, but a variety of second- and third- and fourth-generation antibiotics. You might think that with all these wonder drugs at our disposal, treating illness would be as simple as writing a prescription. But some of these bad germs have proven to be pretty tough customers. After being stunned by one of the broad spectrum "shot-gun" antibiotics, these bugs often will get back up, flex their muscles, and prove they can develop drug resistance.

Doctors have learned that, rather than using shot-gun medications, to try to determine the exact name and nature of the bug that's causing the trouble. This use of culture and sensitivity tests is a more logical method of choosing the proper antibiotic for the particular germ, whether it be a staph or a strep, a bacteria or a bacillus, a fungus or a virus, a parasite or a protozoa. Then we can fire a single bullet, rather than a shot-gun blast of pellets.

The correct name now given to "bad germs" is "pathogens," and our aim in treating disease is to somehow immobilize these pathogens until your body's immune system can complete the job and bring you back to health. As we do this we take care not to upset your body's normal physiological balance; some of the antibacterial medications we use to kill off bad germs may inadvertently kill off "good germs." For example, the normal flora and fauna of good bacteria that inhabit your bowels, which aid in the digestion of food, may be wiped out by a course of strong antibiotics. This can in turn allow the overgrowth of yeast organisms, causing diarrhea, or rectal or vaginal itching.

Really, Mama had the right idea. Clean hands and body: "Cleanliness is next to Godliness." Packs of poultices until the laudable pus drains. Maintain that five foot sneeze barrage. Good preventive medicine, yesterday and today.

2 Pain, Real and Imagined

AT ONE TIME or another you and I have scoffed at a friend's aches and pains, saying, "It's all in his head!" Or we may have complained that "Joe is one big pain in the neck!" Surprisingly, both statements are true, and with scientific proof.

To understand this we need to consider the nature of pain, both what causes it and how we feel it. First we must accept the basic concept of a "mind/body connection," the belief that your "soma" — the Greek root word for "body" — is under the direct influence of your mind/spirit, your "psyche." That's the origin of the term used to describe pain or even illness strongly linked to a mental state, "psychosomatic."

Just what is pain? At a recent seminar at the University of Washington's Pain Clinic, Doctor John Bonica offered us this definition:

"Acute pain is a constellation of unpleasant sensory, perceptual and emotional experience of certain associated reflex responses and of psychological and behavioral reactions provoked by injury or acute disease."

That's a bit much for me to chew on. Most of my patients would simply say, "Pain hurts!" And, yes, pain does gives us distinctly unpleasant feeling. That may suffice as a simple basic definition, but what really happens when we suffer pain?

Let's get down to cases. When Joe's boorish words or actions make us feel uneasy or even irritate us, this gives us a "pain in the neck." In fact, Joe's behavior may have triggered a reflex spasm in the neck spine muscles, similar to the scruff hair on a dog's neck standing up when he's angry.

But the reflex action doesn't stop there. The tightness of those cervical muscles in the neck spasm sets off a physiological electrochemical response which stimulates the sensory nerve endings in that area. These tiny "nerve wires," the afferent nerves — flash messages (at nearly the speed of light) to the spinal cord, where special conduits zing the information on up to the brain.

Once the electrical messages reach that magnificent personal computer of the brain, they're distributed to the various functional departments of the brain — the cerebral cortex, your "gray matter," the mid-brain, the limbic system, the thalamus. It is these neural "regions," and not in the neck, that we actually receive the "pain" message Joe has sent us.

But that's only part of the process. As the computerized messages dart back and forth in your brain, some of these sensory impulses cross over into the action department. Here the special sensory receptors may convey, in addition to pain, a feeling of frustration at what Joe has said or done. Now we have an emotional response to the feeling of pain.

Reacting to this, a group of efferent nerves, the motor nerves, snap into action. They beep out signals that spark you into doing something. You may simply react with a show of disgust, or you may tell Joe to shape up or ship out. Then again, if his acts or words give you great mental pain, you may impulsively throw him a left hook.

In turn, Joe may retaliate by swinging a fist at you. If your personal computer inside your cranium is functioning up to par, in a split-second the sensory nerves in your eyes will tell your cortical gray matter that Joe hasn't taken kindly to your remarks and is preparing to send some knuckles your way. The possibility of impending impact activates your cerebellum to send some quick motor responses to the muscles of your neck and shoulders, enabling you to duck the haymaker.

But if your reaction time was a bit slow, Joe may succeed in sending a fist to your chin landing you on your buttocks.

Now your brain will tell you, yes, the pain you feel is all in your head and not in your gluteus maximus. And the stars you see are not in your eyes but in the occipital lobe in the back of your brain.

Amazingly, all these sensations, actions and reactions, all these sensory and motor transactions, have taken place in the blink of an eye!

Researchers at the University of Washington Pain Clinic inform us that pain takes various forms. There is good pain and there is bad pain. Acute pain and chronic pain. There is organic pain (linked to real, somatic distress) as opposed to psychogenic pain (it's all in your mind).

The acute pain that comes in response to injury can do a body good. A child draws back quickly as his finger touches a hot stove. His personal computer brain stores that memory: Hot stoves are a no-no. Similarly, when we sprain an ankle we voluntarily immobilize it, simply because it hurts to move it. Pain enables healing to begin.

On the other hand, chronic pain resulting from tissue damage, the uncontrolled pain associated with long-term illness, might be called bad pain. And chronic, unrelieved pain can actually retard healing and recovery. For example, too much pain in the post-operative patient can result in bowel distention, reduced urinary output, even delayed healing.

No longer do doctors and nurses rely on the "p.r.n." (pro re nata — translated: "as needed") method of pain control.

Rather than allowing the sensory nerves to send a constant barrage of pain impulses to the brain, we now block these pain signals by regularly administering medications before the pain sets in. Not only does that bring comfort, but it hastens the repair of the surgical wound.

Psychogenic pain, the pain that's "all in his head," carries with it the assumption that it's all imaginary. But if the master organ of our body, the brain, accepts the hurtful sensory impulses as pain, whether they arrive from the psyche or the buttocks, then there's no denying that those unpleasant sensations are very real: pain is what you feel that hurts. We conclude that when Joe gives you that psychogenic pain in the neck, when those muscles go into spasm, that sensation is recognized and recorded by your intracranial P.C. as pain, real pain.

You and your physician can handle such "unpleasant sensory, perceptual and emotional experiences" with a variety of pain therapies, including drug pharmacology, psychotherapy, behavior modifications, acupuncture, hypnosis, even neurosurgery. Each technique is specific to the problem, but all recognize that any pain you feel is "real," even if it's "only in your head."

3 Red-Blooded Health

"MY JOHNNY IS A RED-BLOODED, all-American boy," boasted my neighbor, implying that he's a rough and tumble kid, who regularly during his youth will bash his knee or cut his scalp, spewing out a scary, gory red mess.

Now if "red blood" means vigorous health, how has the term "blue blood," referring to aristocracy, crept into our language? The fact is that all of us, male and female, young and old, have our quota of red, white and blue cells, carrying out our normal, physiological functions. Inspecting your red cells under the microscope, for example, provides physicians with a wealth of information, not about your station in society, but about your health or illness.

The number of red cells present are one indication of whether you are in robust health. In the normal patient the proportionate count of the red blood cells (RBC's, Erythrocytes) is maintained at between four and four and a half million. If for some reason that count falls below that level, it may indicate anemia. An inordinately high count suggests a condition called "polychthemia".

The proper functioning of the red cells depends not only on their number, but also on the intensity of their red color. This ruby redness tells us the amount of iron in the cell, designating the "hemoglobin level." Hemoglobin is the stuff that picks up its load of life-giving oxygen while passing through the lungs, then carrying it to all the tissues of the body.

A loss of hemoglobin is defined as iron deficiency, "tired blood," and may result from an inordinate loss of blood for a variety of reasons, including excessive menstruation, and internal bleeding from ulcers, polyps or tumors. Iron deficiency also could be caused by an inadequate supply of iron in the diet, or from impaired absorption of iron as food travels through the intestine.

Red blood cells, like most all the cells of our body, do wear out and constantly need to be replaced. Each RBC will live for only only about 120 days, after which it will die and be discarded by the body. The "erythrocyte replacement factories" are in the marrow of the flat bones, the breast bone, the ribs, the collar bone, the shoulder bone, the hip, the vertebrae, and the skull bones.

As the bright red RBCs, suffused with oxygen, make their way through your arteries, they drop off their load of precious oxygen, and gradually lose their red coloration. Then, as they float over into venous circulation, they pick up a load of fat and sugar to be stored in the liver. In addition they take on the waste products of metabolism, such as nitrous oxide, the same stuff that comes out of the tailpipe of your car. This venous return side of the circulation is the slow, sluggish side of blood flow, presumably a characteristic of aristocracy.

The human body's circulatory system is truly an amazing

machine. Your heart pumps 5 pints of blood around your body at 70 beats per minute, a total of 105,000 heart squeezes in 24 hours. This works out to one thousand eight hundred gallons of red blood surged through your 60,000 miles of arteries and veins each and every day. And you weren't even paying any attention!

If you think that's astounding, wait until we consider those amazing white cells!

4 White Cells: Microscopic Body-Fixers

PRICK YOUR FINGER and out oozes a sticky red fluid, colored by the more than four million red blood cells in a single drop of blood. Because those erythrocytes keep us alive by supplying oxygen to every organ in our body, we naturally consider them to be the most significant blood component. We pay far too little attention to their fellow travelers coursing through our circulatory systems, the white blood cells.

These hard-working leukocytes go about their duties in a quiet and unassuming manner, and in far fewer numbers: six or seven thousand per drop of blood. But what important tasks they are asked to perform!

Under a microscope, compared to the round and robust red cells, white cells aren't much to look at. Not even white at all, they are transparent, almost colorless. And while red blood cells may live as long as four months, white cells may have a life span of only a few days, a brief but hectic life.

There actually are a half dozen different types of white blood cells, each with a special job to do to keep you healthy. For example, the leukocytes may assume a slightly different role from day to day, rising and falling in number depending on whether they are responding to stress, to exercise, to pregnancy, or to a fever.

The neutrophiles have a very specific and important assignment as your body's number-one infection fighter. Continually cruising through your blood stream, ever on the alert for a 911 emergency call, they act as your first line of defense against the invasion of illness. Once at the infected area they will pounce on the bacteria, kill them and devour them. Neutrophiles may even kill cancer cells.

The main function of the eosinophiles is to assist in the recognition and treatment of allergic ailments, common skin disorders and tumors, such as Hodgkin's Disease.

White blood cells can be good news, but they also can be bad. For example, basophiles predominate in certain leukemias and in a rare condition called "myeloproliferative disorders." (There's a nice word to remember to impress your friends).

Lymphocytes hold center stage in viral disorders such as infectious mononucleosis ("mono," or "the kissing disease"), and still another type of leukemia. Monocytes are seen in certain bacterial infections, as well as in monocytic leukemia.

Finally, the platelets, hundreds of thousands of them in each drop of blood, perform the very vital function of setting in motion the blood-clotting process. Cut yourself and your platelets will rush to the site to form a clot, a thrombus, to seal the laceration. (Sort of like that magic goop you can squirt into a tire to plug a slow leak.)

As a physician for more than fifty years I still often stop to reflect upon the amazing human body, a harmonious constellation of vital organs at work, all nourished, refreshed and protected by blood. Your heart pumping around 72 strokes each minute every hour for decades, whether you're awake or sleep. Those tiny white cells and red cells, coursing through miles of arteries and veins, carrying life-giving oxygen and food and protection against harm. And all directed by the world's most intricate computer, our brain.

5 The Blood Cell Factory Within Your Bones

"Gorbachev Wins Nobel Peace Prize" read the headlines. Then, a few weeks later, "Two Doctors Win Nobel Prize in Medicine for Work on Bone Marrow." Some of my patients were frankly amazed that bone marrow could be ranked right up there alongside world peace.

We can thank Doctors Donnell Thomas and Joseph Murray for sprinkling a little glory dust on an unsung hero — that mushy "stuff" packed inside the hollow cavities of your bones.

Before the Nobel award, most of us didn't give marrow a second thought. Oh we might occasionally glance at that hunk of bone in the pot roast as we readied it for the oven, imagining how the center would be softened to jelly in the next hour or so. And we may have watched old Rover gnaw away at a soup bone from the butcher, trying to get at that (at least to a dog) delicious inner stuffing.

In fact, if most of us gave bones any thought all it was as the interconnected skeleton framework onto which our muscles, tendons and ligaments are attached. As in the song, the neck bone's resting on the back bone, the back bone's hooked to the hip bone, the hip bone's linked to the leg bone.... We sit, stand, walk and run, thanks to our amazing skeletal architecture.

But there is another extremely vital function that our bones perform for us — the constant regeneration of the cell content of our blood. This amazing ability of bone marrow to produce new blood cells is given the tongue-twisting name of hematopoiesis.

All our blood cells — red cells, white cells, and blood platelets — have a limited life span. They are created, they do their job, and then they die. So, if we are to remain healthy, our supply of blood cells must be continually renewed.

And where are the blood cell production factories located? In the spongy red marrow found primarily in the breast bone, the hip/pelvic bones, the ribs, the collar bones, the shoulder blades, and the bones of the spine.

When we consider the vast and vital importance of these blood-producing factories, we can understand why these doctors could be be awarded the Nobel Prize for their bone marrow research. And when we consider the devastating effects when the blood cell production factory gets out of kilter, as it does in the blood disorder called leukemia, the research work of Doctors Thomas and Murray takes on great significance. Leukemia, once a child killer, now can be controlled or cured, thanks to many years of work by these researchers to perfect a technique to transfuse bone marrow.

When these two doctors began their research work some four decades ago, the logical approach for control of this cancerous white blood cell disease was to supply more normal white blood cells through blood transfusions. Unfortunately this technique provided temporary relief, but was not a cure.

The challenge they faced was that in leukemia some of the white cells, the leukocytes, suddenly change into wild, mutant cancer cells. This may be caused by some external irritant such as atomic irradiation, or exposure to chemicals such as benzene. These abnormal, "bad guy" cells reproduce madly, and by taking over the marrow put a stop to normal white blood cell production. That's why blood transfusions were only of temporary value.

After much work these two ingenious oncologists, cancer specialists, hit upon a great idea: They would transfer some bone marrow from a healthy patient directly into a leukemic patient. This was given the name of "allogenic" bone marrow transfusion (BMT).

Early attempts with this technique were again only partially successful. The doctors found that exact matching of blood types was essential. The leukemia patient's body might "reject" the normal cells and marrow, not letting them grow. Moreover, the cancer cells also would gobble up the transfused cells.

Back to the drawing board. Obviously, before they could succeed in transfusing the marrow it would be necessary to get rid of the leukemia patient's diseased marrow, containing the mutant white blood cells. That could be done by irradiation of the bones, or with toxic chemicals.

Now they also increased their efforts to make certain that the marrow donor possessed the exact same blood type and sub-types as the recipient, the leukemia patient. Not surprisingly, they found that most often the best matching donor would be a brother or a sister. If there were no available matching siblings, the search for a donor could be time consuming, often fruitless.

Recently, in an effort to circumvent the difficulties encountered in achieving exact matching, the researchers have resorted to using the patient's own bone marrow for transfusion. This "autologous" BMT involves taking bone marrow from the patient while the leukemia is in remission, then fast freezing it. The healthy bone marrow is later thawed and transfused into the patient, when the need arises.

This idea has suggested several other exciting uses of BMT, for example in some potentially fatal immune deficiencies (AIDS), certain types of life-threatening anemias, and perhaps other forms of cancer.

All in all the use of bone marrow to help the body cure itself is an exciting and promising new direction, richly deserving of what might be better called the Nobel Prize for Health.

6 Fingernails Fully Explained

HAVE YOU GIVEN ANY THOUGHT to your fingernails lately, other than to trim them? Have you accepted the ugly fact those 20 nails on your fingers and toes are — it's mildly painful to remind you of this — dead?

Dead? But every day our nails grow at least a little. And they seem very much alive when they send us a screeching pain signal, when we accidentally bash them with a hammer, or pinch them in a door. A little information about fingernails will resolve this apparent inconsistency.

The outer covering of our body — our skin — consists of two distinct and separate layers. The inner portion, the dermis, is the "living" layer, which contains the nerves, blood vessels, the oil and sweat glands. The outer layer, the epidermis, supplies the hair and the nails and what we think of as skin. This "dead" covering is continuously being added to from the layer below, and just as continuously is being sloughed off or — in the case of your hair and fingernails — snipped off.

It's easier to accept the concept that nails are really dead when we remember that they are composed of an inert protein substance called keratin. As keratinized skin cells are produced in the nail bed, which lies beneath the nail and back toward your cuticle, they are constantly being pushed forward toward the finger tip, there to renew the protective shield that you so blithely clip or file or coat with beautifying paint.

Anyone who has bashed his finger so badly his fingernail turned black knows that it takes anywhere from four to six months for a new nail to grow back. Happily for our barbers and hair stylists, hair cell replacement may take only a month.

Nail cell growth is most rapid during our middle years,

from 20 to 50. Nails may grow more slowly during prolonged illness, malnutrition, and starvation. Deformed nails may result from iron deficiency anemia, emphysema, and other chronic systemic ailments.

On the other hand, pregnancy and warm weather can accelerate how fast your nails grow. Nail-biting, typing or piano playing may also speed up the growth of your fingernails: Mother nature compensates for wear and tear.

Nails serve the obvious function of providing a protective shield for the ends of your fingers and toes. They are a great help in picking up smooth items, and in untangling a knotted shoe lace. Fingernails contribute an important dimension to the sense of touch. And they greatly enhance the fun of scratching where it itches.

Among the most common fingernail problems are hang nails and split nails. Hang nails are torn and ragged ends of cuticle, usually the result of excessive drying or the use of strong detergents. Infection of hang nails at the corner of the nail is called "paronychia."

Split nails may result from chronic illness, but more often are caused by overly long immersion in water containing soap or detergent. The best treatment is prevention in the first place: wear cotton dermatological gloves beneath your rubber gloves. Incidentally, in the past we recommended large doses of gelatin to preserve or to restore nails, but now this has been proven to be without benefit.

Down through the ages, long, colored fingernails have been status symbols among the elite. Egypt's Queen Nefertiti restricted the use of red nail polish to the members of nobility. In some ancient cultures such as China, men of the privileged class allowed their fingernails to grow out to long, grotesque shapes, to show they were not required to do manual labor. As a practical consideration, we can surmise that men with such long and twisted fingernails must have required help with eating, and with their excretory functions. I'm sure they slept alone.

7 It's a Right-Handed World

IT ISN'T FAIR. In fact, it's downright discriminatory. Lefties are branded with a life-long stigma.

In Latin class we learned that the word for "left" is is the root for the English "sinister," which means evil, suspicious, ominous. The French word for "left" is gauche, which in English now means wrong, awkward, tactless. And the Latin root for "right" gives us the words dexterous and dexterity, very positive terms indeed.

Not only is the dictionary against the southpaws, our figures of speech denigrate lefties. A "left-handed" compliment is smudged with insincerity; if a fellow missteps on the dance floor, he has "two left feet."

Our world is definitely set up for the safety and convenience of the majority right-handers. Scissors, hand-saws, can-openers and power tools are designed for right-handers. Only recently have left-handed and counter-clockwise tools become available.

Furthermore, lefties are said to be more accident-prone. A study involving 2000 students at the University of British Columbia found that left-handers are almost twice as likely as right-handed individuals to have serious accidents at work or on the highways.

One of the most surprising findings of this study was that the frequency of death from auto accidents, among drivers under the age of forty, was significantly higher in the population of left-handed people. Why? The researchers theorized that when a driver is startled into making a sudden move to avoid an accident, he'll jerk the steering wheel in the direction of the dominant hand. This would mean panicked lefties tend to swerve into oncoming traffic.

What causes people to favor their left-hand, in a right-handed world? Is the tendency inherited? Does it skip generations? Is it in the genes and the DNA that are "handed" down to use by our parents?

From studies of thousands of children we know that if both Mom and Dad are right-handed, there is less than a one in ten chance any of their offspring will be left-handed. If the father is a lefty there is little change in that percentage, but a left-handed mother raises the chance to one in five. If both parents are left-handed, there is a 40% chance that their children will be lefties.

Some researchers believe left-handers are more subject to nervous disorders such as insomnia, depression, dyslexia and schizophrenia. But, at least so far, such conjectures have been difficult to prove, because of the additional, complex and powerful forces of environment and inheritance.

Our brains are divided into two lobes, or hemispheres, the right and the left. In each of our skulls one of these lobes has a somewhat larger supply of nerve fibers, rather like bundles of tiny wires, leading to other parts of our body, and that side is thought to be the dominant hemisphere. "Motor" nerves carry the impulses that cause our muscles and organs to work, while "sensory" nerves send messages back and forth from our sensory receptors, giving us the sensations of vision, hearing, smell, touch, and taste. At the same time, they coordinate mind and body functions.

As these nerve fibers emerge from the base of the brain, to travel to their designated destinations in the body, they cross over from one side to the other. Thus the nerves from the right lobe control the left side of the body, those from the left lobe, the right. Because of this neural crossover, in lefties the right hemisphere dominates.

In most right-handed people speech is controlled by the left hemisphere. As a result, a stroke affecting the left side of the brain can cause speech loss, aphasia, and possibly motor weakness in the right arm or leg. But in 70% of left-handed people, the speech center is on the right; a left-handed person suffering a stroke usually suffers no loss of speech.

There are some other benefits to being a southpaw. Left-handed pitchers and tennis players, for example, have an advantage against right-handed competitors, throwing or hitting the ball toward their opponent from an unusual angle.

Moreover, the left-handed trait has long been associated with creativity — historic superstars such as Michelangelo, Leonardo da Vinci and Thomas Edison all were lefties. Major southpaw leaders also have emerged over the centuries, including Alexander the Great, Napoleon, Queen Victoria, George Bush and Bill Clinton.

Perhaps it's time we quit looking down our noses at lefties. A left-handed author, with tongue in cheek, offered this waggish observation:

"If the left side of the brain controls the right side of the body, and the right side of the brain controls the left side of the body, then one must concede that those of us who are left handers are the ones who are in our right minds!"

Touché!

8 *Your Quietly Efficient Lymph System*

THE ENGINE UNDER THE HOOD of your car runs on two liquids: the gasoline which supplies the power, and the antifreeze and oil which protect the engine. With a slight stretch of your imagination you can think of your body as a wonderful mechanism which also is dependent on two liquids, blood and lymph.

When we were kids, cut fingers and nose-bleeds introduced us at a (literally) tender age to blood, but this stuff called lymph is a less familiar body fluid. You may have seen a drop of yellow, oily liquid oozing from a skin abrasion, a burn, or from beneath a scab; that was lymph, even if you didn't know what to call it.

Another reason we are more familiar with blood is because you can see the blood vessels just under your skin. For example on the back of your hand, or on the inside of your wrist. Furthermore, most of us know to give blood credit for keeping us alive by transporting oxygen and food to every cell in the human body.

Lymph, on the other hand, goes about its business less visibly, circulating through our bodies almost unseen through a system of tiny, filmy vessels. Lymph makes its presence known only when there's trouble brewing within our bodies.

Lymph contains a specific type of white blood cells, lymphocytes. One primary function of the lymphatic system is to absorb fat and proteins from the digestive tract, then to spread them throughout our bodies to provide nourishment, and to keep the cells functioning smoothly. The fat content of the lymph gives it its oily consistency.

The lymphocytes have two other vital assignments. One is to fortify our immune system against disease, and the other is to combat infection, wherever in your body that may occur. Each of these separate activities is handled by two specialized lymphocyte sub-groups, the beta cells and the T-cells.

The beta cells are protective. They provide us with immunity against bacteria, viruses, even cancer, by manufacturing protective "antibodies" to ward off diseases before they can take hold. This function occurs throughout the lymphatic system; sometimes when you're sick your lymph nodes swell up in your neck, under your arms or in your groin.

The T-cells are a totally different breed of cat, nicknamed "killer cells" by doctors. T-cells continuously move around the lymphatic stream, like hired guns, ready to zap bad bugs wherever they find them. This amazing dual capability of lymphocytes is one of the best kept secrets of human body function.

If your body is confronted by a fulminating infection, or by a cancer cell invasion, an army of white blood cells moves in to answer the 911 call. For example, if a cut on one of your fingers becomes infected, you know it because of the redness, swelling and maybe even pus at the site of the laceration. It may look bad and be mildly painful, but it's just an accumulation of lymph and white cells doing their duty.

If the infection progresses you may see red streaking up your arm, as the inflammation follows the path of the lymphatic vessels, in a condition sometimes loosely referred to as "blood poisoning." As a child you may have received a similar signal that your lymph system was functioning well if, when your tonsils became infected, your lymph glands in your neck puffed up to act as barriers to the spread of the infection.

It is when the beta cells are unable to pump up enough protective immunity that we are faced with such a cruel disease as AIDS, caused by the "human immunodeficiency virus" (HIV). These nasty viruses kill the lymphocytes by making a rear attack (maybe that's why they are called "retro-viruses"), overwhelming the protective white cells before they can fend off the infection.

On comparatively rare occasions the wonderfully beneficial white cells go berserk, producing such deadly diseases as leukemia, lymphoma and Hodgkin's Disease. Fortunately, this happens very seldom. For most of us, most of the time, the white cells in the lymph system are unsung heroes, invisibly keeping us healthy in a disease-filled world.

9 Breasts Versus Brains

IF YOU ARE ABLE TO READ this you fall into the scientific category of Homo sapiens, a term derived from the Latin words for "wise man." Because of our brainpower we have arbitrarily placed ourselves on the top rung of the animal kingdom ranking. But in fact we human beings are grouped with certain other creatures not because of our brains, but because we have breasts.

Sorting all living things into nice, neat categories was a particular passion of a Swedish botanist named Linnaeus, who in 1758 decided that there should be a classification called "mammalia," comprised of the warm-blooded animals who suckle their young.

Almost every school-child knows that cows, dogs and pigs are mammals, but not many know that huge female whales and tiny female bats also breast feed their babies: in this otherwise diverse grouping of animals, size and shape are not determining factors. Neither are legs necessary for an animal to be included in the genus mammalia: whales have fins and swim, bats have wings and fly.

Beyond such logical scientific classification based on breasts, in American culture there seems to be a large amount (no pun intended) of breast celebration. Page after page in Cosmopolitan, Red Book or Playboy features what might be called mammary adulation. As a result of this fixation, grade school girls just can't wait until Mom agrees to buy them training bras.

The basic and laudable physiological function of women's breasts is to supply nutrition for a newborn infant for a limited period of months. After the mother has borne and nursed her children, for the rest of her days she must cradle her breasts in the cups of a bra, discreetly covered with clothing. In warm weather we men can strip to the waist anytime, to enjoy the cool breeze and the sunshine; it doesn't seem fair.

What is the basis for this fascination, this fixation with the female breast? Could there be a lingering emotional attachment dating back to the bonding we experienced when we were nursing? A feeling of loving warmth and privacy as we cozied up to a mother's bosom? A male possessiveness? Even the terms for "mother" in English (as well as in other languages), reflect our association of mothering with the mammary glands, in words such as Mama, Ma and Mom.

In cold, scientific light the mammary glands lose some of their glamour, being derived from the lowly oil-producing sebaceous glands that reside in the skin alongside our sweat glands. And though breasts often are an important part of a woman's self-image, they actually are external appendages, seemingly an evolutionary afterthought.

In spite of their external location, a woman's breasts function in amazing hormonal harmony with the rest of the body, and often in most mysterious ways. Only seconds after a woman has given birth to a hungry baby her breasts respond to the command sent out by the pituitary gland in the brain. A chemical message, in the form of the hormone prolactin, tells the breasts "Make milk now." Then, as the mother's nipples become erect and the infant begins to nurse, the pituitary sends out another hormonal signal to the uterus, forcing it to clamp down in order to expel the afterbirth. Mother Nature thought of everything!

Though female breasts are given a quite noble role, they also are beset with a host of problems, major and minor. Most women are acutely aware of sore breasts and tender nipples at the the time of their monthly period. Some women who choose to breast feed may suffer from breast engorgement or breast abscesses in the post-partum period. Benign fibro-cystic nodules can confuse and worry some women, who fear they have cancer — mammograms can quickly and clearly tell the difference.

Because the human race several million years ago assumed the upright position, walking on two legs instead of four, the female breasts may tend to droop in response to the law of gravity, requiring artificial support. Heavy breasts may cause backaches, as well as bra-strap pain. The bra-less jogger may develop aching breasts called "mastalgia," and sore, tender "jogger's nipples."

In Greek mythology the Amazons were a band of feisty females, whose culture excluded men. Perhaps because of this they held breasts in low esteem, quite in contrast to contemporary American culture. In fact, these Amazons would simply lop off a breast if it obstructed their ability to draw back a bowstring. Now that's true pragmatism!

10 Stuttering

WINSTON CHURCHILL, JIMMY STEWART, Aristotle, Marilyn Monroe and Moses. What could all these people possibly have in common? All were stutterers, and from their youth suffered the anguish of ridicule, the embarrassment and frustration of not being able to easily complete words and phrases in normal conversation.

Today there are at least two million stutterers in the United States, yet scientists still don't completely understand why some people stutter. They can't explain why boys are four times as likely to stutter as girls, and why twins are significantly more likely to be stutterers.

Left-handed people also seem to be more likely to be stutterers, so researchers have tried to find the cause in the nerve pathways connecting their right and left brain hemispheres. In around seven of ten left-handers, speech is controlled on the left side, just as it is in all but a few right-handers. But speech control for the remaining 30% of lefties is shared by both the left and right hemispheres. Just as the cross-over wires connecting AT&T and Sprint occasionally misdirect your message, it's possible the nerve fiber "wires" connecting the speech centers in their right and left hemispheres can get tangled, contributing to stuttering.

Incidentally, in case you're thinking left-handers are somehow deficient, I refer you back to section seven in this chapter, where I note that left-handers are over-represented among the outstanding creative and political leaders of the world.

While nerve specialists search for clues in the brain's wiring, behavioralists believe stuttering is a learned behavior that can be un-learned. One speech pathologist I know, who helps stutterers and was one himself, tells me that 85% of all stuttering can be cured if properly approached early in life.

Speech therapists place part of the blame for childhood stuttering on the family environment, which is to a large extent shaped by parents. They don't feel parents cause stuttering, but say that if a child is predisposed toward stuttering, how mothers and father relate to their children can trigger it.

For example, if parents push their son or daughter to be a perfectionist, when the child speaks his or her tongue, lips and throat may tense up, producing a hesitant stammer or a stutter. Therapists instruct parents, teachers, brothers, sisters and playmates never to ridicule a child's difficulty in speaking, but instead to simply ignore it.

The plight of stuttering is as old as human speech. Aristotle stuttered, but believed the problem was caused by a malfunctioning tongue, which he treated by swirling hot wine around in his mouth — perhaps this relaxation technique worked to some extent. The story goes that Demosthenes, that great Greek orator, improved his speaking ability by striding along the seashore with his mouth full of pebbles, shouting against the roar of the waves.

Speech therapists today teach stutterers to use "starting sounds" before beginning to speak. Winston Churchill used this technique successfully, evident in recordings of his speeches: "M-m-m-m we shall fight them..."

Stutterers use other tricks as well. Some tap out a rhythm with their fingers, or before speaking take a long, deep breath. Another technique that works for some is speaking very slowly, or in an unnatural voice. Interestingly, some people stutter in some situations, but not in others: Jimmy Stewart and Marilyn Monroe didn't stutter when they spoke their lines on the movie set, but did when they cameras weren't rolling. Stutterers don't stutter when they're singing.

If you feel your child is developing a stutter, there's quite a bit you can do yourself to ease the problem. Talk more slowly, use simple language and shorter sentences. Listen patiently, so that your child knows it's okay to take time to talk and to make mistakes.

Avoid commands like "slow down" or "try again." Be careful not to convey subtle disapproval; even a wrinkled nose or a lifted eyebrow can increase a child's insecurity, causing tension which can stimulate stuttering. Above all, don't interrupt; give your child a chance to finish, even though you feel embarrassed by his or her hesitations. The relaxed, patient approach usually succeeds.

This method works with adults as well, but because long-established habits are more difficult to correct, the path to success is more arduous. Yet speech therapists report that, with time and dedication to these various training techniques, stutterers can learn to speak without hesitation.

11 Hernias

As HENRY WALKED into my examining room with a worried look on his face he blurted out "Doc, I think I've got a rupture." His description of the symptoms was simple: "The other day I noticed something pooching out down there," and he pointed to his groin.

Henry's amateur diagnosis turned out to be accurate; he was suffering from what is technically called an "inguinal hernia," one of several varieties of "ruptures" which have afflicted the human race since man assumed the upright walking position.

In most simple terms a hernia is a bulging out of intra-abdominal contents, most usually the bowel, through a weak spot in the abdominal wall. It's like a bulge in a bicycle tire, when the air-filled inner tube pushes out at a weak spot in the tire wall.

The groin is the most common site for hernias, though they may occur in a number of locations. At the belly button they are called "umbilical" hernias, in the upper abdomen "epigastric" hernias. A rupture at the site of an operative incision is called an "incisional" or "ventral" hernia.

Hernias may be present at birth, such as the umbilical or inguinal hernias occasionally seen in infants and children. These hernias may heal spontaneously; if not, they respond nicely to simple surgery.

Ruptures that develop later in life may be caused by a weakening or spreading of the abdominal wall. Obesity may be a contributing factor, and a lack of exercise can induce a softening of the tissues which support the wall and hold everything in. Old age or poor nutrition also can contribute to a weakening of the the abdominal wall.

Henry's inguinal hernia is by far the commonest type of rupture in men. This is simply because, over thousands of years, Nature transplanted the male reproductive apparatus to the outer surface of the body. Male testicles were originally intra-abdominal organs, and this history is evident in the development of a baby in its mother's womb. When the male fetus is three to four months old its tiny testicles begin to grow, then gradually move down to their final resting place in an external bag — the scrotum.

Trailing behind the testicles in their downward course is the spermatic cord, the life-line that carries the blood vessel and the nerves, along with the tube that transports the sperm to the outside. The opening in the abdominal wall through which these structures pass is called the inguinal canal, and this is a spot through which other intra-abdominal contents can "herniate." If there is a weakness in the abdominal wall, ruptures can be induced by increased intra-abdominal pressure, caused by such stresses as a persistent cough, heavy lifting, or straining to urinate or defecate.

As a hernia "pooches out" through the weak spot, it forms a sac which progresses down the inguinal canal, often carrying the a loop of the intestines with it. As time goes on this sac and its contents may proceed all the way down into the man's scrotum, creating serious discomfort as well as some health risks.

Women are less likely to develop this type of hernia because the female groin area presents a different anatomic make-up. There still is an inguinal canal but no spermatic cord, only a ligament that supports the uterus. As a result, in adult women the canal becomes totally obliterated, presenting little potential for herniation.

Women do have a somewhat greater chance of developing a different type of a groin rupture, a "femoral" hernia. This is partly because, in the wider female pelvis, there is a region of greater weakness in the abdominal wall where the large femoral blood vessels pass from the abdomen down into the leg. These vulnerable spots may be further weakened by increased intra-abdominal pressure during pregnancy.

The diagnosis of a hernia is generally straightforward: the bulge can be seen and touched. If the intestine has come down into the hernia a bubbling can be heard. A physician's finger probing into the hernial sac can discern the hole in the abdominal wall. A protruding bowel usually can be pushed back into the abdominal cavity, or it will drop back in spontaneously when the patient lies down.

The treatment is surgical repair, accomplished under local, spinal or general anesthesia. Medicare and health insurance companies now require that hernia operations be done as a "out-patient" procedures, unless there are important medical reasons which might justify hospitalization.

Hernia repair usually can be scheduled as an "elective", operation. But emergency surgery may be required when a loop of intestine becomes stuck — "incarcerated" — in the hernia sac so that it cannot be pushed back into the abdominal cavity. This can result in a bowel obstruction which, if not promptly released, can lead to strangulation of the intestine and its blood supply, ultimately producing gangrene.

Hernias — ruptures — can be simple or they can be serious. Henry was smart to seek help when he saw "something pooching out down there."

12 *Your Skin Has Holes In It (Thank Goodness)*

"PATCHES" ARE A NEW WAY for people to successfully quit smoking. They don't work for everyone, but for many are effective. Yet like so much in modern life, people they've benefitted didn't spend much time considering how anti-smoking patches such as Habitrol and

Nicoderm help in the cure. How can something you stick to the outside of your skin have any effect on your internal cravings for nicotine?

Traditionally we have taken our medicine by popping a pill or downing a teaspoon of syrupy elixir, but in the past few years patches (technically called "transdermal drug delivery systems") have become quite popular. The anti-smoking patches are simply the latest application of this technique. There is a patch that can be placed behind the ear to prevent motion sickness, vertigo and nausea. Some patients wear medicine-dispensing patches to prevent angina attacks. Women can now get their supplementary dose of a female hormone by way of a skin patch.

There are several reasons for using patches in place of pills or shots. People may have trouble swallowing pills, may frequently forget to take their medications, or may simply get tired of taking oral medications day in and day out. As for shots, in most cases they need to be administered by a physician or a nurse...and they can hurt.

It's easy for us to accept that a pill can be absorbed into our blood stream from our stomach or intestine, just as food and liquids are assimilated. (Although one young patient wondered how the aspirin tablet she sent down her throat managed to turn around and travel up to her brain to cure her headache.) To understand how medications dispensed from patches attached to the skin achieve their purpose, let's review the anatomy of our skin.

Your skin has three basic layers, the epidermis, the dermis, and the subcutaneous fat layer. The epidermis is the outer protective covering, composed of tough, flat skin cells. This is a permeable layer which allows the absorption of liquid substances. Below the epidermis is the dermis, a supportive layer containing fibrous strands and jelly-like collagen. It is richly endowed with blood capillaries, lymph vessels and sensory nerves. Beneath this is the subcutaneous fat layer, which supplies padding for the dermis and the epidermis, as well as support for the blood vessels, the lymph ducts, and the nerves.

Medication "released" from a patch enters the body through the permeable epidermis, and then moves to the next lower level into the blood-carrying capillaries. What is unique and especially beneficial about these patches is their ability to release their medication slowly: pharmaceutical companies have devised ways of controlling the rate at which the medications will be diffused through the skin.

For example, a heart medicine may be dispensed over a 12-hour period, making it necessary to apply a new patch only every 12 hours, morning and evening. A motion sickness patch applied behind the ear remains functional for three days. Female hormone patches are applied twice a week. A blood pressure patch lasts a week.

The pharmaceutical industry deserves credit for having gone through extensive animal research to bring us these trans-dermal drug delivery systems. Further efforts are being made to supply other medications through skin patches, always in the hope of eliminating pills and shots.

Patches aren't the only alternative. Already ophthamologists supply medication by eye drops, and gynecologists may use a nose spray for the control of endometriosis. Female hormones can be absorbed into the body from estrogen cream placed in the vagina. For the treatment of asthma or emphysema, medications can be inhaled directly into the lungs, rather than being taken by mouth.

Ah, the wonders of the human body! It's still a mystery to me how the active ingredients in a suppository placed in the rectum can travel up to the brain and then down to the stomach to relieve nausea and vomiting. Yet even though we may not know exactly how it works, we can surely be glad it does!

13 Bravo For Your Bottom

Yesterday I overheard my 10-year old grandson, in a fit of frustration, call one of his playmates a "butt-head." My son, his dad, swiftly reprimanded him, reminding him that such name-calling will not be tolerated in gentlemanly, civilized conversation.

As a grandad several times over, I long ago learned to stay out of family discipline. But as a physician I winced at yet another instance of this important part of our anatomy, the buttocks, being used as a negative metaphor. It's unfortunate that the rump should be the butt of such denigration.

The French more politely refer to our "posterior" as the "derriere," meaning "from the back." Literal Germans refer to our bottoms as "sitz fleisch," literally "sitting meat," hardly a complimentary term for this most important part of our bodies.

Yet in some parts of the world buttocks are accorded more respect, even admiration. The bushmen of Africa are great fans of generous, fatty buttocks on their bushwomen. Such curvaceous physical attributes even have been given a scientific name, steatopygia. Modern anatomists refer to elegantly shaped buns as "callipygian."

But in American English we may tease a person and make him the "butt" of our joke. We may angrily tell someone to "butt out." We condescendingly proffer a "pat on the butt."

Furthermore, we tend to take our derrieres for granted. Do we ever say thanks to Our Creator as we back through a swinging door, "butting" it open as we pass through? In the evening after a hard day's work, as we drop into our chair, do we give a second thought to that magnificent anatomical pillow we carry around behind us?

My well-worn Gray's Anatomy reference book tells me

that "the basic component of the buttock is the gluteus maximus, the most superficial muscle in the gluteal region, and the largest muscle in the body. Hidden beneath this major muscle are two smaller muscles, the glutei media and minimus."

A generous layer of fat lies over these muscles, providing a padding for comfort when sitting on hard chairs. The skin of this area is generously supplied with sensory nerves, making it extremely sensitive to patting, pinching and spanking, plus to what in the vernacular is known as "goosing."

But these muscles are for much more than just sitting on. As they extend to the thigh, the hip bone and the lower back, they help maintain our erect posture, stabilizing our hips and lower back while we are standing or walking. For greater stability we can voluntarily squeeze these muscles, and they also will automatically contract to maintain our balance. And the glutei do help hold our pants up.

Deep within this group of muscles and their protective fatty covering lie the large arteries and veins which provide circulation to the lower extremities. Coursing down from the lower end of the spinal cord and far beneath these muscles is the sciatic nerve, the largest nerve in our body. When this nerve becomes inflamed or pinched we suffer that painful ailment called sciatica.

It is obvious that our posterior anatomy, so often ignored down there behind us, deserves greater understanding and approbation. Only when something goes wrong does our tush demand our attention. Because it is a hairy area, surrounded by warmth, moisture and bacteria, and an area often subjected to trauma, a hair follicle may become infected and produce a furuncle, a "boil." Only rarely the buttocks may develop tumors, abscesses, even hernias. For some unknown reason the skin area between the buttocks, the gluteal cleft, may break out in an itchy, eczematoid dermatitis, especially during periods of extreme nervous tension...and that's an area most difficult to scratch in public!

Now, having said all this, is it not time for us to show a little more respect for our gluteus maximus, media and minimus? To my grandson I will say, "Take not the name of your buttocks in vain, for these three muscles are your powerfully good friends when you shoot baskets or kick a soccer ball."

And you adults, especially if you're sitting down while reading this, might take a moment to say a brief bravo for your bottom.

14 Forgetting to Remember As You Grow Older

THE HEADLINE ON THE COVER of a popular "health" magazine announces, "Finally — A Memory Pill." Hopeful, you buy the magazine, only to find that the so-called "memory pill," with the tongue-twisting name phosphatidylserine, is still in the experimental research stage. Articles that tease then disappoint the reader on such topics of great concern remind me of our preacher when I was a boy, who would say "and finally," a half hour into his sermon, then go on for another fifteen minutes.

Memory loss is a worry I hear almost daily from my patients. "Doctor, Mother is getting so forgetful. Do you suppose she's getting Alzheimer's?" And then the very usual request, "Isn't there something you can give her?" Not only are the family members worrying about Mom, they harbor a poorly-concealed fear that they, too, will someday develop this dread disease.

First of all, let me dispel one common misconception: loss of memory and Alzheimer's Disease are two entirely separate and distinct clinical entities. Alzheimer's is an abnormal, irreversible (so far) disease process. Memory loss is a more or less normal part of the aging process, which an older person can slow by working at remembering.

To understand the mysteries of memory, it is helpful to compare your brain to a computer. A computer stores the information you load into it, and will manipulate that data and output new information when you punch the right buttons. Your brain also can perform those functions, but is capable of an additional and very sophisticated activity called "cognition."

The word cognition is defined as "the act or process of knowing; perception." That is, the activities commonly regarded as thinking, including recognizing, learning, imagining, and problem-solving. And basic to all these activities is remembering: memory.

As fundamental and important as memory is to thinking, exactly how memory works is not completely understood. Psychologists make a distinction between short-term and long-term memory, just as computers do. A computer stores information that's meant to be used right away, and then possibly discarded, on "short-term memory" chips called RAMs, for Random Access Memory. The long-term or permanent memory data goes into the "hard drive" or "hard disc," in the computer's "central processing unit," the CPU.

To make our "human computer" comparison, the Random Access Memory chips in the base of our brain are used for such disposable data as what we had for breakfast. You might consider this information as the kind of stuff we scribble on a scratch pad — the plumber's phone number, or some odds and ends we need at the hardware store. As we get along in years, our "mental scratch pad" information seems to fly out of our minds ever more quickly.

By contrast, the long-term information in your personal memory bank is indelibly imprinted on your brain's hard drive. This would include the vivid memory of your first kiss or, if you are old enough, where you were the moment you heard President Kennedy had been shot. Motor skills learned long ago also are stored on your hard disc — I recently amazed my grandchildren by demonstrating I can still ride a bicycle.

Computer experts can readily identify just where and how your PC uses electricity to store both long-term and short-term memory. But neurology anatomists so far can't do the same for your brain. They can trace the neurons and the synapses that interconnect the various locations in the brain that are thought to be our memory centers: the hippocampus, the limbic system, and the gray matter of the neo-cortex. They believe chemicals in our bodies, along with electrical impulses we produce, are responsible for the phenomenon of memory. But they can't yet explain exactly how it works.

The hard drive in a computer is sealed in a black box. On its spinning disc are electrical charges which represent the information poured into it. Yet so far no scientist has been able to "look into" the human black box at the base of the brain, to determine just where our cognitive abilities find their beginning. Exactly where in the recesses of our calvaria do we think and remember? Where in there do we learn to love, to have human compassion? For the moment, at least, this remains part of the mystery of memory.

15 How The Nose Knows

EVEN IN ADVERSITY WE CAN LEARN. A recent bout with cold-clogged sinuses taught me that I had been taking my sense of smell for granted. The loss of the ability to smell is called "anosmia," the temporary condition I suffered with that bad head cold.

Now that my sinuses have cleared and my nose is unplugged, I have a new appreciation of the need to smell. Until my recent olfactory awakening, my sense of smell ranked a distant last in the importance of my five sensory functions.

Today I can again delight in the aroma of new-mown grass, and enjoy the heady perfume of lilacs in bloom. Once again I find simple pleasure in sniffing that new car fragrance, or in inhaling the rich leather aroma of a new pair of shoes.

Although we may take such pleasure for granted, and relegate them to our subconscious, the advertising folks on Madison Avenue have long appreciated the importance of olfaction. They know that certain fragrances can act like pheromones, body scents that influence the physiology or behavior of other creatures of the same species. The objective of sexual arousal in the male of the human species is reflected in the names they have given perfumes such as Allure, Opium, Innocence, Capture and Temptation. A drop of delicate scent behind milady's ear will quicken a heartbeat, even bring hope of a loving embrace, a beckoning to a more intimate interlude.

Not so long ago, and far distant from such sensual pleasures, a doctor's sense of smell was an important tool in his diagnosis. A trained physician knew that typhoid smells of baking bread, that measles has the aroma of plucked chicken feathers, that a person in diabetic coma gives off a sweet apple scent, and that diphtheria has a pungent odor all its own.

When making hospital rounds the surgeon could smell the bandage to determine whether the wound was clean or infected. When a fecal smell welled up from the open abdomen during surgery he would know that the appendix had already ruptured.

Today, instead of relying on such unscientific observations, we would order a culture to identify the type of infection, and begin pouring in antibiotics. Identifying a disease by the sense of smell is a lost art, and probably just as well. Medical technology has replaced the nose as a way to identify what's wrong with a person.

That may be one reason why our sense of smell has received so little attention from medical researchers. Assisted by operating microscopes, eye surgeons often can restore sight. Ear specialists may use micro-surgery to improve hearing, and highly miniaturized electronic hearing aids now allow the hard of hearing to get back into group conversations, even at cocktail parties.

But medical technologists haven't yet provided rhinologists — the nose specialists — with a "smelling aid" to lessen the plight of the anosmic patient. Those who suffer from anosmia include victims of severe head injuries or of lead poisoning, individuals afflicted with certain rare nervous-system disorders, including some forms of epilepsy.

Nonetheless, nerve specialists have a pretty good idea just how the olfactory system works — or in the case of anosmia, how it fails to work. What we call "smells" are tiny pieces of sensory information, in the form of molecular particles that enter the nostrils as we inhale. Each has its own particular "character" — "Chanel No. 5" or "skunk" or something else. Once inside the nose these molecules stimulate nerve endings in the mucous membrane, which in turn send messages to information centers in the brain.

Some of these messages are fired off to a special little department in the brain called the olfactory bulb, which receives scent directives requiring some action. These specific messages are translated into "You are hungry" or "You are thirsty." Or even "That lady who just walked by has expensive taste in perfume!"

Other split-second olfactory messages are switched to another, very specialized area of our brain's computer, the limbic system. This is the seat of our memory and emotions, from which a particular aroma today may prompt a very graphic image of an experience long ago. For example, that morning more than forty years ago when you walked into your mother's kitchen, just as she took peanut butter cookies out of the oven. Or of that afternoon in the high school chemistry lab when you combined water and sulfer to produce hydrogen sulfide, but which your limbic computer recorded then and recognizes now as "rotten eggs."

This limbic system is given a variety of tasks. Under certain circumstances it may spark electronic messages to areas in the base of the brain, such as the hypothalamus or the pituitary gland, to stimulate the secretion of hormones that control appetite, sex drive, and body temperature. That's how a particular fragrance — of grilled steak, for example — can make us hungry. Or how a woman's perfume can arouse a man's sex drive.

Some limbic messages may flicker their way to the cortex, the outer layer of the brain where we do our "thinking," our cognition. This may give rise to emotions coupled with bodily reactions such as anger, fear or passion, or lead to conscious thought. Or even — with no conscious effort on our part — to release distant memories to bubble up into our consciousness.

My olfactory disability, caused by my plugged sinuses, was a temporary inconvenience. But when a person loses some or all of their sense of smell, their mental powers are proportionately diminished.

Furthermore, those poor people with anosmia have lost some of the precious pleasures of life. I hope that medical technology may soon be able to help them, so that they can salivate in response to the aroma of bacon and eggs frying, can luxuriate in the rich spring fragrance of lilacs, can smile with the pleasure of affectionate recognition at the subtle scent on a loved one's pillow.

16 Hormone Tour

FOR MOST OF US the word "hormone" has a sexual connotation. A woman approaching menopause asks her doctor, "Is it time for me to start taking hormones?" A man in his midlife crisis may begin to wonder if he needs more hormones.

To be sure, sex hormones are essential to our physical and mental well-being, but they are only one of the many natural chemicals which influence and regulate our bodies and minds. We are what we are, and we do what we do, largely because of the secretions of our ductless, endocrine glands.

Anatomists and philosophers in distant history knew about these little lumps of tissue scattered around in our body, and even suspected they had some sort of a regulatory function. They believed that because these glands have no tubes to lead their secretions directly out into the bloodstream or the body, their output is simply exuded throughout tissues like a mist. These wise and intuitive scientists called the secretions "vapours" or "humours," believing that in some ethereal way these substances affected our moods and emotions. They would determine whether we would be in good or bad humor, perhaps even whether we would possess a "sense of humor."

Endocrinologists of today concede that these assumptions were at least partly correct. Indeed, we now accept the fact that these hormonal secretions work their way through our bodies in much the same way as the fragrance of fresh-brewed coffee wafts throughout our house at breakfast time. Doctors know, also, that there are more than a dozen different ductless glands in various parts of the body, secreting over thirty very specialized hormones. Linked together in a feedback system, each gland can have an effect on other glands elsewhere in the body. Via their chemical secretions, the endocrine glands "talk" to each other.

If we were to take a tour of your endocrine glands we would begin inside your head, where we'd first visit the tiny pituitary, about the size and shape of a pea, located at the base of your brain. Then, just above and behind the pituitary, we'd move on to your hypothalamus and pineal glands. These three function as kind of supervisory glands, sending out directives to the other ductless glands elsewhere in the body.

Growth hormones secreted by your pituitary when you were growing up determined whether you would be long-legged or stubby. Another pituitary secretion regulates the body's water level, and the excretion of electrolytes such as salt and potassium from the kidneys. Once a month a woman's pituitary sends out a hormonal signal to her ovaries to release an egg. Another pituitary hormone controls uterine contractions during childbirth and milk production during nursing.

Moving south we come to the thyroid gland, located under your chin at the base of your neck. If you place your finger in the hollow just above your breastbone you can feel your thyroid move up and down as you swallow. This very important gland releases a hormone that regulates your metabolism, the rate your body burns up food to produce energy. Thyroid hormones also help maintain physical growth and mental development.

Buried in the thyroid tissue are the parathyroid glands, about the size of lima beans. These regulates the calcium level in your blood and bones. Too little calcium can cause a weakening of the bones — osteoporosis. Too much calcium can lead to calcium deposits or kidney stones.

Just below your thyroid, behind the breast bone, is the thymus gland, important to the development of our immune system. This gland takes part in the production of white blood cells, the lymphocytes.

Proceeding farther south, down to the pit of your stomach, we come to your pancreas, featured on fancy restaurant menus as "sweetbreads." Like so many of your body's glands, the pancreas has more than one job to do. It produces enzymes that aid in the digestive process, but it also exudes insulin, to regulate your blood sugar level.

Too little insulin results in diabetes mellitus, characterized by an excess of sugar in the blood and urine — hyperglycemia. Conversely, too much insulin can lower the blood sugar level, resulting in a rare condition called hypoglycemia.

Moving through your mid-section, to your flanks on either side of your lower back, we arrive at the site of your two kidneys. These vital organs filter your blood, and produce waste water called urine. Perched on top of your kidneys are two very energetic little endocrine glands, the adrenals. Though each weighs less than an ounce, they pack a hefty wallop, producing several dozen sizzling hormones.

The outer rind of the gland, the "cortex," generates the corticosteriods, cortisone-like hormones. The inner portion, the "medulla," squirts out the "emergency" hormone adrenaline, a substance produced in response to psychological or physical stress — the "fight or flight" hormone. We generate this hormone when we psych ourselves up to ask the boss for a raise, when we finally get up enough courage to ask that special girl for her hand in marriage, or when we react with remarkable strength or speed in an emergency.

Finally, situated down in the pelvic area are the sex organs, the ovaries and the testes, that produce the male and female hormones. These organs, collectively called "gonads," determine the timing and direction of sexual development, sexual capability, and the initiation and completion of the reproductive process.

From this brief tour you can see why the hormonal interrelationship of the endocrine glands is extremely complex, and why it is so vitally important for these organs to "talk" to each other: if one of these ductless glands gets out of whack, your entire hormonal balance can be upset.

Hundreds of years ago, wise men of the day blamed imbalanced minds and bodies on a soul out of kilter. Today we concede that our minds, our bodies (and our souls?) can be affected by hormonal dysfunction, not all that different from what the ancient sages blamed on bad humors.

Today we have tests to evaluate hormonal imbalances, and we have both natural and synthetic hormones with which to correct the problems. But so far science hasn't defined our "soul," or advised us how to test it or mend it. Which is probably just as well.

17 Your Thyroid Thermostat

A PATIENT WITH A HORMONAL imbalance usually is suffering from a deficiency in output from an endocrine gland. An exception is the condition of hyperthyroidism, a markedly increased production of the thyroid hormone, which throws the body's metabolism into overdrive.

No one knows just what causes this peculiar illness, or why it strikes women more frequently than men. In its early stages hyperthyroidism may be misconstrued as an acute anxiety disorder or a nervous breakdown. Occasionally it is mis-diagnosed as bulimia, because of the patient's rapid weight loss, even though they have not reduced the amount of food they are eating. Other typical symptoms of thyrotoxicosis are nervousness, irritability, flushing, and palpitations. Left untreated the disease can cause a bulging of the eyes, called exophthalmos.

There are now several highly technical tests used to clinch the diagnosis. Once that diagnosis has been made, several treatment options are available.

The first is medical management with a substance called "propylthiouracil," a tablet taken by mouth. This approach requires careful calibration of the dosage, and involves follow-up blood tests.

Another alternative would be removal of thyroid gland tissue, an option followed more often in younger people. Though this involves a comparatively straightforward surgical procedure, as with all operations there is some risk.

The third therapy option is the use of radioactive iodine in a liquid form. Iodine is drawn by the body to the thyroid, so when the patient drinks a glassful of a measured dose of the medication, the concoction knocks out the thyroid hormone-producing function of the gland. This treatment is so effective that in many cases the patient will need to take thyroid hormone pills for the rest of his or her life. Luckily, that's not too costly, and is as simple as taking vitamins.

The hormone supplied by your thyroid gland, thyroxine, regulates the rate at which chemical reactions occur in your body. When your chemistry is right and your thyroid is pumping out neither too much nor too little of this hormone, you are totally unaware of this regulatory function, as your body's motor purrs along at its normal rate.

But, when your thyroid gets out of kilter, it can create too much thyroxine, causing hyperthyroidism, described above. Or your thyroid can underproduce thyroxine, slowing down your body's engine in a condition called hypothyroidism. This more common disorder is characterized by extreme fatigue, cold intolerance, weight change, and dry skin and hair.

When a person suffers from hypothyroidism, all of the body's chemical processes slow down. The food you eat is burned less completely and you may gain weight. Even mental functions are slowed — to the point where you may have trouble balancing the check book.

A slower heart rate may lead to impaired circulation. There may be fluid retention, with puffiness around the eyes and in the fingers. Intestinal action may become sluggish, leading to bouts of constipation.

Menstrual periods may change, even stop entirely, resulting in infertility. Sex drive in both men and women may diminish.

It is important to remember that any of these symptoms can result from causes other than a thyroid deficiency, such as emotional or psychological trauma, changes in life style, even changes in environment. Fortunately, we have blood tests which will determine if the thyroid gland is really at fault.

Although it's very rare (about once in 4000 births) a baby can be born with congenital hypothyroidism. Such infants are puffy, lethargic, and difficult to feed. They may have a thick tongue, an umbilical hernia, and may develop dwarfism or mental retardation if their thyroid deficiency is not diagnosed and treated promptly. Fortunately, infant hypothyroidism is easily detectable in routine tests of newborns, and treatment for this rare condition is completely successful.

In a person's middle years there may be a gradual increase in hypothyroidism. In the elderly a low thyroid output may even result in heart failure. But here again this condition is very responsive to treatment with a carefully adjusted administration of thyroid extract.

After reading about these signs of thyroid disorder you might be saying "Hey, I have symptoms just like that — I wonder if something is seriously wrong with me!"

At one time or another in our lives we all have experienced some of the "hyper" signs: anxiety, moist palms, heart palpitations. But these symptoms are far more likely to arise from a temporary social or emotional crisis — illness or death in the family, upcoming final exams, uncertainties in a new job, a stormy love affair.

On the other hand, we all would like to blame weight gain on a "hypo" glandular condition, rather than our overindulgence in calories. But a patient's occasional water retention and puffiness may be due to such factors as hot weather, menstrual periods, or too much salt in their diet. Another symptom of hypothyroidism is unusual sleepiness, but this may be caused by a number of other "normal" factors, including mental and emotional exhaustion, or just plain boredom.

If you are experiencing any of these symptoms on a regular basis, you certainly should see your doctor. But don't fret. Remember that, for most of us and most of the time, our thyroid glands work just fine, quietly and efficiently regulating the speed of that amazing machine that is our body.

18 Those Amazing Sphincters

BY THE WAY, have you within the last 24 hours given any serious thought to your sphincters? I thought not. But you should. These amazing muscular valves (pronounced "s-fink-turs") are performing vital functions around the clock. Your very life depends on them.

For example, up and down your digestive tract a series of sphincters silently and, for the most part unobtrusively, makes it possible for you to eat and to breathe, using a common passage for the start of both processes. Food provides our body's energy, and the air we breathe provides the oxygen. Both life-giving resources enter our bodies through a most interesting valve-like organ, the mouth, which is entirely surrounded by ruby-red lips. Mother told us as kids to close our lips while chewing food, to eliminate those disgusting smacking sounds. We also learned to pucker our lips while sucking through a straw, or while whistling, and to close them when osculating, at least when we were kissing our sister.

Moreover, as infants when we sucked on a nipple we found we could alternate breathing and swallowing. Later, when we began to eat semi-solid food we intuitively knew that we had to keep our mouth shut to initiate the act of swallowing.

When we got our baby teeth and graduated to almost grownup food we knew to chew it, mixing it into a soft, squeezable lump. Our tongue then would push this bolus of food against the roof of our mouth, the hard palate, moving it toward the back of the throat, the area called the pharynx ("fair-inks"). As this happened another valve, the soft palate, would swing up to block off the upper portion of the pharynx, in order to prevent food from entering our nose and sinuses.

Incidentally, if you look in a mirror and "open wide," as the dentists say, you may notice a little dingus dangling from the middle of the soft palate. That's the uvula, which in Latin simply means "little grape." It's that little grape that flutters in the breeze when you snore (which is more likely if you've had a little of the grape before you retired — but that's covered elsewhere in this book).

All these amazing valve closures take place automatically, with absolutely no conscious effort on your part, even when you're eating breakfast and reading the funny papers. Then, as you prepare to swallow, another marvelous automatic event occurs: your breathing stops to allow your mouthful of food to begin its journey toward your stomach. But you just go on reading the comics, giving no thought at all to the intrinsically perfect design of the human body, which can distinguish between food and air, and handle each correctly.

Now as the food slides back over the base of the tongue another valvular gadget, the epiglottis, does its stuff. Just as you begin to swallow, this little flapper, made of gristle (cartilage), claps shut over the opening to your windpipe, the trachea, allowing food to slip by into the swallowing tube, the esophagus. If by chance our signals get mixed and we "swallow wrong," food can get into our "Sunday throat," causing us to choke and cough and wheeze.

Your body doesn't rely on gravity to allow food to drop down to your stomach. Instead, the chewed bolus is squeezed down the esophagus by successive rings of muscular contractions called peristalsis. This is why you can swallow food while lying flat on your back on the beach, and why the astronauts don't starve in space.

While you're chewing and swallowing your lunch up above, your stomach is digesting what's left of your breakfast. Another valve, called the cardiac sphincter, is the "gate" where your esophagus connects with your stomach. It's usually closed, keeping the slightly acidic digestive juices in their place.

But when the swallowful of food or liquid arrives at the bottom of the esophagus, the cardiac sphincter opens to allow the nourishment package to be delivered. Normally this entry goes without a hitch, but sometimes the stomach intake valve misfunctions and goes into spasm, perhaps from nerve tension, or from irritation by coarse or incompletely chewed food. The result is a sharp pain under the breastbone, often mistaken for heart pain. To confuse matters more, because the problem emanates from the cardiac sphincter doctors have named the pain "cardiospasm," a particularly unfortunate term because this digestive pain has absolutely nothing to do with the heart.

On the other hand, this cardiac sphincter valve can get overstretched or weakened, allowing stomach acid to regurgitate up into the esophagus. The resulting burning distress is familiarly called "heartburn," again because it is often wrongly mistaken for heart pain.

Once into your stomach the parcel of food is doused with digestive juices and churned for a time, before it is squirted through the stomach's outlet valve, the pyloric sphincter, into your small bowel. There a variety of juices, enzymes and hormones continue the digestive process.

As the food passes on through your small bowel, which resembles a string of sausages, you are normally unaware of the digestion going on, other than to feel comfortable and satisfied. The process may speed up when we're under stress, which is why when we're reclining white-knuckled in the dentist's chair we may hear a tinkling, peristaltic gurgle.

The most important digestive functions are mainly completed in the 20 feet of small bowel. As the processed food moves on it must pass through another sphincter, the ileo-cecal valve, to gain entry into the large bowel. As the large bowel contents proceed, water is removed to be restored to the bloodstream. Finally the fully processed food, now called feces, is stored at the bottom end of your alimentary canal awaiting evacuation: defecation.

During this time a certain amount of normal bacterial action takes place, as well as some fermentation which produces gas, flatus. Such gaseous distention is given the name flatulence. Unfortunately, this gas is not resorbable, and must be expelled through the rectal outlet, the anus. This very normal act, when it occurs unexpectedly, can cause embarrassment.

As a physician I continue to marvel at the ingenuity of the mechanisms at either end of my alimentary canal. How I can swallow and breathe through the same opening. How I can pay little attention to the movement of food through the digestive process. And finally the amazing function of the sphincters at the terminus of the gut.

Doctor W.C. Bornemieier, writing in the American Journal of Proctology, spoke glowingly of the sphincter ani: "There is not another structure in the body that has a more keenly developed ability to accommodate itself to varying situations. The sphincter can apparently differentiate between solids, liquids and gas. It can tell when the owner is with someone or alone. Whether standing or sitting, with pants on or off. No other muscle of the body affords such protection of the dignity of man, yet is ready to come to his relief!"

19 *The Useless Prostate*

THE PROSTATE IS A RELATIVELY USELESS organ. Sitting there beneath a man's urinary bladder, right in front of the rectum, it's rarely called upon to perform any vital function.

Other glands such as the thyroid, the pituitary and the adrenals are hard at work 24 hours a day, regulating your life support systems, including your heart, lungs, kidneys, stomach and bowels. Thanks to them, your life goes on.

By contrast, a man's prostate has no such vital assignment, and most men are blissfully unaware of this organ, unless or until something goes wrong.

The simple, basic function of the prostate is to provide the lubricating fluid, called semen, that carries and sustains the millions of sperm as they spurt out though the penis when ejaculation occurs. That's about it.

These days most couples plan to have no more than two, maybe three children. Since only one sperm is needed to initiate a pregnancy, from the standpoint of reproductive efficiency the prostate is an organ of comparative futility.

Not only that, this indolent little gland, about the size of an apricot, can stir up a fair share of mischief. A painful, fulminating infection, prostatitis, can bring beads of sweat to a man's brow, while it sends chills running up and down his spine. Because of the gland's remoteness, and because of its anatomical structure, many antibiotics fail to pierce the capsule in which it's encased, to snuff out the infectious fire.

An even more common disorder occurs when the prostate begins to grow, as a man passes middle age, to the size of an orange. This is what's called "benign prostatic hypertrophy," or BPH. With time the enlarged prostate may put pressure on the urethra, the tube in a man's penis through which urine flows, making it difficult for him to begin to go, and to need to go more often. If the urethra becomes nearly or completely blocked by the enlarged prostate, the urine retained in the bladder may become infected. Eventually, if the gland continues to expand to a troublesome size, it may need to be removed surgically.

Another nasty habit of the prostate is its tendency to become cancerous in a man's Golden Years. Prostate cancer is the third most common cause of death in men, exceeded only by lung and colon cancer. After the age of 80 almost all men will have a tiny nest of cancer cells in their prostate, lying dormant.

Even though BPH in its early stages may cause no symptoms, and even though prostate cancer may be very slow to grow, it is still important for men in their middle years to have their prostate checked as a part of their annual physical examination.

The basic part of that procedure is the palpation of the gland with the finger through the rectum. This digital exam is virtually painless, and the minor insult to a man's dignity is far outweighed by the benefits.

The finger of an experienced examiner usually can identify a cancerous nodule. But a very early cancer, or a cancer deep within the gland, may be difficult to detect. It is here that a new diagnostic blood test, the Prostatic Specific Antigen test (PSA), can be of great value. Yet, like so many other lab tests, this evaluation has several shortcomings. Careful interpretation by your physician will assist in planning further diagnostic procedures.

It would be exciting news for all men over fifty if there were a pill that could shrink an enlarged prostate gland. Not long ago a headline in the magazine Medical World News hopefully announced that "Drugs May Replace Surgery For BPH." Unfortunately, it isn't quite that simple.

For some time a blood pressure medication called Hytrin has been used with modest success in reducing the size of the gland. A newer drug, Proscar, appears to hold more promise for shrinking an enlarged prostate. As with any medication, a patient's physician will watch carefully for any side effects.

The poor little old prostate, with not much to do most of the time, has a bad reputation for causing problems. What's a man to do? Don't waste time worrying about your prostate, but do have it checked regularly. If detected promptly, most prostate maladies can be managed and treated.

20 Go Ahead, Have a Good Cry

The young man who has not wept is a savage
George Santayana

ACROSS FROM ME SAT A YOUNG MAN, strong and healthy, six foot four inches tall. But he was weeping. A soft, gentle cry, a few tears trickling down his cheeks.

His tears had been caused by our discussion of a sad event that had touched his family. Then, the conversation over and his tears dried, his smile said, "Now I feel better." For him it had been a good cry.

Crying in private, crying in public. At a recent Mothers-and-Daughters breakfast meeting of a local women's group, a member read her winning essay on "Why I Love My Mother."

Not long into her rather sentimental reflection she choked up and halted to shed a few tears. So did many of her listeners. After she was finished there were smiles of happiness all around. The members of the audience somehow had been welded together by those few emotional teardrops.

As I walked out of this meeting into the bright sunshine, my eyes still were blurred with tears. I reached for my sunglasses and some Kleenex, to mop up the teary drizzle.

Driving off, settled and composed behind the wheel of my car, I pondered on the complexity of crying. I wondered about the mystery of tears, little drops of salty fluid that can flow from sadness or from pain, or from joy, or from a strong shaft of sunlight.

Later I found that many serious researchers at various eye clinics also are trying to unravel the mystery of tears. For example, Dr. William Frey of the St. Paul Dry Eye and Tear Research Center is a nationally recognized authority in this field, and has even written a book entitled, "Crying, the Mystery of Tears."

Biochemists, psychiatrists and behavioral psychologists have accumulated a great deal of information about the cause as well as the composition of tears. Even so, they're still not sure just why we shed tears when we are sad, happy, or angry. Or why we cry when we peel an onion or look up into the sun. But here is some of what we do know.

Ordinarily we think of tears only as the freshet of fluid flowing from the eyes and down the cheeks. The fact is, however, that tears are being secreted constantly by two small lacrimal glands, located just above the eyeball. As the tears flow across the eye they lubricate and wash the surface of the eye, just as your tears have been doing as you have read this, and as you have helped the distribution of these lubricating tears by unconsciously blinking.

We all have at one time or another tasted our tears, or the tears of a child or other loved one, so that we know they contain salt. From more formal research we know that our teardrops carry other vital chemicals — protein substances to keep the surface of the eyeball healthy, anti-bacterial agents to control inflammation and infection, plus some hormonal secretions.

The saline solution of tears is very important to those of you who wear contacts. The lenses actually float on tears, and soft lenses must absorb water from the tears in order to function properly.

Not everyone can naturally produce tears. The unfortunate people who suffer from Sjogren's Syndrome — the "Dry Eye Disorder" — must bathe their eyes with artificial tears. Fortunately, they are available over the counter, without a prescription. In this dry eye syndrome Mother Nature has shown significant sexist discrimination. For reasons unknown, nine time more women than men are afflicted.

Dr. Frey and his associates think they know pretty much about tear production for the routine physiologic functions — to keep the eye washed and lubricated. Much less well understood by these scientists are the causes and functions of emotional tears, a phenomenon so far dealt with mainly by songwriters and poets.

Rather remarkably, chemical analysis has found that the content of emotional tears actually differs from that of physiologic tears — the kind that flow when you pinch your finger in a drawer. The way researchers produced the two different types of tears is itself an interesting story.

First of all, the dedicated workers at the Eye Research clinic recruited volunteers who expressed a willingness to cry on demand — would you be willing to be in that group?

To produce "irritant tears," they exposed their subjects to the familiar fragrance of freshly cut onions. To generate "emotional" tears the researchers showed the volunteers several tear-jerker movies: "Brian's Song," "The Champ," and "All Mine to Give." Here is a brief summary of their findings.

♦ Women excelled over men in the total volume of tears produced when they watched the three-hanky movies. (Of course, any husband or boyfriend could have supplied that information, but scientists prefer complicated answers.) The researchers also found that female tears contained 60% more of the hormone prolactin, as compared with the male tears. It seemed logical to deduce that, in addition to producing milk, this hormone can stimulate the production of tears. That's why women are better criers than men.

♦ Emotional tears also contained a 25% higher concentration of protein, increased amounts of the body's natural opiate endorphin, and more of the stress-related hormone ACTH. This suggested that emotional tears may have a function in stressful or depressive disorders.

♦ In addition, the researchers at the clinic found that during a sobbing session the tears of these volunteers contained thirty times more of the chemical manganese — effectively eliminating it from the body. Interestingly, manganese has been implicated in mood alterations of the mentally ill.

So it just may be that the old-fashioned doctor was wise beyond his time when he advised his troubled and depressed patients to "cry it out," hoping thereby to remove the body's "bad humors."

Many men of an earlier generation were taught that little boys and macho men do not cry. Perhaps I as much as implied that to my sons as they grew up. But now this tall and strong man sitting before me, my son David, had demonstrated as he unloosed those gentle tears that he is not a "savage," and that yes, it's okay to shed tears.

Washington Irving confidently put crying into perspective:

There is a sacredness in tears. They are not the mark of weakness, but of power. They are the messengers of overwhelming grief, of deep contribution and of unspeakable love.

"Not feeling so good…"

Introduction

WE FLOSS, WE JOG, WE AVOID FATTY FOODS. We ride stationary bikes, we buy shiny exercise machines. We pop vitamins and eat health foods.

Newspapers and magazines devote pages to health and nutrition, most TV newscasts carry a medical information segment.

Physical fitness is in, good health is our goal. "Health maintenance" is the presumed objective of managed health care. "Wellness" is the buzzword of the nineties. Just the other day my patient Agnes Castle called the office for an appointment, informing my assistant Kelly that she wanted "a wellness examination — my insurance plan covers it."

There was a day when doctors wrote your prescriptions in Latin, and sternly told you to "do as I say and don't ask questions." Today you want to know just exactly what it is you've got, what you're taking for it, and why?

That's why essays such as these can be written for you, and read by you. There are a few physicians who might long to go back to the good old days, when no questions were asked and no explanations given. It would be much less trouble, and save a lot of time.

Obviously, I'm not one of them.

1 "It Must Be a Virus…"

OFTEN WHEN WE PHYSICIANS are struggling to cure a stubborn illness, we'll tell our patients "it's a virus." Or we unscientifically advise them that "you've got a flu bug — there's a lot of that going around." We admit our defeat in dealing with an adversary that refuses to drop, even after being pounded with round after round of antibiotic bullets.

Doctors prefer treating diseases we can get a handle on, so viruses especially frustrate us. Up until recently, these nasty bugs didn't even have scientific names. They refused to grow on ordinary culture mediums, and couldn't be seen through the lens of a standard microscope.

But now, after years of frustration, there is some light at the end of the virology tunnel. Ultra-magnification with electron microscopes has made it possible to identify many species of these viral critters. Moreover, new and more sophisticated culture techniques have enabled scientists to grow and study these viruses in the clinical laboratory.

Using these new techniques, we've discovered there are perhaps hundreds of varieties of viruses, ranging from the simple cold or flu bug to those which cause herpes and AIDS. And, more important than simply cataloging the many different viruses, we now are beginning to understand what really makes them tick.

Just for fun, the next time you strike up a conversation with your favorite virologist, ask him to describe the flu bug. He will gladly tell you that it is "a pleomorphic enveloped virus with highly characteristic surface spikes of nucleoprotein, anchored in the lipid envelope by a sequence of hydrophobic amino acids."

Got that? Now you know why you felt so lousy and ached all over the last time you were laid low by the flu!

To put it more simply, a virus is a tiny, ultra-microscopic organism that attacks your body's immune system, and has the ability to multiply wildly in your blood stream, joints and muscles. It can cause you to be mildly ill for 24 to 48 hours, or to be very, very sick with fever, malaise, vomiting, diarrhea, and generalized weakness. Only rarely is it fatal.

Up until recently, slow and steady progress was being made in understanding how viruses operate, and how to counteract their affects. Then the epidemic growth of AIDS, along with genital herpes, stimulated much more broadly and better funded virus research.

One research outcome has been the growing understanding of the range and relationship among virus-caused diseases. We have known for years that specific viruses cause mumps, measles and chicken pox, "childhood illnesses" to be tolerated as part of growing-up.

But recently researchers awakened to the link between the chicken pox (varicella) virus and the bug that causes shingles (herpes zoster), that ugly disease that mainly afflicts older folks.

They also learned that infectious mononucleosis ("mono," the "kissing disease") is related to the cytomegalovirus and Epstein-Barr, the "glandular fever" viruses.

Sound a little complicated? It gets worse.

Now the virologists have given names to these newly found viruses, and have catalogued them according to which part of our anatomy they pick on.

"Rhinoviruses" give us those sneezy, runny nose colds.

"Adenoviruses" cause our sore throats and "pink eyes."

"Enteroviruses" produce "summer colds" and "stomach flu."

And the "RSVs" — respiratory syncitial viruses — are supposedly the culprits that initiate chest colds.

Then we come to the influenza viruses A and B, responsible for making thousands feel crummy every winter, with a sudden onset of fever and aches, and a general feeling of weakness and exhaustion. The exasperating thing about these flu viruses is that they change their characteristics from year to year, requiring annual changes in the composition of the preventive vaccines.

But it was the rapid spread of two sexually transmitted diseases, herpes and AIDS, which accelerated virus research. The public panicked, and the government was forced to get into the act. It's difficult to say whether recent breakthroughs were the result of bureaucratic pressure and government funds, or a product of of planned research programs. The important point is that there now is hope for those suffering from AIDS and herpes, as well as many advances in finding specific medications for the treatment of other viral diseases.

For example, Zidovudine (generically called AZT, short for azidothymidine) has been found effective in treating patients with AIDS, and Acyclovir is being used in the treatment of herpes. Interferon can minimize the symptoms of the common cold.

Other new anti-viral drugs include Trifluridine, which has been successful in treating certain serious types of conjunctivitis (pink eye), and Ribavirin, beneficial in RSV chest infections. Amantadine and Rimantadine can prevent or modify influenza Type A, and are especially valuable for those people who failed to get their flu shot.

Confused? So am I. First of all, as our experience with these drugs grows we may find they are not all they are cracked up to be. Also, in the wake of all these medication breakthroughs, there is a need to balance costs with benefits. For example, the immense expense of treating the common cold with interferon would be totally out of proportion to the benefit gained.

Another positive outcome from this intense attention

on viruses has been some important progress in the prevention and treatment of cancer. For some time, we have believed that viruses cause certain types of cancer. Recently, and somewhat to their surprise, medical researchers discovered that the AIDS and the herpes viruses are remarkably similar to viruses that are assumed to cause cancer.

Could it be that they are genetically related? Might it be possible that some of this new virus research will lead us to a hoped-for cancer control? Sure, we've been disappointed before, and we'll not get our hopes too high. But now we at least have room for optimism.

2 Those Not So Harmless Childhood Diseases

NOT LONG AGO a headline in our local paper blared "Two Women Die of Childhood Disease. Measles Encephalitis Takes Lives of Two Adults." Several of my patients asked me "What's going on here? I thought we had these childhood illnesses pretty well under control."

Could it be that we are getting complacent about immunization against infectious diseases? Maybe we imagine that it's not so important anymore because we have all those potent antibiotics and other wonder drugs to fight all manner of illness.

Unfortunately many infectious diseases, particularly those occurring in childhood, are caused by viruses, and therefore are not controlled by antibiotics. The surprising and sad headline reminds us that a disease such as measles, relatively mild in childhood, can develop into a very serious illness, even cause death, in adults.

Several years ago my son Dave, at age 39, broke out with chicken pox. Of course, everyone teased him about getting "a kid's disease." But for him it was no joking matter. This husky six-foot-four fellow was laid low by this "childhood illness." You can be sure that this dad was grateful that my son didn't develop any of those potentially serious viral complications, such as encephalitis, inflammation of the brain.

Every so often we physicians see a sharp increase in strep throat infections. It happens that the streptococcus bug also causes rheumatic fever, and such minor epidemics bring back memories of the days when strep throat and rheumatic fever struck down many otherwise healthy young sailors who were thrown together in "boot-camp" training at the nearby Farragut naval base. Today, thanks to penicillin and a wide array of second and third generation antibiotics, most of the streptococcus critters no longer present a serious threat.

On the other hand, and much to our dismay, the majority of childhood diseases are caused by viruses which are resistant to antibiotics medications. Therefore, vaccination is the best way for us to control these illnesses. Unfortunately, however, at least in northern Idaho during the past ten years, fewer parents have been having their children vaccinated with DPT, MMR and polio vaccines. This is a disturbing trend because complacency about vaccination could allow these viral diseases to creep back into prominence, in adults as well as well as in children. And the dangers, especially to adults, from "childhood diseases" are far more than just embarrassment. Here's a brief summary of possible complications:

- ✓ Red Measles (Rubeola) can result in fatal pneumonia or encephalitis — inflammation of the brain.
- ✓ Mumps, an infection and inflammation of the

- ✓ salivary glands, may affect the testicles or the ovaries, with possible loss of fertility.
- ✓ Whooping Cough (Pertussis) is characterized by uncontrollable bouts of coughing. These coughs can be so severe as to rupture blood vessels in the eye or the brain, or they may even burst the bronchial tubes, leading to pneumonia.
- ✓ German Measles (Rubella) is usually a relatively mild illness, but if a woman contracts the disease during pregnancy, her baby may be born with serious congenital defects. This is why premarital rubella tests are required.
- ✓ Diptheria — Toxins produced by the diphtheria organism can damage the heart, the kidneys and the nervous system. The thick, tenacious diphtheria membrane can block the airway, causing suffocation. To allow the patient to breath, a tube is inserted through their throat to their trachea.
- ✓ Tetanus — We all know about the horrors of lockjaw. This disease is easily prevented by the administration of tetanus vaccine.
- ✓ Polio — Poliomyelitis, or "infantile paralysis," is largely a forgotten disease in the United States. But polio is still rampant in parts of the Third World, and could very well spring up in this country once again. And to be immunized against this terrifying illness, all you do is suck on a sugar cube!

Immunization of infants and children is a bit of a nuisance for parents, especially when an injection is required. Soft-hearted mothers and dads hate to subject little Johnny and Susie to needle pricks. There is a slight chance (very slight — one in 150,000) of a significant reaction to the immunization shot, and often there may be a temporary redness and swelling at the site of injection, plus a low-grade fever. But that's a small price to pay for giving your child the protection afforded by a complete immunization program. Furthermore, in doing this you have given the adult members in your household an added measure of protection against those kid diseases that can turn into vicious, even fatal illnesses in us grown-ups.

3 You May Have More Than Just "A Common Cold"

FOR THE PAST TWO WEEKS you've been fighting what you thought was "a common cold." You've had all the usual symptoms, including a sore throat that just won't go away. Your doctor told you that the "strep" test was negative. The medications you've tried haven't helped. What's going on here?

There is a good probability that you've been tussling with one of the newly identified "pharyngitis viruses." This group of nasty critters includes the influenza virus, the rhinovirus, the adenovirus, the cytomegalo virus, the herpes simplex "cold sore" virus, and the Epstein-Barr virus, or EBV.

Medical researchers are now finding that the EBV is the most common and widespread of these cold-causing culprits. The Epstein-Barr virus has been identified in sore throat victims in Europe, Asia and Africa, as well as in the U.S. Epidemiologists now believe that EBV causes the acute illness known as "infectious mononucleosis," and the relapsing ailment called "chronic fatigue syndrome."

The perplexing chronic fatigue syndrome commonly affects young, Caucasian, well-educated, affluent adults — which is why it is sometimes called "The Yuppie Syndrome." Those afflicted complain of "a cold I just can't shake," or "a flu that keeps coming back."

Mononucleosis or "mono" is characterized by the sudden onset of a sore throat, low grade fever, swollen glands, and generalized aching: the patient just feels lousy. This illness often occurs in teenagers and college students, and has therefore been nicknamed the "kissing disease."

Mono usually is mild and self-limited, with no serious after effects. The sore throat subsides, the swelling of the glands recedes, and the feeling of well-being gradually returns. Doctors usually just tell their patients to get extra rest, and to avoid physical exertion, rather than prescribing high-powered medications. Antiobiotics may be used, however, to fight a secondary bacterial infection.

Diagnosis of the acute form of mononucleosis is relatively straightforward. Indications are a clinical history of sore throats, swollen glands and extreme malaise, along with a positive antibody screening test.

Diagnosis of the chronic form of mononucleosis is more difficult and less accurate. Medical researchers estimate as many as nine out of ten adults have experienced a relatively mild EBV infection by the age of 40. Because of this they may carry the Epstein-Barr antibodies in their blood stream indefinitely, making a positive diagnosis of any present illness uncertain.

To make an accurate diagnosis, your physician will look for certain kinds of changes in the blood cells, shifts which typically occur when a patient has this viral disease. There may be an actual decrease in the white blood cell count, accompanied by an increase in the "abnormal" sizes and shapes of those particular white blood cells, the lymphocytes, which indicate the EBV infection.

Because symptoms of illnesses caused by the Epstein-Barr virus are often vague, and because the laboratory tests do not always provide us with a conclusive diagnosis, your physician may wonder "Is this really an illness, or is it all in the patient's head?" Are we dealing here with a hypochondriac? Or does this person have a immune system deficiency that prevents his or her body from successfully combatting this persistent, sub-clinical infection?

The patient feels rotten and naturally expects treatment — a pill or perhaps a shot, and his or her family begins to wonder why the doctor doesn't do something. Unfortunately, there is no antibiotic which acts specifically on the Epstein-Barr virus. Yet the physician may be concerned that the patient has a mixed infection, with a superimposed bacterial illness, and so feels justified in ordering an antibiotic.

Recently several anti-viral medications have been under intensive study. Zovirax (acylovir), the drug used in herpes infections, may be of some benefit in the treatment of EBV-caused illnesses. Corticosteroids are of limited value, but may be used in those rare instances when the patient's throat is so badly swollen they are having trouble breathing. Obviously, we have a lot more to learn about these pharyngitis viruses. While we're waiting for some good news from medical scientists, we'll fall back on the art of medicine, laying our trust in that good old healing remedy, "the tincture of time."

4 Not Enough Iron

MOST OF US WHO TOOK HIGH SCHOOL CHEMISTRY can remember that the symbol "Fe" stands for the element iron and that O_2 means oxygen. But few of us realize how important these two molecules are to the maintenance of good mental and physical health. For your heart to continue to beat and your lungs to continue to pump, your body must have an abundant supply of Fe to transport O_2 to every cell in your brain and your body.

How this works is itself a bit of marvelous chemistry. A soluble form of organic iron, a deep red pigment called "heme," is stored inside your red cells. This particular pigment has the ability to hook up to the oxygen molecule as the red cells circulate through the lungs.

To accomplish this life-giving function, the heme with its absorbed oxygen attaches itself to a protein called globin, creating "hemoglobin." This is the stuff that makes your cheeks pink, the vital compound which enables you to do anything and everything physical and mental, from holding this book and turning the pages, to your making sense of these black marks on paper called words.

Pink cheeks are just fine, but even more important is the ability of the iron in the red blood cells to transport oxygen through your circulatory system, to the muscles of your arms and legs, your diaphragm and your heart.

The life span of these hard-working red cells is about 120 days, after which they are disposed of in the spleen. But in a neat bit of internal recycling, the heme is transferred to the bone marrow, to be used again in the production of a new batch of red cells.

When for some reason there is an insufficient supply of iron to replenish the hemoglobin in the red cells, the result is "anemia," the "iron poor blood" we hear about and read about. This iron deficiency anemia, by far the most common form of anemia, is particularly common among teenage girls and women in their reproductive years — sex discrimination in nature!

A recent study of 16- and 17-year-old high school girls concluded that their mood swings and lassitude, as well as their inability to concentrate, could be traced to an iron deficiency. The researchers determined that the girls became deficient in iron due to poor diet, loss of iron during menstruation, and during periods of active growth.

Up to 45% of American women of all ages suffer from iron deficiency at one time or another. This is the price a woman pays for the privilege of procreation — loss of iron when the potential placenta sloughs off during monthly menstruation, and during pregnancy when her body's iron is depleted to support the development of her growing fetus.

This is not to say that only women experience iron deficiency anemia. Both men and women can suffer from bleeding from the gastro-intestinal tract, the leading cause of iron loss. Additional serious problems include bleeding from ulcers, and from polyps and bowel pockets (diverticula) and cancers.

Often the discovery of such an anemia in a routine blood test will alert your doctor to order other diagnostic exams to pinpoint the cause. Bleeding high in the gastro-intestinal tract will usually cause the bowel movements to be grayish or black. Red blood in the feces suggests bleeding from lower in the GI tract — anemia coupled with a change in bowel habits could indicate cancer of the colon.

A less common cause of an iron deficiency anemia is bleeding from the kidneys or bladder. Blood in the urine may be caused by kidney stones, tumors or infection. A person with a low hemoglobin count in a blood test, coupled with such bleeding, will be asked to have specific x-rays of their bladder and kidneys.

To distinguish iron deficiency anemia from less common types of anemia such as pernicious anemia, analysts study hemoglobin levels and the size, shape and number of blood cells. This is important to determine which treatment is most appropriate.

The first step in treating an iron deficiency anemia is, of course, to determine the fundamental cause of the patient's anemia, then to correct this problem. Once this is done, iron replacement is essential, which is provided with tablets, capsules or liquid, containing such compounds as ferrous sulfate or ferrous gluconate. In extreme cases, transfusion of blood cells may be necessary.

Usually oral iron supplements will restore the Fe, the heme, in the red cells so they can again absorb adequate amounts of O_2 to relieve the fatigue, the breathlessness and the palpitation. The patient's thinking and concentration will be improved, and there will be pink again in their cheeks.

And from this brush with iron deficiency anemia they certainly will appreciate one lesson in basic chemistry, the vital link between Fe and O_2, iron and oxygen.

5 New Ways to Treat Ulcers and Stones

"BUT DOCTOR, I READ SOMEWHERE that you can dissolve gall stones with medicine, so you don't have to have an operation." I had just told Sue that ultrasound pictures had revealed stones in her gall bladder, and advised her to consider having an operation to have them — and her gall bladder — removed.

The presence of these gall stones, called "cholelithiasis," was giving Sue repeated attacks of indigestion with colicky pain, but now she was digging in her heels, not very happy at the prospect of major surgery. She was hoping to find an easier way to get rid of those stones.

Several weeks before I saw Sue, my good friend and patient Clyde was awakened at 3:00 AM by an agonizing, lancinating pain in his left side. Like so many people who experience left-side pain, Clyde thought he was having a heart attack.

But when a shot had relieved his pain, and blood appeared in his urine, a diagnosis of kidney stones (nephrolithiasis) was quickly confirmed.

Clyde, like Sue, reads everything he can get his hands on about the latest medical advances. He had seen somewhere that kidney stones now can be pulverized by shock waves in a process called "lithotripsy," then flushed away without the use of surgery. This sounded like a first-rate idea to him — anything to avoid being cut into by the surgeon's knife.

Another patient, Don, came in to the office a few days after Sue's visit, complaining of a vague, gnawing discomfort in the pit of his stomach, which usually got worse when he was hungry. Eating something or drinking milk seemed to help a little, but Don admitted that he was "popping Tums all day long."

I ordered an X-ray of his upper gastro-intestinal tract, but I knew Don was having problems at the office, and that his finances were a little shaky. The two sets of symptoms fit together. I tried to be gentle when I broke the news to him that the shadow on his X-ray indicated an ulcer. His natural response was, "Jeez, Doc, does that mean I gotta have it cut out?"

Ten or fifteen years ago, surgery to remove an ulcerating patch of stomach lining might have been the required treatment, especially if the ulcer was causing bleeding, or was obstructing the passage of food during digestion. Or if the ulcer was becoming "intractable," no longer responding to medication and to other non-surgical management.

Stomach surgery for ulcers is a comparative rarity in the U.S. today. Instead, ulcers are treated with rather remarkable drugs such as cimetadine, brand name Tagamet. This medicine, along with related compounds — Zantac, Carafate, Pepcid, Axid — has made the medical management of ulcers eminently successful.

Non-surgical medical techniques aren't quite as effective alternatives for Sue and her gall stones and Clyde with his kidney stones. Two medications are available to dissolve gall stones, Chenex and Actigall, but they have some serious limitations.

- The stones must be less than an inch in diameter.
- The medicines work slowly. You must take two capsules each day for up to two years.
- The medicines are expensive, about $1,500 a year.
- The medications may cause diarrhea, skin rashes, elevated cholesterol.
- You may still have gall stone attacks during the course of the treatment.
- With your gall bladder still in place, you can make more gall stones.

Cracking gall stones with ultra-sound shock waves has been tried with mixed success. But not only may more stones form after the shock treatment, there is a continuing danger of infection in the gall bladder, which could spread to the nearby pancreas, causing dangerous pancreatitis.

Cracking up kidney stones by lithotripsy now is an acceptable procedure, though it also has some limitations:

- The stones must be small.
- To fit into the shock wave machine, you can't be too tall or too short or too fat.
- You must not be pregnant, have heart disease, or be taking certain medicines.
- These shock waves may have a long-term deleterious effect, such as possible damage to the ureter, the tube leading from the kidney to the bladder.

Should Sue, Clyde and Don go under the surgeon's knife? The surgical procedures are well-practiced and have proven effectiveness, but are understandably scary. Or should they correct their problem using a non-surgical approach? The techniques are newer, and have their limitations, but the patients don't need to "go under the knife."

Their doctor can't decide for them. Each of the three arrived at his or her decision after a full discussion with me, their primary physician, and after consultation with the surgeon. We provided them with all the necessary information upon which to base a judgment, in a process called "informed consent." Then each decided whether their doctors should dissolve, crack or cut.

6 Gout No Longer "Rich Man's Disease"

KING HENRY THE EIGHTH was a slob. He overate and he drank too much. He was a mean man with a nasty temper. And he had a deplorable habit of disposing of his wives by lopping off their heads.

It's a safe bet that Old Hank had the gout. You've seen pictures of him with his florid face, his rotund belly, his swollen legs. Historians tell us that he ate voraciously of meat, and that he quaffed off long draughts of wine from silver goblets. Based on this reported behavior, we might assume further that the pain from his gouty arthritis contributed to his mean disposition.

Gout has been around for centuries. Hippocrates called it "the unwalkable disease," and gave it the Greek name of "podagra," literally "pain in the foot." Because gout often is a byproduct of overindulgence in food and drink, in England and Europe it was considered a disease of the upper classes. Cartoonists delighted in drawing pictures of paunchy noblemen gorging themselves from a table loaded with rich food and jugs of wine. Those afflicted would be depicted with one foot resting on a "gout stool," to ease the pain in their joints, and with a bandage around their big toe.

Gout is caused by a dense accumulation of uric acid crystals, usually in a single joint, most often the great toe. We all have uric acid in our blood stream, as a by-product of the metabolism of purine foods, particularly meat. Gout was looked upon as the rich man's disease because the diet of the wealthy was loaded with purine-producing foods such as liver, kidney, heart, sardines, anchovies, fowl and seafoods. The poor man's diet, on the other hand, consisted mainly of low-purine foods: cheese, dairy products, vegetables and bread.

Uric acid normally is excreted from the kidneys in the urine — hence the name. But when a person's urine becomes too concentrated; or when there is overproduction of uric acid; or when there is decreased uric acid excretion; these tiny, sharp crystals are formed. Then a cloud of these salty little snowflakes may float through the blood stream to be deposited in a distant joint. Or they may accumulate in the kidneys to form stones — calculi — which may go on to produce renal colic.

The first attack of gout most often occurs in the great toe, probably because that appendage frequently suffers an accidental or unnoticed injury. Gout may also affect the ankle, the knee, the hand or wrist, and the skin.

Incidentally, gout is guilty of sex discrimination, affecting males over females in a ratio of 20:1. Men in the over-40 age group are especially vulnerable, though occasionally women will develop gout in their post-menopausal years. Older age groups are more likely to be affected, simply because the offending crystals accumulate over the years.

Those of you who have experienced gout know the symptoms. You may have had chills and fever, headache and malaise. Your skin became red and swollen, and felt hot and exquisitely tender. No one dared touch that throbbing toe. Even the weight of your bedcovers was unbearable.

What causes gout? An intercurrent illness such as pneumonia, a urinary tract infection, even a surgical procedure may precipitate an attack. Also, certain diuretic medications may lead to high levels of uric acid — hyperuricemia. Obesity increases uric acid production. Alcohol binges may precipitate an attack of gout. Repeated trauma may make a joint susceptible to the deposition of uric acid crystals.

The first step in coping with gout is to properly treat the initial attack. This is done quite successfully with an anti-inflammatory drug such as indocin, with the time-tested drug colchicine, or with corticosteroids. Aspirin is of little help and may be contraindicated.

Prevention is the best remedy. These days my patients are quite happy to follow healthier diets, especially those low in cholesterol. They know over-indulgence in alcohol is a no-no, and most who need to shed a few pounds are trying to do so. And to protect the great toe from contusions, as well as just to feel better, they wear sensible shoes, and otherwise treat their feet well.

If you've experienced any of the symptoms of gout, your doctor can measure the uric acid content of your blood. If necessary and appropriate, he or she will prescribe medications to decrease the amount of uric acid you produce, to prevent the formation of crystals.

So, though gout may not be curable, it's controllable. Furthermore, by controlling gout we may also prevent the formation of kidney stones, and there even is some evidence that reducing the excess output of uric acid may help prevent hypertension and heart attacks.

Just think, if Henry the Eighth had lived in the 20th

Century, he wouldn't have suffered from gout — and could have been a better husband and a more benign ruler. Plus, Anne Boleyn might have lived out her normal life span!

7 Gas Is No Laughing Matter

FLATULENCE IS NOT FUNNY. Yet as I sat in a group of around a hundred doctors attending a continuing education lecture titled "Gas and Related Problems," I watched many of my colleagues giggle nervously, some nearly roll into the aisles.

I didn't happen to be laughing, but I was wondering why the apparent malfunctioning of our digestive tract, our amazing food factory, can seem somehow ludicrous. Other systems, such as our heart and lungs, we take seriously but most of the time for granted, as they chug away through 24 hours of every day.

But we are acutely conscious of the excreta and effluvia that escape from our stomach and bowels, and all too often we treat them with scatologial derision.

Gastroenterologist Michael Levitt, a professor at the University of Minnesota School of Medicine, has made a special study of the problems of flatulence, burping and belching, subjects that have been given little serious scientific attention. In his wide-ranging study of historic references, Dr. Levitt found that "gas" has caught the attention of authors down through the ages.

Mid-Victorian writers spoke of the "rumbling of the bowels," and the painful "gaseous torment." The Knights of King Arthur's Round Table reportedly would gorge themselves with food and drink and "therefore there would be great bursts of laughter with much belching and pharting."

Far from being funny, gas and flatulence can cause great personal discomfort, both physical and mental. The cramping, gut-twisting pain can be very real, as we all know. And the inadvertent release of a malodorous bolus of gas can be a mortifying experience.

In my youth, I remember times when my very sensitive Aunt Mathilda would suddenly hasten from the room in the midst of a conversation, after modestly excusing herself. A moment later, we would hear a distant rumbling; my father and my Uncle Hubert would nod knowingly.

Unfortunately, there haven't been too many science researchers who have taken flatulence very seriously. But a high percentage of a physician's patients will admit to having frequent bouts of uncomfortable gas and bloating.

We do know that there are two general sources of intestinal gas. The simplest form is composed of the air we accidentally swallow, through a process called aerophagia. This can occur if we eat too rapidly, gulp our food or guzzle liquids. Gum chewing also can be a cause.

Some people actually swallow air, consciously or unconsciously, to try to induce burping, hoping to relieve gaseous distention. But the inert nitrous gases swallowed in this way cannot be absorbed through the intestine, and must pass on through.

The other form of gas is produced by the fermentation of food, specifically fats, sugars and proteins. This fermentation is accomplished through the action of the friendly bacteria which normally inhabit our large bowel.

Some foods, such as the simple sugars called monosaccharides, are absorbed directly through the intestinal lining. More complex foods must be broken down by this digestive process before they can be absorbed. These include the high-fiber foods I encourage my patients to eat for their good health, including wheat products, cabbage, onions, beans, asparagus, celery, carrots, Brussels sprouts and, yes, broccoli.

It is this fermentation that generates the gases — hydrogen, nitrogen, carbon dioxide, and methane — which cause the bloating. The fermentation of several of these veggies, especially cabbage, onions, and asparagus (they're given the high falutin name of "fructo oligo saccharides") produce a gas with a distinctive odor, ultimately released through the breath or flatus.

A few of my patients suffer gas and cramping because they have difficulty digesting milk products. This condition is caused by a lack of lactase in their systems, the enzyme which aids in the digestion of lactose, the "milk sugar." Because of this deficiency, dairy products give them indigestion, bloating, even diarrhea. Fortunately supplementary lactase is available in many grocery and health food stores.

It's not widely known that these digestive gases are explosive. The methane produced by our internal fermentation is chemically identical with marsh gas, and with "fire damp" in mines. A certain gentleman of Boston once was ignorant of this fact, but no longer.

As reported in the New England Journal of Medicine, this individual happened to be enjoying a cigarette as he leisurely accomplished his excretory functions. Just after expelling a large bolus of methane he flicked his lighted cigarette into the toilet. The highly respected journal recounted that the ensuing blast shattered the toilet bowl and made an ugly mess on the bathroom floor. It also reported that for the next three weeks the Bostonian ate his beans standing up, and gave up cigarettes for good!

There are a few medications your doctors may prescribe if flatulence is a continuing problem. There are several over-the-counter preparations, such as Beano, that might help. Charcoal, available in capsules, is an often effective old-time remedy.

The simplest way to avoid gas is, of course, to avoid those no-no foods. But for many of us that would be difficult; those fructo oligo saccharides are our staff of life!

8 Liposuction: A Costly Way To Improve Your Looks

YOU SAY YOUR FRIEND constantly complains her hips are too hippy, her buns are too bulgy, her lovehandles too droopy? Well, here's some good news. You can tell her that help is on the way, and it's called "liposuction," a relatively new surgical procedure that will permanently remove those ugly deposits of body fat.

I first learned about liposuction more than ten years ago, at a surgical meeting in Los Angeles, where plastic surgeons demonstrated how this procedure could remove unwanted fat pads to aesthetically shape the body. Fat from the abdomen, hips or buttocks was simply sucked away.

Because these procedures were being done mainly in the Los Angeles area, where the movie and TV celebrities boast of their face lifts and tummy tucks, I thought that this was a passing fad, limited to the Beverly Hills bunch.

I was wrong. The liposuction technique, imported from France more than 15 years ago, has become the fastest-growing cosmetic surgical procedure in the United States. Liposuction has largely replaced older and more dangerous operations for the removal of excess fat.

Although "liposuction" is the name most widely applied to this procedure, I'm afraid we physicians sometimes like to complicate, obfuscate and bewilder with our terminology. As a result this surgical technique has been variously referred to as suction-assisted lipectomy, lipodissection, suction lipectomy, lipolysis, lipoplasty, suction curettage, aspiration lipectomy and lipexheresis.

Just how does liposuction work and why is it successful? A lot like the vacuum cleaner pipe you use to suck dust balls from behind the sofa. Or, to speak a bit more clinically, like the suction tube or "cannula" your dentist uses to remove the saliva from your mouth as he drills.

Liposuction uses a similar vacuum device. A cannula with a sharp tip, connected by a tube to a suction pump, is inserted into the fat pad through a tiny skin incision in your skin. The surgeon quickly sweeps the tube back and forth through the adipose lump, swiftly vacuuming out the fat globules.

Fat is not, by definition, bad. We all have been endowed with a certain number of fat cells, tucked away beneath the skin of our body. When we "get fat," we don't make more fat cells; we only add more oily fat to the existing cells. When we slim down, we deprive these same cells of fat.

Liposuction is a process that actually sucks out globs of fat cells; none will re-grow to take their place. This permanent loss of fatty tissue results in a lasting change in the contour of that particular part of the body. I must emphasize that liposuction is not an acceptable way to lose weight, but is instead a way to smooth and streamline particular parts of the anatomy.

The areas most commonly chosen for such anatomic reduction are the hips, abdomen, breasts and buttocks. In nonscientific vernacular, the liposuction procedure is undertaken to correct "riding breeches," "saddle bags," "droopy bottoms," "pot bellies" and "love handles." Even chubby cheeks, double chins and "widow's humps" may respond to this suction pump procedure.

A patient undergoing liposuction plastic surgery usually has been given a light general anesthetic and will go home the same day. A stay in the hospital is necessary only when extensive surgery is to be done in several areas of the body.

Up to this point, it would appear that liposuction might be just the thing for your friend afflicted with hippy hips or overdone buns. A pleasant visit to the doctor's office on Friday, then back to work on Monday, sleek and svelte. Please pass the message on that liposuction has serious difficulties and drawbacks.

First of all, during this procedure a great deal of blood and body fluid can be lost, along with the fat. To promote good healing and to assure a favorable long-term result, pressure must be maintained over the operative areas with elastic supports, which must be kept in place for weeks, even months. The prolonged use of a girdle may be required.

Furthermore, although the surgical technique sounds simple, it is anything but that. Liposuction must be performed with great care, usually by a doctor who has had special training, most often a plastic surgeon.

Finally, the extremely high cost of liposuction is rarely covered by health insurance, because it is considered "cosmetic" surgery.

So if your friend is determined to get rid of some fatty bulges, my initial advice would be for her to exercise more and to eat less and better. But if she still insists on permanently whittling down those love handles, you may assure her that liposuction is a safe and satisfactory procedure. But tell her to start saving her pennies.

9 Diabetes: A Serious But Controllable Condition

THE WORDS "WATERSPOUT OF HONEY" have been translated from Egyptian papyrus documents dating from around 1550 B.C. to describe the ailment we know today as diabetes mellitus. Not only had those wise ancients designated diabetes as a specific disease, they knew that the urine of a person so afflicted was sugary sweet.

Barefoot doctors in medieval China, traveling out into the provinces, also knew about this metabolic disorder, and accurately listed the typical symptoms: unusual thirst, increased frequency of urination, and increased hunger, especially for sweets.

In modern medicine these three symptoms are called by the scientific names of polydipsia, polyphagia and polyuria. To help me recall these three tongue-twisters, my medical school professor said with a smirk, "Just remember the three 'P's, no pun intended."

That same professor explained to our first-year class in physiological chemistry that the disease originally was diagnosed with a very simple test. To demonstrate, he held up a beaker of golden yellow liquid and announced dramatically: "Ladies and gentlemen, this jar contains the urine of a diabetic patient here in the hospital." With that he thrust a finger into the fluid, then licked it exclaiming "How sweet it is!"

Then he asked us all to try this simple test, "so that you can learn how the diagnosis of glycosuria, sugar in the urine, was originally made." And because each of us wanted to do well in that tough P-Chem course, every one of us stuck a finger in the diabetic urine, and tasted the sweetness of it.

After we all had done so the professor continued: "My young friends, you have learned not one, but two lessons. First you now know that diabetic urine contains sugar; second, that to become a good physician you must develop your powers of observation. You should have noted that I used my forefinger to dip into that beaker, but it was my middle finger that I placed in my mouth."

Reading about diabetes mellitus in Sir William Osler's venerable text, "Principles and Practice of Medicine," we also learned that "He who understands diabetes, understands medicine."

What he meant was that diabetes is a complex disease that touches upon the physiologic functioning of every organ in the body. The diabetic patient might feel the impact of this disease in his stomach, his kidneys, his eyes, his legs. Even in his or her reproductive system.

It is important to understand that there are two separate and distinct diabetic conditions. One affects younger people, usually under 40, another form is seen in older people. The symptoms — the Three P's — are the same in both types, but there the similarity stops. Type I, the young person's diabetes, has been called the "thin type." Roman physicians characterized this disease process as "the melting down of the flesh into sweet urine."

Mature-onset diabetes, Type II, is thought of as the "fat type." Centuries ago physicians listed the symptoms as "torpor, indolence, and portulence." The older diabetic of today has the same listlessness, laziness, and pudginess.

Just as the characteristics of these two diabetic conditions differ, so do the causes and treatment. The younger Type I patient has diabetes because his pancreas does not secrete the insulin his body needs to burn up the starches and sugars in the food he eats.

His body attempts to compensate for this metabolic dysfunction by burning up fat. The Type I diabetic patient becomes very thin, and his body produces too much acid, a condition called ketoacidosis, which can lead to coma.

The pancreas of older diabetics may secrete some insulin, but for unknown reasons their body tissues are unable to use it properly in the metabolic process.

Because of this causal dissimilarity, treatments differ for Type I and Type II diabetes. Diabetes in young patients is usually controlled with injections, while Type II diabetics use oral medications.

There are similarities in management, however. Those afflicted with either type of diabetes must carefully regulate their weight, their diet, and their exercise. Because of the complexity of the disease and of its treatment, the care of any diabetic patient can be rather complicated, involving the patient and the family, the doctor and health care professionals, particularly dieticians.

Diabetes is usually discovered by accident, during a routine physical, when a urinalysis tests positive for sugar. This finding alone does not indicate diabetes mellitus because several other conditions may allow sugar to pass through the kidneys.

But a positive test for sugar, called "glycosuris," does alert us to the possibility of diabetes, prompting your doctor to proceed with more definitive tests. Blood samples drawn when the patient has been fasting, and then after eating, will lead to a more accurate diagnosis.

You would think that after more than 2000 years of experience with sugar diabetes, and with all our contemporary research capabilities, we would have by now come up with a cure. But we haven't, though we do know that viruses, infections, our body's immune system and the genes we inherit all are part of the complex puzzle of diabetes.

Yet even if we have no cure, we've made progress in controlling diabetes. Well over thirty different brands of insulin are now available, each with different capabilities, plus seven brand name anti-diabetic oral medications.

Patients can test their own blood and urine samples at home, and learn how to regulate their medications. We even have automatic insulin pumps, and pancreas transplants are possible.

Many years have passed since the 1921 isolation of insulin by the Canadian physicians Banting and Best, for which they won the Nobel Prize. Until this discovery, only the mildest forms of diabetes could be treated. We can hope that in a not-so-distant tomorrow a researcher will discover a cure for diabetes mellitus.

10 Amazing New Aids For The Hard of Hearing

IF FATE DECREED that tomorrow you would lose either your sight or your hearing, which would you choose?

Helen Keller, both blind and deaf, wrote that she thought the loss of hearing far worse than the loss of sight. But I imagine most of us would feel just the opposite. We use our eyes so much each day to read, write and watch television, to lose our eyesight would be a great catastrophe. To lose our hearing would be a major inconvenience, but a handicap we could cope with.

These attitudes are reflected in how we relate to the blind and the deaf. Toward sightless people we feel sympathy, and perhaps want to assist them. But we may become impatient with the person who is hard of hearing. Significantly, when someone who hasn't been paying attention to what we've been saying asks "What did you say?" we might shoot back "What are you, deaf or something?"

Furthermore, we even sometimes make jokes about those who are hard of hearing...

Three old codgers, each of them deaf, were riding the bus. When they came to a stop the first one asked "Is this Wembley?" The second fellow responded "No, this is Thursday." Prompting the third one to comment "So am I, let's get off and go for a drink."

Yet when a blind person bumps into the furniture or misjudges the curbing, rather than laughing, we hasten to help him. We give him a measure of both self-reliance and dignity with a white cane, and with seeing-eye dogs.

The hard-of-hearing person, on the other hand, receives little sympathy (and less empathy) for his invisible handicap. Small wonder that many of these people carry a chip on their shoulders, and allow their false pride to prevent them from seeking help to hear better.

Furthermore, many people maintain the unfortunate and incorrect belief that hearing aids don't work, or that they "just make things worse." Even that the hearing-aid business is a rip-off, designed to take advantage of folks with hearing difficulties.

Another even more unfortunate misunderstanding is that if a person has "nerve deafness" (technically referred to as sensorineural hearing loss), he simply cannot be helped. Now we know that's not necessarily true.

I recently had the privilege of addressing a meeting of an organization called SHHH — Self Help for the Hard of Hearing. I knew several in my audience were "stone deaf," victims of this so-called "nerve-deafness." And yet they listened to me and responded in a perfectly normal manner.

After the meeting I expressed wonder as to how this could be possible. They explained that I was within the circumference of a Carron Audio Loop, an electric device that transmitted and amplified my voice so that every person in that group, regardless of the type or degree of hearing loss, could tune me in. Amazing!

I later learned that this Carron Loop was only one of many new and promising technological advances on the hearing horizon. The SHHH people proudly tell us that they now have available hearing helpers — they call them "Assistive Listening Systems" — that enable the hard-of-hearing to attend church, the theater, cocktail parties, even to go square dancing!

Examples of ALS include hearing aid-compatible telephones in hotels, hospitals, and other public facilities. At the same time, ever more compact and powerful hearing aids, with a wide range of specific applications and effectiveness, continue to be perfected and made available.

I hope that these technological marvels, combined with a greater level of public understanding, will encourage the hard-of-hearing to break out of their silent, resentful, withdrawn world. The SHHH people want the hearing-impaired to once again be able to walk — or dance — out into the mainstream of life, displaying their shiny Assistive Listening Systems just as proudly as the blind display their white canes.

11 Unhappy Facial Maladies

WE ALL TRY to put our best face forward. Our face is that part of us that tells the world who we are and what we are. Our face is the switchboard that lights up to bring messages of sight and sound and touch, and it can produce scowls of anger, smiles of happiness, even a flow of tears.

When there is discomfiture deep down in our body, we may be able to hide it. But when there is dis-ease in our face, it shows.

There are two peculiar ailments of the face, both derangements of the facial nerve, that can be personal tragedies to the unfortunate victims. Marjorie has trigeminal neuralgia and Mildred has facial palsy.

Marjorie's facial neuralgia hurts because it is an affliction of the sensory, "feeling" fibers of the facial nerve. On the other hand, Mildred's dis-ease, also known as "Bell's palsy," doesn't hurt in the usual sense. But it ablates the motor or "action" function of the facial nerve, paralyzing half the muscles of the face. That hurts her pride.

Because we don't know exactly why these two disorders occur, and because we have no quick and easy cure, they are a frustration for both the patient and the physician.

Trigeminal neuralgia is an acute inflammation of either the right or left facial nerve, resulting in an excruciating, stabbing one-sided pain, which can affect the chin, the cheek, the tongue, the teeth and gums, and the forehead just above the eye. The pain can be so severe it can cause a wince or a twitch. French scientists gave it the name *tic douloureux*, "painful twitches."

The pain from trigeminal neuralgia may come in brief bouts, but as time goes on the anguish may be almost constant, severe enough to literally immobilize the patient. Specific trigger points usually can be identified, and the pain may be brought on by touching the face, washing, shaving, eating, drinking, kissing, talking, even sitting in a draft. You can well understand how those afflicted with trigeminal neuralgia can become unhappy and dysfunctional.

Diagnosis is usually straightforward, but because infections of the sinuses, ears and teeth can cause similar facial pain, doctors check these areas first. If tests confirm trigeminal neuralgia, the condition can be managed with carbam azepine (Tegretol), in carefully adjusted doses. Unfortunately, the patient may develop a resistance to the drug, or be unable to tolerate doses high enough to suppress the pain.

When that happens, surgery is the last resort. Using an a extremely delicate technique, the sensory segments of the affected portions of the nerve can be divided. This produces numbness in the corresponding part of the face, but to relieve the pain, this is a loss most patients are willing to accept. Marjorie had run the gamut of medical management without a complete resolution of her pain, and so was ready to undergo definitive surgery.

Mildred's Bell's palsy is different from trigeminal neuralgia in several important ways. This disfiguring paralysis of the facial muscles is painless, and usually lasts only three or four weeks. Yet even though physical pain is not a factor, the embarrassment and emotional hurt brought on by this disfigurement can be very real. Mildred was an unhappy lady until we were able to correct the condition.

The loss of muscle function on one side of the face causes the cheek to sag and the mouth to droop. Facial expressions such as smiles or frowns are grossly distorted. A person suffering from Bell's palsy can't completely close his eyelid, and no longer can whistle.

Fortunately, complete recovery usually can be accomplished within two months. Medical measures may include cortico-steroids, artificial tears, and a patch over the affected eye. Antibiotics may be indicated occasionally, and in rare cases, surgery may be required to relieve pressure on the nerve.

Most human dis-eases can be hidden from public view, but these maladies can't be concealed. The unhappy victims must face the public. Marjorie or Mildred would quickly tell you they'd gladly trade their facial disfigurements for a slipped disc or a kidney stone.

12 Hyper/Hypo, Too Much/Too Little

TWO OF THE MOST PERPLEXING EMERGENCIES in medical practice are hyperventilation and hypoglycemia. And they aptly illustrate the prefixes hyper and hypo, from the Greek words for "over" and "under," which often show up in medical terms describing some imbalance in the body.

A few days ago Marilyn came home after a long day of shopping. As she unpacked her parcels she began to feel faint and dizzy, with numbness and tingling in her hands and face. She then had a scary sensation of not being able to get enough air into her lungs, as if she were suffocating. To compensate she began to breathe more quickly and more deeply, until she suddenly slumped to the floor. Her frantic husband Fred called 911, and soon Marilyn was whisked off to the hospital emergency room.

For a patient experiencing trouble breathing, it wouldn't be unusual for a physician to immediately order oxygen. But the alert doctor carefully considered the details of her symptoms, and noted her otherwise normal pulse rate, blood pressure and other key signs. Instead of hooking her up to oxygen and high-tech monitors he had the confident insight to ask Marilyn to first breathe into a paper bag. In less than a minute she regained full consciousness, the color returned to her cheeks, and she began to breathe normally.

The explanation of what happened is quite simple: Marilyn panicked, and in her frantic attempt to pump more oxygen into her lungs she caused an acute imbalance in her systemic oxygen/carbon dioxide levels.

We all know the life-giving power of oxygen — on television we see football players breathing deep breaths of it on the sidelines. Knowing its vital role in preserving our bodily life, it's difficult to imagine we ever could get too much O_2. On the other hand, we remember that carbon dioxide is a noxious substance, a by-product of metabolism that is disposed of through respiration — we might imagine our body wants constantly to eliminate all CO_2.

Yet our body chemistry requires a certain level of carbon dioxide in our blood circulation, to activate and to regulate our breathing center in the brain. Under ordinary circumstances the O_2 and the CO_2 proportions are automatically maintained in a delicate balance. Rapid over-breathing — hyperventilation — upsets that balance by flushing out all the necessary carbon dioxide.

For some unknown reason this hyperventilation syndrome occurs most frequently in otherwise normal, healthy women such as Marilyn. It may be touched off by anxiety, stress or panic. The treatment is, of course, reassurance and support — plus the paper bag breathing trick.

Hypoglycemia, low blood sugar, is another unusual metabolic disorder, which may present similarly alarming symptoms: weakness, a feeling of overwhelming warmth, dizziness and profuse perspiration. If you're suffering from hypoglycemia you may feel a tingling in your lips and hands, and a temporary blurring of vision. Someone suffering from hypoglycemia may even wobble and stagger as though he were drunk.

Early one morning not long ago a local physician hastened to the hospital, to meet a patient brought in on a medical emergency. He didn't have time to grab breakfast and, when the operation turned out to be longer and more tedious than anticipated, the surgeon developed the hypoglycemic syndrome. His surgical partner, observing the doctor's pallor, weakness and profuse perspiration, imagined he was having a heart attack.

The real reason was the surgeon's low level of energizing blood sugar, blood glucose. A glass of orange juice and a sugar donut quickly restored the surgeon's normal blood sugar level, and the operation was smoothly concluded. To avoid that same hypoglycemic experience, marathon runners load up on carbohydrates, usually in the form of pasta, the night before racing.

Hypoglycemic reactions occur not infrequently in diabetics who may have accidentally taken a larger dose of insulin or more hypoglycemia pills than necessary. Or they may have burned up more glucose through extremely strenuous exercise.

In these instances, once again the treatment is simple — restoration of a normal blood sugar level with fruit juice, sugar tablets or candy. It is vital, however, that the family and friends of a diabetic be aware of these symptoms, and know what to do about them. Most diabetics wear bracelets to identify their disease, giving emergency medical personnel a head start in arriving at a diagnosis and beginning treatment.

To paraphrase the old saying, "the Greeks had words for it," in this case for "too much" and for "too little." Prompt recognition of these two unusual and frightening conditions deserves our attention, because home remedies can be so simple, safe and successful — in rare instances even life-saving. If Marilyn's husband had been tuned in to her condition, that 911 call could have been avoided.

13 Maybe You Have Lupus, Most Likely You Don't

WHEN I WAS IN MEDICAL SCHOOL, I suffered all the symptoms of the illnesses I was currently learning about. From syphilis to TB, from cancer to diabetes, my fellow medical students and I were certain we had somehow or other contracted each new disease.

Over my years in medical practice, I have seen the same phenomenon in the adult population. A few years ago, patients would come in worrying that they had contracted herpes. Next, they worried about AIDS. Following that, it was Epstein-Barr.

These periodic waves of concern about specific diseases are largely generated by the mass media. This was especially true in the case of lupus. All it took was the appearance on "Larry King Live" of an actress who proudly proclaimed that she had had this disease, and that she was a survivor. As she recited her symptoms — tiredness, achiness, low-grade fevers, joint pains — it became obvious to many of the millions watching the program that they too had experienced those very same symptoms, and so also must be suffering from lupus.

Furthermore, this young woman complained that she had been to "at least a half dozen doctors" before one finally was able to come up with the correct diagnosis. She was implying, of course, that we docs need to sharpen our diagnostic abilities. Let me protest that perhaps it is the nature of this unusual disease that makes diagnosis so difficult.

Lupus is what doctors refer to as a chronic multi-system inflammatory disease. Its technical name is "systemic lupus erythematosus," or SLE. Lupus can affect the skin, the heart, the kidneys, the muscles, the joints — any organ of the body.

It has a way of attacking the strong fibrous tissues, the connective fibers that hold every organ of our body in place. Those are the tissues which contain collagen, the "glue" that holds our body structures intact for a lifetime.

Doctors don't yet know what causes lupus, but the disease apparently strikes when a person's immune system is in a downswing. Nine out of ten of those suffering from lupus are women between the ages of 20 to 45. Because this period coincides with a woman's reproductive years, researchers suspect a hormonal link.

Initial lupus symptoms include a fever, a skin rash on the cheeks and nose in the shape of a "butterfly," accompanied by extreme tiredness, and possibly aching joints.

A person with lupus might also experience chest pain, lung congestion, and an upset stomach. Their kidneys may be affected, resulting in blood and albumen in their urine. A lupus suffer might also have extreme muscle weakness, and her nervous system may be dulled, producing mild mental symptoms, even depression.

On the basis of these clinical indications, it's pretty obvious that both the patient and the doctor can easily be confused as to the exact diagnosis, because a wide variety of infections also can cause the same symptoms. Which is why Larry King's lupus guest drifted from one physician to another.

In making a diagnosis, various blood tests can be helpful. Common laboratory examinations such as the sedimentation rate and the blood platelet count may be used for screening purposes, but the antinuclear antibody test is more often of positive help. Yet it is not infallible because, while most lupus patients will have a positive ANA test, a positive ANA does not necessarily mean the patient has lupus. In fact the test can give "false positives," even to syphilis. Surprisingly, the ANA test may prove positive in certain elderly patients who are in good health. Suffice to say, the test requires careful interpretation.

Once a diagnosis of lupus has been made, what about treatment? Here more skilled help is needed. Careful and continuous surveillance is essential. Lupus is not controlled by a short course of pill-taking.

The mainstay of treatment is acetylsalicylic acid — good old aspirin. If aspirin proves inadequate, certain drugs used in the treatment of malaria have proved useful. Also, some of the new anti-inflammatory medications can be used, and cortisone-type medications are helpful during acute flare-ups.

A number of studies suggest lupus is linked to stress, and there is reason to believe that getting rid of stress can actually induce remissions. Maybe it's true that, in the case of lupus, laughter is the best medicine, that happiness is healthiness.

Oral contraceptives are contraindicated during the acute phase of lupus, apparently because of their high hormone content. Pregnancy is advised only under careful management. Finally, because sunlight can lead to an eruption of skin rashes, lupus sufferers should wear wide-brimmed hats, long sleeved shirts and sun screen when they're outside.

Up to this point, that's the bad news. The good news is that the next time you have a fever, malaise, a skin rash and aching muscles or joints, the odds are that you are being attacked by a flu bug or a strep or a virus — that you're not suffering from lupus — and that in a week or two you'll be yourself again.

If you are a man who has survived the teens and the twenties, you are now probably home free as far as lupus is concerned, yet another instance where Mother Nature is guilty of sex discrimination.

If you are a woman in your 20s or 30s, and you happen to experience these symptoms, remember that the chances are 96 to 4 that you are not coming down with lupus. Those are pretty good odds.

In the unusual instance where a diagnosis of lupus is actually confirmed, it's reassuring for the patient to know that the disease is treatable, rarely fatal, and usually has long periods of remission.

14 *Lou Gehrig's Disease*

LOU GEHRIG WAS A GREAT and strong baseball player in the 1930s, but is best known today for the terrible, wasting disease which took his life in 1941. In one of the most poignant newsreels of that era, Gehrig saluted his fans and said farewell, knowing he would soon die of amyotrophic lateral sclerosis. What he did not know is that his name still would be linked to this disease a half century after he hit his last home run.

Fortunately, Lou Gehrig's disease is quite rare; in more than fifty years years of medical practice I have had only two patients who suffered from this irreversible nerve and muscle degeneration. But both times I had to sadly stand by, knowing there was no way to halt the progress of this illness, as it relentlessly numbed then paralyzed the nerve fibers of the central nervous system.

Unfortunately, Lou Gehrig's disease is one of the few illnesses in which a physician can make an absolutely certain prediction of its outcome: after a gradual, inexorable deterioration of the patient's physical powers, death will come within five years.

Just what is the nature of this terrifying disease process? Its scientific name describes its symptoms. Amyotrophic means the loss of muscle and the loss of muscle strength; sclerosis refers to the degenerative changes that are taking place in the nerve fibers that activate the muscles.

What the patient feels is like our feelings in that nightmare most of us have had, when we are trying desperately to walk, run or swim away from a threatening person or thing, but our legs seem to be made of lead. When we waken in a cold sweat we're happy to realize it was all a bad dream.

But Lou Gehrig's bad dream was very real, and it wasn't going to go away. In the beginning the powerful ballplayer felt a vague weakness; his arms and legs felt heavy. He noted with irritation that he was losing his quickness at the plate, and didn't have his old stamina when running the bases. Gehrig at first thought he simply had the flu. But when the weakness steadily increased he consulted his doctor, who diagnosed amyotrophic lateral sclerosis.

Your spinal cord is a like a bundle of tiny wires which transmit electrical impulses from the brain to various parts of your body. Some of these organs are under voluntary control, things we think about, and are performed for the most part by the muscles of the arms and legs, neck and back. The involuntary functions are those automatic and continuous activities of vital organs such as your heart, kidneys, intestines of which we are blissfully unaware.

The sad irony of Lou Gehrig's disease is that the involuntary functions continue while the voluntary capabilities shrivel. Those who have the disease continue to see and hear, to think and understand, while their muscles become immobilized. These poor people are emotionally and cognitively alive, trapped in the cocoon of a wasted, lifeless body.

Can we who are hale and healthy even begin to comprehend the terror this knowledge would evoke in the mind of a person afflicted with Lou Gehrig's disease? Visualize, if you can, the scenario that would unfold in the home of a man who has contracted ALS. His wife and children would have to confront the certain reality that her husband and their father was going to die in a few years. And that, until he did pass away before their very eyes, this strong and dependable man would gradually become a helpless, emaciated invalid.

If Dad had had a heart attack or a stroke, or had been given a diagnosis of cancer or leukemia, the family would have at least been given the hope of palliation, if not a cure of the disease. Amyotrophic lateral sclerosis, on the other hand, gives no such comfort. Not only do we not know its cause, we also know there's no cure.

As is so often the case in such hopeless medical situations, the patient and his family frantically grasp at straws. They try all manner of remedies with a shadow of hope, including some quackery. Pancreatic extracts, amino acids, anti-viral injections, even snake venom — but all in vain.

The truth sinks in. No matter what is done for a person with ALS his arms and legs will wither, his chest muscles will waste away. Breathing will become labored and swallowing begins to be difficult, almost impossible.

To keep life-giving oxygen flowing into his blood stream, the patient is hooked up to a ventilator. A tube is slipped into his stomach to allow food to by-pass the faulty swallowing mechanism.

Through all this frenzied activity the ALS patient lies in his bed, anguished and immobile, totally aware of all the effort being expended to extend his life, but unable to say anything. He can't even express a "yes" or a "no" with a nod or a shake of his head.

Amazingly, a person afflicted with Lou Gehrig's disease still can move his eyes, and so is able to spell out a few words with the aid of an alphabetical eye chart. This is his final and only means of communication with the people around him.

The sadness, the hopelessness deepens. The wife is physically and emotionally exhausted. A home nurse brings some relief, but she, too is drained by the stress she feels. The family physician, knowing that science is of no avail, falls back on the art of medicine, giving freely of his wisdom and his compassion.

The patient is fully and cruelly aware of all this. His heart and mind still function. At long last, with the flickering of his eyes, he spells out on the alphabetical chart: "Let me die."

The doctor assembles the family with the pastor, priest or rabbi; the family lawyer is consulted. The physician asks the opinion of several of his colleagues. Then the wife, the children, the entire family reach a heart-rending decision to end the agony of their loved one.

Finally, when all the words have been said and all the tears have been shed, the doctor complies with the patient's and the family's request. He administers a gentle sedative, and then withdraws the life support systems. Both the family and the patient are relieved of the burden of this cruel disease.

15   *Anxiety, Fear and Panic Attacks*

WHEN ELLEN CALLED WITH TERROR IN HER VOICE, I knew she was having another "panic attack," similar to those she had been having for nearly a year.

"Doctor, my heart is pounding, there's a tight feeling in

my throat, I'm light-headed, and I just can't get enough air into my lungs. What'll I do?"

Much has been written in the psychology and psychiatric literature, as well as in the mass media, about these mysterious panic attacks. Several television news programs have explored this condition with the clinical name of "agoraphobia," literally fear of open spaces.

Such attacks invariably are related to two other emotional disorders, anxiety and depression. The symptoms of an acute panic attack such as Ellen was having are easily recognized, but it's more difficult for doctors to accurately define the other two conditions.

All of us have anxieties from time to time. For example, when we worry about a speech we need to make, or a final examination we have to take in a few days. If we react to this kind of stress in a healthy way it can propel us to rehearse that one extra time for that talk, or to take the extra step of outlining our notes before the big test.

But the overwhelming and irrational anxieties, the mounting fears that are symptoms of agoraphobia, not only are abnormal and unproductive, they may totally disrupt a person's life. For example, Ellen is a devout Catholic, but her fear of going into public places prevented her from attending mass, a deeply comforting experience for her.

Because standing in line at the supermarket once had brought on a panic attack, Ellen's friends and relatives now do her grocery shopping for her. Because she fears suffering humiliation in a public place, Ellen has become a recluse, a prisoner in her own home.

The anxious person who becomes agoraphobic obviously feels and acts depressed. But while the anxious patient becomes overly dependent, the depressed patient becomes withdrawn and reclusive. Beverly Mead of the University of Oregon Medical School illustrates the difference with the anxious patient saying, "Don't leave me," while the depressed patient mutters "Leave me alone!" Doctor Mead further clarifies: "Anxiety is when you see a cop car trailing you; panic is when you see those flashing blue lights in your rearview mirror!"

Some 12 million Americans suffer from a variety of phobias, unexplainable and unreasonable fears. Some are as predictable as ophidiophobia, the fear of snakes. Or as ombrophrobia, fear of rain; aerophobia, the fear of flying; or mysophobia, the fear of germs — both Howard Hughes and Napoleon incessantly washed their hands. But fear of open spaces is by far the most common phobia. Of all people who seek professional help to deal with their phobias, 60% suffer from agoraphobia.

Fortunately the chance of cure is excellent. Psychologists use several successful therapeutic approaches, all of which are aimed at demonstrating that there is nothing intrinsically fearful about the dreaded object or situation. Therapists carefully guide the afflicted person through a "desensitization" program, to communicate that his or her fears are unfounded.

In the case of agoraphobia, psychologic therapy rarely fails. If it does, drug medication may be tried. If this becomes necessary, three general categories of medications are employed: The benzodiazepines, a form of tranquilizer; the amino oxidose inhibitors (MOA); and a newer drug called alprazolam. Only recently has this drug been certified by the Food and Drug Administration as the drug of choice, if medications are to be used.

As is so often the case with new medications, drugs that are supposed to help patients may also cause complications and adverse reactions. Those using the benzodiazepines may become drowsy, so these drugs aren't good for people engaged in skilled or hazardous occupations. Monoamine oxidase inhibitors (Parnate or Nardil) may have cross reactions with certain foods or medications, resulting in serious blood pressure elevations. Alprazolam (Xanax — spell it frontwards or backwards) can make a deep dent in your pocketbook in those instances when it must be used in high doses.

To summarize the condition and current treatments,
- Anxiety and depression are complex clinical disorders, often difficult to define.
- Agoraphobia is a very real nervous ailment, intermingled with both anxiety and depression.
- Panic attacks are a well-defined nervous disorder, often of a hysterical nature. They are frequently experienced by persons afflicted with agoraphobia. They respond well to psychologic or psychiatric treatment.
- Drug therapy is available, but must be used under careful supervision.

16 Arthritis: Painful, Usually Treatable

YOU'VE PROBABLY HEARD that old story about Granny Green, who lived alone in a little old house on the hill. When asked if she got lonely living up there all by herself she replied "Oh no, I have lots of company. Each night I go to bed with Ben Gay, and I wake up in the morning with Charlie Horse. Then I swing my legs over the side of the bed and walk to the bathroom with Art Ritus."

My diagnosis would be that Granny was afflicted with the common, garden-variety rheumatism called degenerative osteoarthritis. It will afflict most all of us, both men and women, if we live long enough. But not all Seniors are affected in the same way, or to the same degree, perhaps due to the genes they've inherited.

By the way, the term "degenerative" has nothing to do

with your morals. It simply refers to the gradual wear and tear on the joint surfaces of the bones of your back, hips, hands, arms and legs.

People in joint-stressing occupations may get arthritis when they're comparatively young. Ballet dancers often do, after so many years of dancing on their tippy toes. Many football players are penalized quite a few yards in their later years, for the pummeling they subjected their bodies to in exchange for million-dollar salaries.

The symptoms of osteoarthritis are well known: the "hitch-in- the-gitalong" called "sciatica," or the "lumbago" so often blamed on the kidneys. The slowed or slightly stooped gait, the morning stiffness, the difficulty in getting in and out of bed, or up out of an over-stuffed chair.

Effective treatment for osteoarthritis includes weight loss and rest and relaxation, plus regular but not excessive exercise, and heat on the painful joints.

Aspirin in its many forms is the gold standard of medication. New and fancy (and expensive) non-steroidal anti-inflammation medications can be used when the symptoms are severe. Brand names include Indocin, Motrin, Clinoril, Nalfon, Naprosyn, Tolectin, Meclomen and Feldene.

Cortisone injections are reserved for episodes of unbearable pain, especially when the inflammation is concentrated in one joint.

The aches and pains of arthritis are invariably worse in cold and changing weather, and in these instances physical therapy and heat applications can bring relief. For some that can mean getting out of town for a while in the winter. My dear friend and patient Helga summarized the benefits of this therapy, with her typical Scandinavian directness: "Ve like always to go South in the vinter. My Olie, he always feels better when he is in heat."

Surgical joint replacements are used only as a last resort. Recent advances in orthopedic surgery have brought us artificial steel, rubber and plastic replacements for certain joints that no longer respond to conservative measures.

Rheumatoid arthritis is the other most common bone and joint affliction. In contrast to osteoarthritis, RA occurs in the younger, 20 to 40 age group, more commonly in women. There is even a form of juvenile rheumatoid arthritis.

Osteoarthritis is apt to strike only one or two joints, in the hips, the back or the knees. Rheumatoid arthritis in its initial phase acts more like a systemic disease, giving the patient a generalized aching, tiredness, and vague muscular pains.

When the joints, especially the hands, are attacked they will be swollen, red and tender, with pain on movement. These symptoms may subside, only to return a few days later.

In osteoarthritis the disability results from a grinding away of the opposing joint surfaces, as the cartilage which acts as a cushion between the bones is slowly eroded.

In RA the entire joint is involved. The joint capsule and the synovial fluid — the oil that lubricates the joint — become inflamed and thickened. This inflammation extends to the tendons and the bones until the whole joint is involved and deformed, often to the point of being useless. This results in grossly misshapen hands, a typical sign of rheumatoid arthritis.

Diagnosis of RA in its early stages is not always easy. But the swollen knuckles and distorted joints of the hands and feet give physicians a strong hint that our patient is suffering from systemic rheumatoid arthritis. Special blood tests may help confirm this.

Early treatment is essential to minimize the destructive process, and aspirin in large doses is the first line of defense. Slow-release aspirin is now available, and has the advantage of causing less stomach irritation.

To control an acute episode, non-steroidal anti-inflammation drugs may help. Resting is an important treatment, and splinting the affected joint is often successful.

Gold therapy, administered by injections or pills, has brought welcome relief to many patients. And when these forms of treatment bring no relief, doctors may prescribe one of several more exotic drugs, with tongue-twisting names like penacillamine, hydroxychloroquine, azothioprine, and sulfasalazine.

Recently research workers found by accident that a drug called methotrexate brought relief to some RA victims. Cancer and psoriasis patients undergoing treatment with methotrexate were pleasantly surprised when their swollen, aching joints showed remarkable improvement. Apparently this drug can help the body heal itself in several different ways, by giving a boost to the body's immune system.

As is so often the case with many of the new and improved magic medicines, wonder drugs all too often have side effects. Because of these adverse reactions, physicians carefully and constantly monitor patients using any of the arthritic medications. Even aspirin is not entirely harmless.

There is some good news for people afflicted with RA. Half of them will recover completely after one or two acute flare-ups. Only one in ten RA sufferers will become disabled. Apparently, the immune systems of the other nine respond effectively when challenged.

Older folks, victims of osteoarthritis, can assume a philosophic attitude and accept the creaking of their joints as a badge of honor at having survived the many battles of the advancing years. They join Granny Green in their day-to-day companionship with Ben and Charlie and good old Art Ritus.

17 "My hand keeps going to sleep..."

YOU'VE PROBABLY OCCASIONALLY "SLEPT WRONG," perhaps with your wrist cramped under your chin, then awakened with a numbness in your hand, a burning and tingling in your fingers You shook your hand vigorously, or perhaps just hung your arm down over the edge of the bed. Very likely the discomfort disappeared, and you gave it no further thought.

But for some people these peculiar sensations return again and again, and they begin to wonder "what's going on here?" Their physician likely would tell them that they are suffering from a rather common condition called "carpal tunnel syndrome."

Just behind the palm of your hand, at the crease of the wrist, is a tough fibrous band called the carpal ligament. It's there to hold together and stabilize the bones in your wrist, collectively known as "the carpals." Passing through the tight compartment beneath this ligament, on the way to your hand, is the median nerve.

Any swelling or inflammation in or around the little tunnel beneath that ligament squeezes the nerve, giving you a feeling of numbness and tingling in your hand.

Carpal tunnel syndrome may clear spontaneously, without treatment. Although not a life-threatening condition, if it persists the thumb muscle may be atrophied and weakened.

Mother Nature's sex discrimination again: women are five to ten times more likely to suffer from CTS than are men. Also, occupations or sports that involve constant flexing and extending of the wrist may lead to carpal tunnel syndrome. As a surgeon, I've had it myself.

CTS may occur during menstrual periods, or in pregnant or menopausal women, presumably because of a hormonal imbalance or water retention. There are other systemic disorders such as rheumatism, diabetes, obesity and thyroid dysfunction that in rare instances may be associated with this syndrome.

Diagnosis is not always easy. For example, the same sort of numbness in the hand can be caused by pressure on nerves in the neck in advanced arthritis, or from a bulging intervertebral discs. To confirm the diagnosis your doctor will do nerve function tests, or will order nerve conduction tests.

Often the symptoms disappear as quickly as they came, but if the pain, numbness and tingling persists a wrist splint may give relief, especially at night.

If the numbness doesn't disappear in response to these more conservative treatments, cortisone may be injected directly into the ligament. This also can serve as a diagnostic test: if the cortisone shot brings relief it is proof positive that the problem is swelling or inflammation in the carpal ligament, not a nerve problem somewhere else in your body.

Finally, if all these measures are unsuccessful, even after several injections, surgery is indicated. This entails cutting across the ligament to relieve the pressure on the nerves and vessels that pass through the carpal tunnel. The good news is that this procedure is 80% to 90% successful.

18 A Successful Fix for Dupuytren's Contracture

MY PATIENT BILL BJORNSON recently retired from his job out at the sawmill. He and Ron Reagan, not my patient but also retired, have something in common. Both were afflicted with a peculiar condition called Dupuytren's contracture, and both had the condition corrected by successful surgery.

Named after a famous 19th-century French surgeon, this disorder causes the ring finger and the little finger to be permanently bent at the knuckles.

To imagine this deformity, ask your hand to make a "V-for-victory" sign. As you do this your ring finger and your pinkie are both sharply flexed, and a deep wrinkle has formed across your palm.

This is exactly how Bill's right hand and Ron's left hand looked to them. The difference is that now you can return your fingers to a straight and outstretched position. But their last two fingers in the afflicted hand stayed clenched, and the deep wrinkle in their palm remained.

Though the condition is painless, it can be mighty inconvenient. For example, in the right hand it interferes with the handshake, in the left it may trap a wedding band.

Dupuytren's contracture is most commonly seen in white males over 40, rarely afflicts women, and tends to run in families.

Repeated trauma to the palm of the hand may or may not be a contributing factor. For nearly thirty years Bill Bjornson used his hands to pull the levers on the big steam rig that sliced logs into lumber. But President Reagan certainly hadn't made his living wielding a hammer or an ax with his left hand.

This is one of those afflictions where we doctors know the condition in the body which causes the patient's problem, but aren't sure of what led to the condition.

Dupuytren's contracture is caused by a build-up of scar tissue in the fascia in the palm of the hand. Your palmar fascia is the heavy-duty padding, the "heel" of your hand, that overlays the tendons that activate your five fingers. When something causes the palmar fascia to thicken and contract, the fingers gradually draw up into the flexed position.

Conservative management by splinting may bring temporary release of the clenching tension. Injection of the palmar fascia with a cortisone solution also may be tried. But eventually nothing short of surgical removal of the scar will bring relief. Both Bill and Ron elected to have this surgery.

The surgical procedure consists of a careful dissection and removal of the scar tissue. The surgeon must work in a bloodless field, because important nerves and blood vessels pass through that area, so a tight tourniquet is applied.

Bill told me he wanted to be asleep during the procedure: "Doc, no way do I want to know what's going on!" The President, on the other hand, didn't want to miss a chance to swap stories with the surgeon, so he had the job done under "local."

Ron and Bill's experience differed in several other ways. To greatly reduce the expense, Bill's operation was done as an out-patient procedure. His wife bundled him into the car and took him home as soon as he had awakened from the anesthetic.

On the other hand, President Reagan stayed overnight at Walter Reed Hospital, in a room that he had visited on a number of occasions during his eight years in the White House.

But, happily, they have this in common: both made an excellent recovery. After a period of physical therapy Ron was ready to swing his leg over the saddle and grasp the reins of his favorite horse at his California ranch. And Bill was again able to firmly grip a golf club, so that when spring rolled around he was back out there pitching and putting with the best of them.

19 Vertigo

My patient Mary Rowland was miserable: "I get dizzy all the time, and even when I'm lying down the room spins around if I move my head. All the time I feel like I'm just about to throw up."

Just my telling her that these were the symptoms of an irritating disorder called vertigo seemed to ease her fears that she had a mental problem. I took this opportunity to explain how the ear — particularly her inner ear — functions to allow us to keep our equilibrium as well as to hear.

The tiny hearing mechanisms in each side of our head are truly wonderful. Sound waves jiggle the eardrum, which vibrates this message through bones familiarly called the hammer, anvil and stirrup. This physical agitation passes through the cochlea, then is translated into electric impulses in the auditory nerve, which routes these bits of energy to the hearing section of the brain. The pattern of these pulses allows us to identify these neural signals as a particular kind of sound.

We may not often consciously appreciate our ability to hear, but all day long we react to sounds, enjoying a melody or a conversation with a friend, being irritated at loud music being inflicted on us in public, or covering our ears as a fire truck roars by, its siren blaring. Yet few of us give any thought to the amazing computerized device within our inner ear and brain that continually allows us to steadily keep our balance. Unless, of course, like Mary, we suffer from vertigo.

And, while others notice when someone loses even a little of their hearing ability, the vertigo victim is alone in his or her experience of a life of total misery, a giddy, whirling world.

The locus of our equilibrium lies within the part of our

inner ear called the labyrinth. This delicate structure consists of three interconnected semicircular tubes, each bent at right angles to the other two. These tubes or "canals" contain fluid, and the movement of this liquid as we move allows our brain to constantly monitor the position of our head and body. These positional impulses, coupled with our eye movements, enable us to maintain or regain our balance, whether we're walking along a level sidewalk or across the deck of a pitching ship.

But when the pressure of this fluid changes markedly, or when the inner ear becomes inflamed, its messages to the brain become confused, and we get dizzy and nauseated, even to the point of vomiting. Beads of sweat form on our foreheads, and we feel faint and may fall.

These distressing symptoms can be caused by such comparatively simple disorders as an acute sinus infection or a viral inflammation in the middle ear. Vertigo also may be caused by a sudden drop in blood pressure or low blood sugar. Or vertigo may be a symptom of a far more serious condition, such as transient ischemic attack, a small stroke, even a brain tumor. Fortunately the incidence of these latter conditions is relatively infrequent.

Whatever the cause, the sensation of dizziness and a loss of balance that Mary experienced can be agonizingly real. The feeling of spinning, along with nausea and vomiting, are devastating. Even milder symptoms of vertigo — feelings of faintness, brief blackouts, or a fleeting weird sensation that the patient describes as "not being quite with it" — discourage a person from leaving home and certainly from driving a car.

Successful treatment depends on finding the cause. A sudden onset of vertigo, and a fairly prompt response to treatment, suggests a less serious condition. Infection, often from a virus, is by far the most common cause in these cases. A more gradual development of symptoms, including a weakness in the arms and legs or visual changes, is cause for greater concern.

Happily, Mary's vertigo responded well to conservative measures: medications, bed rest, a low salt diet...and the tincture of time to allow the body to heal itself.

And as Mary slowly recovered from her bout with vertigo, both she and her family now knew that her dizziness was indeed "all in her head," right there in her inner ear.

20 Depression: It's Not Just "All In Your Head"

SNOW AND NIPPY WINTER WEATHER bring pleasure to many of us who love our four seasons. But for others, dark clouds of sadness and depression inevitably move in during the winter months. For a few, feeling blue leads them to attempt to end it all: depression-related suicides are especially high during January and February.

Depression, like the common cold, has long frustrated medical researchers. In the United States today over 15 million citizens suffer from depression severe enough to require treatment. And there are millions more who endure what psychiatrists term "masked depression," people who don't realize that their physical aches and pains actually are symptoms of depression.

What is depression, and why is it so widespread? First of all, depression takes many forms. The American Psychiatric Association's "Diagnostic and Statistical Manual of Mental Disorders," lists 319 differential diagnoses, each with its own code number.

For you and me that's much too complicated. Instead, let me share three true-to-life vignettes, to illustrate the three general types of depression. They involve patients of mine whom I'll call Rita, Molly and Rebecca.

Rita suffered from the common, everyday type of depression that can result from emotional, psychological or even physiological disruption of a person's lifestyle. This particular variety of depression usually is precipitated by the events and pressures that impact directly upon a person's life.

That traumatic, stressing event in Rita's life was a devastating divorce proceeding. For someone else the "exogenous" event could just as well have been distress over a son arrested for drunken driving. Or the extraneous factor might have been a major business loss, the death of a loved one, a break-up of a love affair. Even something as simple as a flunked college entrance exam.

Symptoms of this form of depression include vague aches and pains, a frequently upset stomach, and abrupt and extreme mood swings. Also, loss of interest in work or play, called "dysphoria," the inability to work, learn or concentrate.

Fortunately Rita's recovery from her depression was quite rapid. Her family gathered around her, she accepted her doctor's assurance that she wasn't going crazy, that with a little more medical help she would soon be on the road to recovery.

Rita's problem could be called a neurosis — a mild, usually temporary disorder of the nervous system. On the other hand, Molly's depression was a manifestation of a more serious biological disorder.

The cause of Rita's depression lay somewhere "above the neck and between the ears," while Molly's affliction was truly an internal, organic dysfunction.

By contrast, Molly's whole body was involved, presumably because of a malfunction in her mind-body electro-chemical interaction. Biochemical substances such as the hormone norepinephrine, or electrical conductors such as serotonin, were being over- or under-produced, upsetting the nervous system's delicate balance.

This chemical imbalance in her body caused Molly to withdraw from family and friends, and to abruptly begin weeping for no apparent reason. She seemed to lose all interest in life — there was nothing to live for. Her husband was deeply concerned, fearful that his wife was losing her mind.

Incidentally, these symptoms closely resemble the mental and physical anguish, the dysphoria and torment experienced by the PMS patient, or the woman suffering from "menopausal melancholia." This similarity seems to lend credence to the hormonal, biochemical theory of depression.

In the Sigmund Freud era this patient would have repeatedly reclined on a couch, in a long and costly course of therapy, aimed at unearthing suppressed memories of infant or childhood unhappiness, especially sexual experiences. This was known as the "talk cure."

Today to treat depression the talk cure has been largely replaced by anti-depressant medications that have a more reasonable price tag.

The third mental disorder under the general heading of depression is the so-called "manic-depressive psychosis," more properly termed a "bipolar affective disorder."

The term "bipolar" refers to the peculiar nature of this depression, characterized by wide swings of mood. For a time the patient will be in a "high," in a wound-up, hyperactive state of "euphoria." He or she will function at a vigorous pitch of activity and productivity, often working at a frenzied pace.

But then they fall into the depressive, dysphoric phase, the state Rebecca was in when she was brought into the hospital emergency room by her sister.

A few days before she was in a tizzy of activity as she prepared to leave her home in Utah, to visit her sister's family in north Idaho for the Christmas holidays. She was so busy and feeling so good she completely forgot to take her anti-depressant medications, lithium and potassium. And driving that long distance to the family get-together, she hadn't bothered to stop for her regular meals.

The first night after her arrival at her sister's home Rebecca carried on a steady stream of conversation, far past midnight. But then she began lapse into long periods of silence, punctuated by hysterical weeping spells.

At times she was had delusions and was paranoid. She repeatedly cried out to her sister "You don't love me anymore, nobody loves me. Oh why can't I die?" She was obviously sinking into a deep depression, rapidly losing her contact with reality. Her sister saw it was time to seek help.

There's a happy ending to this story. After Rebecca was admitted to the psych unit at Kootenai Medical Center her medications were quickly reinstated, bringing her potassium and lithium levels back to normal. That, coupled with compassionate counseling, gradually led Rebecca back to reality, restored her self-esteem and her ability to make an emotional adjustment. Truly a remarkable transformation.

So far we don't have a good scientific explanation how this comes about. But we know that depressions — from the minor to the manic — are an electro-chemical phenomenon. And we do know that anti-depression medications can make a difference.

No longer do we simply rely on a "talk cure," knowing that depression does not stem only "from the neck up and between the ears." We have learned, moreover, that the treatment, to be successful, must be aimed at the mind and the body.

It's significant that even Medicare, Medicaid and most

insurance companies now accept depression as not just a mental disorder, but a biological illness, with 319 different identifying code numbers.

Incidentally, please excuse the coincidence of my selecting three female patients to illustrate the three different types of depression. By no means is this malady limited to women. Abraham Lincoln suffered from a deep, dark melancholia. Edgar Allen Poe wrote "The Raven" during one of his sodden periods of depression. Franz Liszt, Robert Schumann and Hector Berlioz wrote some of their most brilliant compositions while in the manic phase of their depressions.

21 To Sleep, Perchance to Dream

We spend around a third of our lives in the arms of Morpheus, the god of dreams. Most of us usually enjoy a "good sleep," and awake refreshed. But one of every three adults has trouble falling asleep or staying asleep, which in its extreme form is called insomnia. Even people who only occasionally have difficulty sleeping regularly use sleeping pills, which is why sleeping potions are a bonanza for the pharmaceutical industry.

One of these is Halcion, a clever brand name derived from the adjective halcyon, for "calm, peaceful, tranquil." This mild sleeping pill has been widely used by people the world over to drift off to dreamland, including former President Bush. Halcion belongs to an important family of drugs called the benzodiazepines, which are used in the treatment of anxiety, stress, depression and on occasion prescribed for patients with insomnia. These medications change or reduce chemical interchange between nerve cells in the brain by lowering brain-wave activity, and by reducing the rate of brain-cell metabolism.

As we slumber through the night, the deepness of our sleep rises and falls. It's when we are sleeping lightly that we dream and, perhaps to "see" things when we are dreaming, our eyes quickly move behind our closed lids. That's why this lighter phase of sleep is called "rapid eye movement," or REM. When we are "dead to the world" researchers term this type of sleep "non-rapid eye movement," NREM.

Dreaming stimulates an increased blood flow to the brain, as well as an increased metabolism and stepped-up brain activity. Anything that interferes with that process, such as a sleeping pill in the benzodiazepine family, could theoretically have an adverse effect.

Sleep labs have determined that there is a wide variation in how quickly various sleeping medications take effect, and how long they last. Halcion, for example, goes to work quickly, but its effectiveness lasts only about five and a half hours. Other benzodiazepines that are effective longer are more likely to cause a "hangover," daytime drowsiness or nerve function impairment.

A few years ago some researchers tentatively linked the extended use of Halcion to psychiatric disturbances. Because so many people relied on this sleeping pill, including the president of the United States, this possibility received extensive media coverage, especially when a study of inmates at a Michigan prison found that those who were given a one milligram dose for 42 consecutive nights were more likely to have memory problems.

Unfortunately, the study was flawed in several ways. For one thing, the prisoners had not been given a psychiatric evaluation before the study. Also, many of the prisoners admitted they slept poorly because they feared being assaulted while they were in a sound sleep. Finally, the one milligram dose is higher than most doctors recommend. After a thorough review the drug was approved by the

Food and Drug Administration, in revised dosage recommendations.

There is plenty of evidence that long-term sleep deprivation may result in diminished mental alertness. If you are having trouble sleeping, and your problem isn't severe and chronic, any one of many over-the-counter, non-prescription sleeping pills may help you get a good night's sleep.

The active ingredient in practically all of the medications is diphenhydramine, an older antihistamine. In its basic, generic form it is relatively cheap, but when compounded in various trade-name drugs such as Sominex, Sleep-ease, Exedrin PM, Nytol and Tylenol OM, the cost mounts.

The sleeping medications most commonly prescribed are Halcion, Prosom, Restoril and Dalmane. While scientific studies have determined the benzodiazepines are both safe and effective, extended and uninterrupted use of the drugs diminishes their efficacy. This may then cause the patient to increase his dosage, in turn leading to the negative side effects.

A safe and gentle sleep remedy that has stood the test of time is milk, taken either hot or cold. The reason is that milk contains tryptophan, an amino acid that the brain converts into the neurotransmitter, serotonin. This is the chemical that influences our moods and works in conjunction with the brain's natural analgesic, endorphin. It is important to note that the synthetic tryptophan does not have that capability – it may, in fact, be harmful.

"To sleep, perchance to dream. Aye, there's the rub!" Do you suppose Shakespeare was an insomniac?

To Sleep, Perchance to Dream • 181

"After A Long Illness…"

Introduction

"I THINK I'M FALLING APART — IT MUST BE OLD AGE!" I hear variations of this a dozen times a week from patients coming into the office with a multitude of complaints. It's as if Age is automatically equivalent to aching, hurting and being tired.

It is quite true that advancing years bring more chronic illness: arthritis, diabetes, heart disease and an increased incidence of cancer. Because of the increasing population of older Americans, medical schools are now training specialists called "geriatricians."

At the same time, mature Americans are being urged to improve their own health by practicing preventive medicine through regular exercise, careful diet, and a sensible life style.

And we are facing the increasing need to house and to care for the seniors who no longer can be cared for at home. The "old folks home" and the county poor house have been supplanted by nursing homes, foster homes and extended care facilities. Simultaneously, modern technology has means of prolonging life, and all too often is able to prolong the process of dying.

On the positive side, to that grumbling patient who gripes that "it's tough to grow old" I might counter with the comment that at the turn of the century people didn't "grow old," at least not by today's standards. Life expectancy was around 50, and diseases such as smallpox, polio and TB wiped out thousands each year. Pneumonia was a sure killer, but now we have a half dozen antibiotics that will stop the pneumococcus bug in its tracks. Research scientists are making steady headway against diabetes, cancer, Alzheimer's and Parkinson's diseases.

Today, as we live our expected average span of nearly eighty years we are happy to wake each morning to the gift of a new day, remembering the words to that old hymn, "Let us count our blessings, and name them one by one."

1 Smile...It's Only Cancer!

I CHOSE THIS TITLE NOT TO BE FACETIOUS, but simply to emphasize that the time has come to talk abut cancer in the same terms we use for other chronic illnesses — diabetes or arthritis or heart disease. Fortunately, this is happening more and more these days, such as when we physicians are invited to speak to groups of concerned citizens, or when news stories honestly state that a public figure is being treated for a particular type of cancer.

But this was not always so. Not long ago we and our patients tried to hush up a diagnosis of cancer, as if it were a venereal disease. "Cancer" was the nasty "C" word, and when a person died of cancer, the obituary said only that the deceased "died after a lengthy illness."

Much of the credit for the healthier attitude toward cancer must go to the American Cancer Society's Public Education Program. Also, the media now talks about cancer much more openly. Obituaries come right out and say, for example, that Rex Harrison died of cancer of the pancreas. And when Sammy Davis Jr. died from the throat cancer he got from smoking three packs of cigarettes a day, People Magazine devoted four pages to this cancerous connection. Such honest and open discussion helps discourage people, especially young people, from starting or continuing this destructive habit.

Now it's even all right to smile when you say the "C"

word, and no longer is it necessary for a doctor to lie to the patient who has been diagnosed as having cancer. These days, when I must tell a patient they have cancer, their response is more likely to be, "Okay, let's get busy and do something about it!"

That's a healthy response, making treatment easier and probably more effective. Certainly such a positive approach to trying to get well makes my relations with these patients more positive and enjoyable. I like that because, without apology, I'm a happy and upbeat person, following the example of whoever it was who said "I never met a man I didn't like..." (Let's see, was that Mae West...or was it Liz Taylor? Of course it was Will Rogers.)

Laughter can help fight cancer and other diseases. It has been established that people who are happy have stronger immune systems, and so are more able to withstand infection. There is reason to believe they are less likely to get cancer; if they do, they have longer survival rates.

To test this thesis the Royal College of Physicians studied two hundred women with inoperable breast cancer. Half of the women in this group were randomly selected and given routine care in ordinary cancer clinics.

The other one hundred breast cancer patients were given the same appropriate cancer therapy, whether radiation or chemotherapy, but they were treated in "happiness clinics," where the nurses and doctors wore smiles, and the rooms were bright and cheerful. Also, all the patients attended "laughter therapy" group sessions, where they swapped funny stories, exchanged hilarious experiences, or watched happy videos. In this carefully controlled scientific experiment, members of this "happiness group" lived an average of 18 months longer!

I am convinced that such "happiness therapy" can help in the treatment of any illness. Perhaps I first began believing this when I was in medical school, when my father, a

German Lutheran minister, gave me this advice: "Son, as you take care of patients, God does not like a long face."

I think this would be good advice for all young doctors. When some of us physicians begin practice after so many years of training, I'm afraid we may take ourselves too seriously. We go around with a frown on our face instead of a smile. Out at the hospital the other day I overheard one patient say to another, "Your doctor surely is a sourpuss — he never smiles. Do you suppose he has an ulcer?" The other replied, "No — but I think he's a carrier." To fight this tendency in myself, I long ago adopted a kind of 11th Commandment: "Thou shall not take thyself too seriously."

Norman Cousins, former editor of the Saturday Review and a highly respected writer on many non-medical topics, documented the great curative power of laughter in his book "Anatomy of An Illness." His observations are based on his own experience when he was in the chronic disease wing of the Los Angeles General Hospital, being treated for a serious and very painful illness called "spondylitis."

This hospital was a dull and dreary place, without happiness and smiles. Cousins, trained as a psychologist, thought this was all wrong, and decided he would lighten things up a bit. As a prank, he filled the urine specimen glass left by a student nurse with some of the apple juice brought in by his wife the night before. When the young trainee returned, she inspected the "specimen" and commented that it looked a little cloudy. Cousins took a look himself and agreed, saying "You know, you're absolutely right, maybe I should put it through again." And with that, he drank it. The poor student nurse ran out to tell her supervisor what this crazy fellow in room 501 had done. When they returned, Cousins confessed, and they all had a good belly laugh. Remarkably, Cousins found he was without pain for the rest of the morning.

This experience convinced him that he might be doing

more psychologically to help himself overcome his ailment, so he checked out of the hospital and into a hotel room, where he began reading humorous books, and watching Groucho Marx and Abbot and Costello comedies, using a projector his son had brought him. Cousins' condition gradually improved, and he ultimately recovered. I'm not arguing that we should abandon standard medical care for cancer, only that we all should take full advantage of endorphin, the natural "happiness hormone" that our bodies produce. To stimulate its production, if we are a cancer patient or if we are around cancer patients, we should live each day to the fullest, and make laughter a regular part of our life. To stay healthy and perhaps to get well, follow the simple advice of the person who said "I think my day wasted if I haven't laughed at least fifteen times."

2 Good News About Cancer in Women

THERE IS GOOD NEWS ABOUT CANCER, especially about female cancer. Take for example cancer of the cervix, the lower, vaginal portion of the uterus. Before we began to do routine Pap tests, physicians often would discover advanced cervical cancers, most difficult to treat with extensive surgery or with prolonged radiation treatment.

Not any more. Thanks to Pap smears we now are able to pick up very early cancers of the cervix which can be successfully eliminated with surgery, "burning" with lasers or using "cryotherapy," a freezing technique.

Because women are living longer, these days we're seeing more cancers of the body of the uterus, the inner portion, the "baby carriage." Fortunately, when detected early these cancers have a high cure rate. My patient Geraldine, for example, had her uterus removed with a hysterectomy, and she's cured.

And when we operated on Geraldine we also removed both her ovaries, just to be on the safe side, because ovarian cancer is a particularly treacherous form of female cancer. I routinely advise any woman aged 40 or over, who is going to have a hysterectomy for any reason, to have her ovaries removed at the same time. Today hormone replacement is very safe and effective.

The news about breast cancer, the other major female malignancy, is not quite as happy. We are seeing only slight improvement in breast cancer statistics, for which researchers cite several reasons:

- More and more women are coming into the older age group, and it's in these later years that breast cancer is most likely to occur.
- Thanks to mammograms, we are finding more breast cancer at an early stage of development, which increases the statistics on the number of cancers. Of course the good news is that these early detections are more treatable and curable.

What can a woman do to improve her own personal cancer statistics?

- She should have regular mammograms as recommended by her doctor. Fearing radiation, many women are reluctant to have mammograms, but new techniques use tiny doses of X-rays. Other women resist this important diagnostic test because they've heard mammograms squeeze your boobs until they hurt. But again, with the newer techniques that's really not as bad as it sounds.
- She should make sure she was born into a family where the women have a low incidence of breast cancer; if one woman member of a family has had breast cancer, this increases the statistical incidence in other close female family members.
- Having babies early in life provides a measure of immunity to breast cancer. The fact that nuns have a relatively

high incidence of breast cancer is a real-life demonstration of this statistical fact.

❦ She should stick with a low-fat diet. Not only does this help with weight reduction, and not only is it good for her cholesterol count, recent studies link high-fat diets with both breast cancer and colon cancer.

❦ She should regularly examine her breasts, between menstrual periods, for lumps or other irregularities. And she should make sure her physician examines her breasts thoroughly when she has a physical.

❦ If she smokes, she should quit; if she doesn't, she shouldn't start. Lung cancer caused by smoking is one of the most preventable of cancers. Sadly, the incidence of lung cancer among women is rising rapidly, especially in young women and in teenage girls, paralleling the increase in smoking by young women. This trend must be blamed in large part on seductive cigarette ads, depicting women puffers as slim, svelte and sexy.

And she should laugh, observing that 11th Commandment: "Take what you do very seriously, but take yourself lightly." Not only do women look prettiest when they're smiling or laughing, happiness builds up their immune system. So, men as well as women, let's all learn to laugh — just for the health of it!

3 Cancer in the Entertainment Business

COULD IT BE THAT PUBLIC FIGURES have a particularly high risk of getting cancer? Michael Landon, Lee Remick, Sammy Davis, Gilda Radner and Tip O'Neill all were front page news when they announced they had the Big "C."

Lee Remick succumbed at a much-too-early age of 50, after a two-year battle with lung cancer.

Michael Landon received a great deal of sympathetic news coverage when he refused to have any medical treatment for his cancer of the pancreas.

As Sammy Davis waged a long but losing battle against cancer of the throat, his life and death struggle was brought into our homes via television.

Perhaps saddest of all is the story of Gilda Radner and her courageous fight with ovarian cancer, a tragedy played to hundreds of thousands of fans on TV, and in newspapers and magazines.

Tip O'Neill retired from Congress after many years of productive public service, because he had contracted colon cancer. Yet soon, this grandfatherly fellow was back in the public eye, in television commercials.

There is no proof, of course, that a movie star or public figure has a greater likelihood of getting cancer, but their life-styles might be a contributing factor.

Michael Landon, the chubby-faced Little Joe Cartwright of Bonanza, portrayed an upright, kind and loving family man. But Landon admitted that in real life he drank too much, and that he smoked two to three packs of cigarettes a day. NBC publicist Bill Kelsey joked that "We used to bet his socks smelled smokey, because he inhaled so deeply."

Landon's refusal to undergo treatment for his pancreatic cancer is understandable, knowing that this particular variety is 97% fatal. It takes a certain kind of courage to proclaim to the world, "I'll go down fighting."

Cancer of the lung, the tumor that claimed the life of that versatile character actress Lee Remick, has a similarly bleak prognosis — 85% to 95%, depending on how early the diagnosis is made.

Though he now has passed away, I retain a clear mental picture of talented and charming Sammy Davis, cigarette in his hand, smoke curling up, as he sang those lovely melodies. Did his throaty voice sound a warning of his cancer battle that lay ahead?

Gilda Radner's death from ovarian cancer had nothing to do with her lifestyle, but she might have lived if her tumors had been detected sooner. She and her husband, Gene Wilder, suffered through many months of anguish, coping with a cancer that had been overlooked in its early, curable stages. After her death Wilder admitted that "The fact is, Gilda didn't have to die. But I was ignorant...she could be alive today if I knew then what I know now."

Wilder was unaware of the strong history of ovarian cancer in Gilda's family. Unknown to Gilda, a grandmother, a cousin and an aunt had had ovarian cancer. If she and her husband had been aware of this, they and her physician would have been specially alert to early warning signs of ovarian cancer. A cure might have been possible, and we might still be laughing with Gilda.

These are the sad, postmortem lessons left to us by Lee, Michael, Sammy and Gilda. A more positive message is sent by a happy, living cancer survivor, former Speaker of the House Tip O'Neill. Each time he appears on your TV screen he implicitly says "We caught my cancer early and, shucks, having a colostomy really isn't that bad!"

If by chance these stories and messages are heard down here on Earth, and as a result, some people can beat the odds against cancer, there are going to be some smiles and joyous singing somewhere up there in Entertainer's Heaven!

4 Who Needs Those Pap Tests and Mammograms?

WE CALLED HER "TANTA," the German equivalent of "Aunty." She came over from the old country to help take care of the five kids in our family. I was the youngest, and by the time I was a pre-medical student in college, she was ready to return to Germany.

It was at about that time, and apparently because I was preparing to become a doctor, that she asked for my help. With an embarrassed blush she confided her secret, that she had a lump in her "bosom." Would I get a bottle of tincture of arnica for her to apply to this lump, to make it go away? In my young innocence, I complied. But Tanta later died in her old home in Nuremberg, of ulcerating, metastatic cancer of the breast. My tincture of arnica didn't work.

Another true story...

Early in my practice in north Idaho, a sturdy Scandinavian women came into my office, reluctantly complaining of a watery, slightly bloody discharge from her "privates." She allowed me to perform a pelvic examination, in which I found a large, fungating tumor of the lower uterus, obviously an advanced cancer of the cervix. By the time she had overcome her shyness, and sought professional help for her problem, the tumor had already spread, and treatment was of no avail.

What a remarkable change has taken place during the past several decades in the health care of women, and in women's awareness of their own bodies, as they have shed their false modesty. Only rarely in this enlightened era do we see such advanced tumors, thanks to the work of Doctor Papanicolaou, and the popularization of his Pap test by the American Cancer Society. Physicians now routinely diagnose and effectively treat pre-malignant lesions discovered in pelvic exams.

Likewise, few medical students today ever will have the opportunity to see an ulcerating cancer of the breast. Fortunately, Tanta's false modesty and her ignorance about her body are things of the past. Now women regularly examine their breasts and, when indicated, have routine mammograms.

All this didn't happen overnight. I can well remember how, when the Pap test first became available, many physicians were skeptical of its usefulness. And only in recent years have mammograms become widely accepted by the public.

Who needs Pap tests? Occasionally a woman past menopause will ask me, "Why should I get Pap tests? Aren't I through with all that stuff?" As a physician I have to tell her that "You're still a woman, and so still have all the potential for female disorders, including cancer, infection and hormonal imbalance." And I'm likely to add that "Pap tests are just good preventive medicine; by having examinations regularly you can take advantage of the latest medical diagnostic advances."

Pap tests also are a good idea for younger women who are sexually active, especially those who have had several sex partners. Viral infections and sexually-transmitted diseases may place such people at increased cancer risk. Early diagnosis and treatment of pre-cancerous conditions can allow a woman to retain her child-bearing capability.

I was recently reminded of the importance of mammograms, when these tests on two of my female patients detected two breast cancers too tiny for me to have felt by manual examination. Yes, mammograms do flatten and squeeze a woman's breast, often to the point of discomfort, so the tests should not be scheduled when a woman's breasts are tender, such as around her menstrual period. But surely the protection mammograms provide far outweighs the temporary discomfort.

Who needs mammograms? Women in their later childbearing years who have never been pregnant are thought to be at special risk, as well as women who had their first pregnancy in the late thirties or early forties. Also, women whose mother, sister or aunt have had breast cancer. Ideally, all women over the age of 35 or 40 should afford themselves of a "baseline" mammogram.

And the answer to the larger question "Who needs all these Pap tests and mammograms?" is quite simply "More women than we thought." This year as many as 16,000 women in the United States will die of invasive cancers of the uterine cervix, tumors that have spread beyond easy control, but which very well might have been discovered at an early stage by a regular Pap test. And in the next twelve months around one in nine American women will develop breast cancer, even though it is widely known and accepted that early detection carries with it high hopes for a cure.

In recent years our cancer diagnosis skills have increased greatly, as has our ability to successfully treat cancers we've detected early. Yet physicians remain faced with a serious challenge: persuading our patients to take these tests.

5 *Hope for a Leukemia Cure*

LEUKEMIA IS A WEIRD DISEASE. First of all, this cancer affecting the body's white blood cells is actually several diseases. It encompasses different types of acute and chronic leukemias, varying forms of Hodgkin's disease and lymphomas, each with its own symptoms, and each with its own degree of hope for cure.

Not only that, the symptoms of leukemia are not always apparent to the patient; often this sneaky, stealthy disease is discovered by sheer accident during a routine physical examination.

Almost without exception the various forms of leukemia are characterized by a wild over-production of white blood cells in the bone marrow. This occurs by a process called "mutation," during which the cells divide repeatedly in a helter-skelter proliferation. The substantial increase in the white cell population gradually crowds out the normal cells, resulting in a reduction of the red cells, the platelets and the "good" white blood cells.

The loss of the red blood cells leads to anemia. An inadequate supply of platelets can interfere with the blood's ability to clot, resulting in easy bruising or various forms of insidious bleeding. Loss of normal white blood cells reduces the body's ability to withstand infection. Any of these leukemia insults can ultimately lead to death.

The diagnosis of red cell anemia is relatively straightforward. By contrast, diagnosis of white blood cell disorders can be a head-scratcher for the physician. Moreover, differentiation between the acute and chronic forms of leukemia is of significance in making a prognosis. And whether the leukemia occurs in children or in adults also can change the outlook.

Which of the two main types of white blood cells that can be involved in leukemia, lymphocytes or myelocytes, must be determined. Additionally, there needs to be a differentiation between lymphomas and the two types of Hodgkin's disease. At times it may be necessary to do a bone marrow biopsy, by taking small snippets of marrow from the hip bone or breast bone in order to arrive at a diagnosis.

Fortunately, leukemia in all its forms is a rare disease. This year there will be only 6 or 7 cases of acute leukemia for every 100,000 U.S. inhabitants. The chronic forms are even less common, with an occurrence rate of 4 or 5 per 1,000,000 population.

What causes a white blood cell to start cranking out

multiple copies of itself? Medical researchers believe this wild and disorganized mutation can be set off by a virus, similar to the one that causes AIDS. They have indicted solvents such as benzene, formerly used in dry cleaning. Nuclear accidents or explosions — such as occurred at Chernobyl and Hiroshima — are rare causes. Some researchers have even linked genetic factors to the incidence of leukemia.

Whatever the cause and whatever the diagnosis, the basic treatment is usually chemotherapy or radiation therapy, often both. Steady refinements in accuracy and dosage have greatly minimized the side effects.

Unfortunately, bugaboos about these types of treatment still persist, prompting cancer sufferers to seek alternatives. Occasionally a misinformed patient will desperately grasp at straws, foregoing accepted, standard treatment, relying on herbs and tonics, coffee enemas to "flush out the toxins," or cottage cheese and flax seed oil to "dissolve the tumor." These well-meaning efforts are usually physically harmless...unless they delay or replace prompt, effective and medically accepted treatments that could be life-saving, especially in children.

Not too long ago a diagnosis of leukemia sounded a death knell. Acute leukemia, untreated could be fatal within weeks. Today we are gaining on controlling and conquering this frustrating disease; current treatments can bring long periods of remission, even cures.

Animal research on viral disease is progressing at a rapid pace. Wouldn't it be wonderful if AIDS research could, by serendipity, bring us a life-saving cure or even prevention of this weird white blood cell cancer!

6 Three Mothers and Their Cancer Kids

HERE ARE THE STORIES OF THREE MOTHERS who, if asked, will tell you, "Yes, kids do get cancer."

One is Erma Bombeck, who wrote a beautiful book about children who have cancer.

Another is a mother who, forty years ago, lost her only son to childhood cancer.

The third is a mother who cherishes each new day of her life with a son who survived cancer.

When cancer strikes a young person, parents and friends may be sad and even bitter at the prospect of a life that may be tragically ended before it reaches its potential. But these days there is cause for some happiness too, because medical advances are enabling more of these young lives to be saved.

That funny lady, Erma Bombeck, went out of character to write her book about kids who are surviving cancer. Fortunately she approached this potentially heavy topic with her patented light and gentle touch. The tone of the book is optimistic, with a hope for tomorrow. She manages tenderness without being maudlin.

The book is called "I Want to Grow Hair, I Want to Grow Up. I Want to Go to Boise," and is based on her observations of cancer kids at Camp Sunrise, a most unusual rehabilitation center for cancer kids, near her home in Arizona.

What she learned from these youngsters makes for easy reading about gutsy kids who walk with artificial legs, race around in their wheel chairs, or paste decals on their bald heads. Lots of laughs and very few tears.

Adults get cancerous growths of organs such as the

uterus, breast or prostate, but the majority of childhood cancers are an affliction of the blood cells, such as leukemia, lymphoma or Hodgkin's disease. Furthermore, adult cancers are linked to the aging process; the longer we live, the greater the chance we'll develop a cancer. To some extent we can accept such ailments as the price we pay for the gift of a long life.

But childhood cancer strikes out of the blue. One day we see a happy, jumping-jack of a child; the next our little one is pale and listless. We wonder why, until a study of the blood cells under the microscope brings us the horrible diagnosis: cancer.

Erma Bombeck tells the cancer stories of well over 200 young people, as they undergo treatment for this vexing disease. And, because more and more of these kids are living on into adulthood, she is able to express a spirit of hope and optimism.

There is some sadness, of course, as these youngsters undergo chemotherapy and radiation treatments and marrow transplants. But there is happiness too, as these courageous children cope with their nausea, their hair loss, their utter exhaustion, as they battle to achieve a remission — even to attain a hoped-for cure.

Over 40 years ago our second mother — call her Marge — was given that terrifying explanation of what was ailing her four-year-old son: leukemia. In those days such a diagnosis sounded a death knell, and also carried with it the stigma of the word "malignancy," that somehow was associated with a sense of shame and a feeling of guilt. Back then we talked about cancer in a hushed voice, as if it were somehow dirty. Now, thankfully, we can speak about cancer openly, treating it as just another disease.

Sadly, forty years ago treatment of childhood cancer was rarely successful, and soon Marge's only son was dead. Yet this personal tragedy led to much good for others: this heartsick mother vowed to devote her time and energies to the cancer cause through the rest of the days of her life, and was founding, charter member of our local cancer society.

The third mother's story is a happy one, in which an earache turned out to be a life-saver. When little David complained of a sore ear, his mother Barbara took him to the doctor. The physician astutely looked beyond the offending ear and, noting the child's distended abdomen and his sickly appearance, hardly typical of an ear infection, obtained blood tests. The conclusion: David's earache was purely incidental; he had cancer!

By good luck David's earache brought him into early and successful cancer therapy. The young boy struggled through the miseries of cancer treatment, undergoing surgery and then enduring chemotherapy. Now he is the picture of health, a happy five year-old boy who plays ball as vigorously as he strokes his little fiddle. Chances are excellent that David will grow to manhood, and live out a normal life.

In their own way each of these mothers has rendered a service to the cancer cause.

Through her book Erma Bombeck has given us new insight into the hearts and minds of cancer kids. Plus, according to the publisher, "all the monies earned by the author from the sales of this book in the United States will go to the research work of the American Cancer Society."

Marge, through her four decades of work in the local chapter of the American Cancer Society, typifies the devotion all volunteer workers contribute to the growing success we have in the early diagnosis and treatment of malignant tumors.

Barbara, as a woman who has suffered the fears and the heartaches as the mother of a cancer kid, now symbolizes the hopefulness and optimism that have replaced the pessimism and despair that a diagnosis of malignancy used to bring.

7 Doctor Parkinson and the Shaking Palsy

IMAGINE THE THOUGHTS THAT MUST HAVE PASSED through the mind of Dr. James Parkinson, an English physician in the early 19th century, as he became aware of the degeneration of his own nervous system.

As his hand trembled, and his handwriting was reduced to a tiny scrawl, he must have wondered "Am I becoming paralyzed?" Yet with scientific courage and candor, he took up his pen and wrote "An Essay on the Shaking Palsy," published in 1817.

"There are involuntary tremulous motions with lessened muscular power in parts not in action and even when supported; with a propensity to draw the trunk forwards, and to pass from a walking to a running pace. The senses and the intellect remain uninjured."

Nearly two centuries later his initial description of his own symptoms remains essentially accurate today, though his name "shaking palsy," paralysis agitans, is not precisely correct: Parkinsonism is characterized by a shaking, but there is no true paralysis.

Neurologists usually speak of "early," "moderate" and "advanced" Parkinson's. Early symptoms are hand tremors and what Parkinson called "glacial slowness" in performing such everyday tasks as washing, shaving and dressing. At this stage, the change in handwriting may become evident.

In the next moderate phase, there may be a rhythmic shaking of the head, legs and hands, as well as a continuous rubbing of the forefinger against the thumb — the "pill-rolling" motion. The patient's gait becomes slow, shuffling and forward-leaning; in this second stage, the person suffering from Parkinson's often appears about to break into a run.

As the disease becomes more advanced, the patient

wears a mask-like, expressionless face. His speech may be sluggish, and his muscular rigidity increases, interfering with his voluntary motions.

The progression of Parkinson's through its several stages may take as little as five years or as long as fifteen. Because the disease is not life-threatening, and because it does not affect mental acuity, the patient literally observes his own physical decline.

Men are afflicted somewhat more often than women, and the symptoms usually don't appear until a person is in his 60s to his 80s. Parkinsonism is relatively rare, attacking little more than 1% of the population over 50 years of age. There is no good evidence to suggest that the condition is inherited.

Nearly two centuries after it was first described, the exact cause of Parkinson's disease remains a mystery. Some theories hold that it is simply the result of a deterioration of the brain cells, perhaps through hardening of the arteries.

Other researchers believe that a "brain fever," encephalitis, contracted in the patient's 20s or 30s, leads to a delayed onset of this condition in later years.

A Parkinsonian symptom complex also may be induced by toxins such as carbon monoxide, maganese, or the prolonged use of phenothiazine tranquilizers. In almost all cases such symptoms disappear when the toxic substance is removed.

Even though we are unsure of the direct cause of this disease, we now understand the chemistry of the brain's misfunction in Parkinsonism. Under normal conditions, certain chemicals, dopamine and norepinephrin, act as high octane additives, enabling our nervous system to spark on all eight cylinders. In patients suffering from Parkinson's, for some unknown reason these chemicals are in short supply.

The obvious therapy, therefore, would seem to be to supply these lacking substances, and we can do that by administering the medicine levodopa (Sinemet). Antispasmodic, muscle-relaxing medications such as Artane, Cogentin and Kemandrin are used with some success to reduce stiffness and rigidity.

A new drug, brand name Eldepryl, is now being used with good success. Congress has passed a bill which will allow research on the transplantation of aborted fetal tissue in the treatment of Parkinsonism.

So far, a solid cure remains elusive, though researchers remain optimistic. For the time being, even though we cannot cure this rare ailment, at least we can slow its progress and relieve its symptoms.

8 Skin Cancer Caused by Child Abuse?

IMAGINE THAT YOU'RE A MEDICAL RESEARCH SCIENTIST who has made a breakthrough of earth-shaking proportions: you've discovered how to significantly reduce the incidence of the world's two most common cancers — skin cancer and cancer of the lung.

Anticipating your announcement, television crews have set up their lights and cameras outside your laboratory where reporters cluster with their pens and pads at the ready. You emerge from your office, and step forward to explain your discovery: "Ladies and gentlemen, after considerable research in our laboratories we have concluded that the principal causes of skin cancer and cancer of the lung are, respectively, sun and cigarettes."

A collective hush falls over the group, then a groan, and then a lone voice pipes up: "You mean you got us here just to tell us that? Hey, man, there's nothing newsworthy about sun and cigarettes causing cancer!"

The kind of "medical breakthrough" newspeople prefer

usually involves a pill or a vaccine, not a call to change personal behavior. Furthermore, citing cigarettes as cancer-causers is beating a dead horse. And as for skin cancer — that concerns other people, mostly aging adults.

You might have done a little better with your story on the link between sun and skin cancer if you had come out with it during a summer heat wave. But not much better, because we human beings have such short memories.

A more effective way to interest reporters in your skin cancer story would have been to announce that you've discovered a new form of child abuse. That parents are actually increasing the chances their children will contract a life-threatening malignancy, when they let them get sunburned.

In the past the public has been taught to regard skin cancer as a rather innocuous disease, 98% curable, afflicting mainly old folks. To a certain extent that's true, but now we are learning that the seeds of a very serious type of skin cancer, malignant melanoma, may be planted in the skin of children when they are very young, probably before the tender age of ten. Now that's newsworthy.

The two most common types of skin cancer, the basal cell carcinoma, along with the less common type, squamous cell cancer, are both slow-growing and related to sun exposure. The rays of sunshine that warm your skin also may be activating carcinogens — the producers of skin cancers. These are the same rays that, when we're on the ski slopes or at the beach, increase deposits of dark pigment called melanin in our skin, giving us "a healthy tan." But at the same time, these rays may be setting the stage for future malignant changes in the skin cells.

Perhaps because the first two types of skin cancer are slow-growing and 98% curable, there has been too little concern or urgency about the prevention of basal cell and squamous cell carcinomas. The third type, malignant melanoma, has been given less attention because it was believed to be quite rare.

But in the last two decades we have seen a dramatic upsurge in the frequency of melanomas, apparently due to the steady increase in sun worshipping.

In the United States in 1991, 32,000 individuals were newly diagnosed with melanomas, and of those 6,500 already have died. Medical researchers estimate that 80% of those melanomas were the result of excessive sun exposure during childhood.

Such statistics will cause 21st century historians to be puzzled by this peculiar phenomenon of sun worshipping, so popular in the 1960s, 1970s and 1980s. Back then people would deliberately burn their skin in the sun, to produce a thick, brown hide. Northerners, to create an image of being "rich and famous," vacationed for weeks in California, Arizona or Florida, spending hours in the sun to acquire a "beautiful tan." When they returned home, they'd retain their color by cooking their epidermis under ultraviolet lamps, in places called "tanning parlors."

Such is the nature of fads. In contrast, some of you older readers may remember when a pale, pearly skin was considered a thing of beauty. To avoid the tanning rays of the sun, milady would wear long white gloves and a wide-brimmed hat, and carry a parasol (a word meaning, literally, "guard against the sun") as protection against the burning and browning rays of Old Sol.

That's ancient history. Today old and young — mostly young — yearn for that "healthy tan." But here's the rub: skin cancer is no longer an affliction affecting mainly Seniors. Now these skin tumors, particularly melanomas, are being diagnosed among Yuppies and Middle-Agers. Dermatologists feel certain that many of these cancers can be traced back to severe sunburns, especially those resulting from exposure to sudden bursts of hot midday sun. They believe that such burns increase by around one third a person's chance of developing a malignant melanoma within the next 10 to 20 years following the intense exposure.

Realizing that we and our children will continue to be naturally drawn to the sun's warming rays, here are some basic rules to reduce your chances of having a sun-linked skin cancer:

(1) Avoid midday exposure, when the sun is high in the sky.

(2) Avoid heavy bursts of burning, especially in children.

(3) Wear protective clothing, hats or caps.

(4) Always use sun screen with a Sun Protective Factor (SPF) of 15 or better on all exposed areas. Use the same strength for kids and adults. Use a double amount on the edges of your bathing suit, on the back of your legs and on the top of your feet. Re-apply every 3 or 4 hours.

(5) Use special sunglasses, marked for sun protection.

(6) Remember that you can burn even on overcast days, and from water reflection while boating, or from the snow during winter skiing.

What about recognition and diagnosis of skin cancers?

(1) Carefully observe any skin bumps or blotches, especially if there's a change in their appearance, or if they are aggravated by sunlight.

(2) Remember, malignant melanomas need not be "black," but can be red, blue, tan or brown. Be particularly aware of an irregularly-shaped growth on your skin, especially if it is crusting and growing rapidly.

(3) Your risk of developing skin cancer is higher if you are fair-skinned, a red-head, or if blood relatives have had melanomas.

Maybe there's nothing "newsworthy" about skin cancer being caused by the sun, but this new information about the dangers of sunburn in youngsters should be a shocking reminder that parents are responsible for protecting their children against excess exposure to the sun. Not to do so amounts to a form of child abuse.

9 Heart Attack, Hot Brash or Hiatal Hernia?

"Do you suppose I was having a heart attack yesterday while I was grubbing in the garden?" My patient Marie Parsons was fidgeting nervously in my office, telling me in a worried voice about chest pains she'd had the day before. "For most of the morning I had been bending over, weeding. Then suddenly I got this boring, burning sensation in my chest!"

After taking a more complete history, performing a thorough physical examination, including some special tests, I was glad to assure Marie that she hadn't experienced a heart attack but rather a condition called "reflux esophagitis," resulting from a "hiatal hernia." Actually, Grandma knew about this irritating malady, and often suffered from it after weeding the cabbage patch or the strawberry bed, but she simply called it "hot brash."

It really did not require exceptional diagnostic acumen on my part to diagnose a possible hiatal hernia. All of Marie's bending over working in the garden had forced acidic stomach juices up into her swallowing tube — what Grandma called the "gullet" — precipitating an attack of "heartburn."

Physicians regularly consider the possibility of reflux esophagitis and hiatial hernia in patients who complain of acute stomach distress and chest pain. And, because the symptoms of one disorder can mimic the symptoms of another, doctors take special care in making their final diagnosis.

As it turns out, we are able to treat the gnawing pain of stomach ulcers at the same time we relieve the burning, hot brash discomfort beneath the breast bone, arising from the backflow of stomach juices up through a hiatal hernia, where the esophagus meets the stomach.

At this point, a muscular, two-way valve automatically opens when you swallow, allowing food to pass into the stomach. When it's working properly, that valve prevents the backflow of any food or liquid already in the stomach.

But when this valve is weak or relaxed, gastric contents can be regurgitated back up into the swallowing tube. When this happens it's called "esophageal reflux," and the irritation this causes can result in a painful inflammation of the esophagus, called "esophagitis." If such inflammation persists, it can cause scarring, and may even change the nature of the cells that line the lower end of the esophagus. Moreover, if stomach acid is constantly regurgitated through this widened opening, the esophagitis this causes may eventually cause swallowing difficulties.

In some instances, this weakened valve allows a portion of the stomach to balloon through the valvular opening, creating a hiatal hernia. This, unfortunately, is a rather common condition.

Men develop more ulcers — we males are certain that it's because we carry the weight of the world's worries on our shoulders! But, surprisingly, more women than men have hiatal hernias. Obesity may contribute to this condition, but I would be more ready to believe that differences in female anatomy (and thank heaven for those differences!) are the real reasons for these anomalies.

Other than heartburn, the symptoms of hiatal hernia and esophagitis are hoarseness, laryngitis and sometimes a chronic cough that may result from acid irritation in the upper throat. Older people, who have suffered from the condition for many years, are more likely to have the cough.

You can prevent such gastric reflux by following a few simple rules. Eat slowly, chew thoroughly, don't wolf your food. Lying down on the sofa to watch that football game right after you've eaten may not be a good idea. Likewise, don't go to bed right after a heavy evening meal.

For those suffering from reflux esophagitis, cigarettes are a no-no, because nicotine raises the level of stomach acid. Also, alcoholic drinks should be reduced to a minimum, and should be well diluted. Coffee, onions, chocolate, peppermint and excessively fatty foods may exacerbate reflux. Sleeping with your head slightly above your feet may help.

In the past, anti-acid medications were widely used to treat reflux esophagitis, but have fallen from favor because of side effects such as diarrhea, and their tendency to interfere with the effectiveness of other medications the patient might be taking. Plus, on a long-term basis, they are not very cost-effective.

A more logical approach would be to find medications to block acid secretion. A decade ago it was discovered that a particular class of drugs called "H_2 Blockers" could effectively reduce the ability of that old acid pump, the human stomach, to over-produce the corrosive hydrochloric acid that is responsible for so much of this gastric mischief. The prototype drug was cimetidine, with the brand name Tagamet. This drug therapy resulted in a dramatic and welcome reduction in the need for stomach surgery.

Since the introduction of Tagamet, several additional H_2 Antagonist medications have been developed, including Zantac, Pepcid, and Axid. More recently, a super, gangbuster pill called Prilosec (formerly Losec) has become available, and it is by far the most effective in absolutely wiping out all acid production.

But all these drugs, like so many new medications in use today, have their drawbacks. First of all, they're expensive: many of these pills cost around three dollars each. Research and testing required to meet the Food and Drug Administration's rigorous requirements can cost millions of dollars for a single preparation.

However, put in an overall health cost perspective, the cost of these medications is considerably less than hospitalization for ulcer management, control of bleeding, or for surgery.

We have been using the H_2 Blockers long enough to be confident of their short-term safety, but research continues on Prilosec to determine any problems with long-term use of this medication. Among the concerns are effects on the blood and iron counts, or even the possible eventual production of stomach cancer.

Although I was able to reassure my patient Marie that she wasn't having a heart attack, I was, at the same time, careful to remind her that chest pain of any kind is not to be ignored. We know, for example, that angina — the pain of heart vessel spasm — can co-exist with the pain of reflux esophagitis.

Surely if Marie actually had been experiencing the early symptoms of a true heart attack, a myocardial infarction, then immediate medical attention would have been life saving.

And, conversely, swallowing some baking soda or antiacid pills, or popping some of her neighbor's Tagamet pills, just might have been foolhardy.

So if you're having chest pains, you may have stomach problems, not heart problems. But don't take chances; find out for sure from your doctor which it is.

10 When is a Heart Attack Not a Heart Attack?

CHATTING WITH MY NEIGHBOR GLADYS, in the produce section of the supermarket, I mentioned that our mutual friend Art Rowland had suffered a heart attack a few weeks back.

"Oh, my goodness," she said, "did he die?"

That's a normal reaction to the diagnosis of "heart attack." We consider our heart to be a very special, even a mysterious organ. Heart problems are automatically thought to be serious, with the potential of a fatal outcome.

So I was glad to tell her that Art had spent a couple of days in the hospital, and while there had had a minor operation. After a short vacation, he was already back at work.

It happened we both were picking up broccoli for dinner, and were in a hurry to get home. I would have liked to have had the time to talk with Gladys about "heart attacks"— what they are and what they aren't. Many of us are so worried about heart failure that we're apt to self-diagnose chest pains in any form as a heart attack.

For example, a gentleman farmer of my acquaintance recently spent a strenuous half-day bucking hay bales. The next morning he awoke with a severe pain beneath his breast bone, his sternum. Worried that he was having "a coronary," he rushed off to the hospital emergency room. To his great relief he was diagnosed as simply having "chest wall pain," a muscle strain totally unrelated to his heart.

Martin Malden is one of our most successful and hardworking real estate brokers. A few months ago, after a long and strenuous day, he and a colleague went out to Tony's Surf 'n Turf for dinner. The two had several drinks, then got ready to devour a couple of large steaks. But as Martin happily chewed his first bite, he suddenly felt a deep, boring pain in his mid-chest. His panicked friend ran to the phone and dialed 911, to report a heart attack in progress. Still imobilized by the pain and by worry, Martin was whisked by ambulance to the hospital. Various tests confirmed that his heart was functioning fine. The final diagnosis was "esophageal spasm," a temporary tightening of the swallowing tube, which prevented him from swallowing that steak.

Angina is another temporary, non-fatal condition sometimes wrongly construed as a "heart attack," the type of sub-sternal pain that may occur after exertion. An agina attack is simply the heart muscle crying out for a greater supply of oxygen, so it can pump blood faster. The coronary arteries on the surface of the heart are unable to deliver enough oxygen, because of a spasm or a narrowing of those blood vessels. The pain of angina disappears when the stress on the heart is stopped, or when the person takes a vascular dilator such as nitroglycerin.

When enough fatty deposits slow the flow of blood through a coronary artery, this increases the chance of a low grade heart attack, as the body sends a signal that its heart function is less than 100%. Luckily, this is just what happened to my friend and patient Joe Long, who called me at the office one afternoon, complaining of chest pains. The next day an X-ray picture of his heart, an arteriogram, revealed an obstruction in a single coronary blood vessel. His arteriogram showed numerous other functioning blood vessels located in that area, which provided collateral circulation.

To correct Joe's condition, a few weeks later doctors inserted a long, flexible catheter with a balloon at its tip in his leg, and ran it up to his heart to perform what is known as an "angioplasty." Once the balloon had reached the obstructed spot, it was carefully inflated to dilate that area, thereby restoring the normal flow of blood.

Also, in some cases chemicals can be used to dissolve the fatty cholesterol plaques on the vessel wall, remotely like pouring Drano down a clogged kitchen sink.

When these methods are insufficient, more extreme measures must be used to restore circulation to the heart muscle. One is to transplant short strips of blood vessel, taken from the patient's leg, to bypass the blocked area. This is the source of the reference you often hear to a "double" or "triple" bypass heart operation. This stops the process of "coronary infarction," the dying and ultimate death of a localized area of the heart muscle, caused by a lack of blood.

Another method of cleaning out plugged blood vessels, is the use of a pencil-size tube with a spinning cup-shaped cutter at its end which, like the angioplasty device, is pushed up to the heart through one of the patient's major blood vessels. In the same way your plumber might run an electric "snake" through a drain, this "atherocath" shaves away fatty plaques, atheromas, unblocking the vessel.

This corrective technology is truly amazing, and more is on the way. Yet by far the best way to cure heart disease is to prevent it in the first place. Avoid fatty foods, exercise regularly, quit cigarettes, and think happy thoughts. And, oh yes, be sure you selected parents who will die of old age at 95.

11 How a Black Egg Helped Me Kick the Cigarette Habit

I USED TO SMOKE CIGARETTES. I smoked not because it was something I really enjoyed or really needed, but because at that time it was the "in thing;" everybody did it.

Then one day I gave it up. My decision to quit probably came from my maturation into a somewhat wiser physician. I finally came to the realization that smoking cigarettes was a dumb, unhealthy, expensive habit.

But what actually pushed me into that final break with the cigarette habit was, believe it or not, a black egg.

It happened at a reception held at the beautiful Mandarin Hotel in Hong Kong, where our traveling medical group was being welcomed by the local medical society. Hard-boiled black eggs were among the hors d'oeuvres we were urged to sample. We were told they obtained their ebony hue, and were transformed into a delicacy, by being buried undergound for a year. I downed one to please my host.

In the wee hours of the next morning I was rudely awakened by an urgent call to the nearby bathroom. For the next half dozen hours, both ends of my gastro-intestinal tract saw a lot of action.

As my distress slowly lessened, and I began to believe that I wasn't going to die on the 12th floor of a hotel overlooking Hong Kong harbor, I reflected on the sins of my past with an earnest wish to somehow make retribution. My life restored, some sort of penance seemed in order.

My most odious habit was cigarette smoking. What better time than this to give it up? I resolved then and there to quit, once and for all. That was nearly 25 years ago, and never again have I reached for a coffin nail. Simple as that.

Since that decisive moment for me, I've observed with special interest the steady increase in public sentiment against smoking. At first, the impetus came from wide acceptance of the scientifically proven link between cigarette smoking and lung cancer, in spite of the loud protestations of the tobacco lobby.

A little later, emphysema caused by smoking began to get its share of public attention. But for most of us, lung cancer and emphysema are intangibles — they happen to other people, not to me. We've heard that lung cancer doesn't hurt, and emphysema isn't a reality until we finally puff and wheeze when we climb a fight of stairs. Plus, these vague illnesses happen only to old folks, and old age lies in the far distant future.

But when a couple of years ago we were told that smoking can be a major contributor to heart disease, that struck closer to home, because so many different groups were cited as being at risk.

For example, women over 35 who take birth control pills shouldn't smoke, because the combined effects can precipitate coronary problems. Cigarette smokers who jog or play racquet ball are in danger of suffering a sudden, fatal heart attack. And if Dad or Mom, sister or brother had ever had a heart condition, you should think very seriously about giving up smoking.

Furthermore, we now know that heart disease can strike young people, athletes, mountain climbers, golfers, TV comedians, even Larry King — it took an angioplasty and bypass surgery to keep him Live...and to convert him to a stalwart foe of smoking.

Moreover, we all know that when you have a "coronary" it hurts, and hurts bad. Heart attacks strike suddenly, without warning, and you may not survive to tell your friends how much pain you were in. The relationship between smoking and coronary disease is at last pushing people to quit. Smoking definitely is no longer the "in thing."

Peer pressure is a strong force. Smokers now are made to feel uncomfortable when they light up, and by law are sequestered in public places. Domestic flights are non-smoking, as are some entire office buildings. In years past, medical meetings were held in rooms blue with smoke. Now, to my knowledge, none of the more than one hundred doctors in our community smokes.

Sadly, this healthful message hasn't penetrated two segments of our society: teenagers and young women. Attempting to get them hooked while they're young, and to a disturbing extent continuing to succeed, the tobacco industry relentlessly promulgates several lies: Ladies, cigarette smoking will keep you slim, beautiful and sexy; Hey macho guys, cigarette smokers are he-men with hair on their chests.

Which is just so much baloney! Cigarettes stain your teeth and your fingernails, wrinkle your skin and give you bad breath, cut your wind and your stamina. Plus, there's a serious chance that cigarette smoking will lead to such life-threatening ills as lung cancer, emphysema and heart disease.

If you happen to be one of the small minority of Americans who still smoke, consider your heart and the job it has ahead of it. If you don't make it too difficult, it will continue to beat as many as a couple of billion more times through the rest of your long life. Give it a break and throw away those coffin nails. Just say no — you don't need to go to Hong Kong and eat a black egg to give you the determination to quit.

12 Love and Disinterest in Nursing Homes

"ONE THING I WANT YOU TO PROMISE ME, Doc, don't ever let them put me in a nursing home!" The speaker was my patient Jim Fluitt, in the hospital recovering from a serious heart attack, but this is a plea heard over and over by physicians with patients who are elderly.

As I walk the corridors of one of the extended care facilities in our community, and see some of my ailing and helpless friends, I often find myself agreeing. Here time seems to stand still, here people are waiting for their lives to end.

Ninety-year-old year old Margery croaks to me, "I want to get out of this place. Hey, doctor, why can't I just die?"

Walter wanders about aimlessly, periodically roaring, "Nurse, nurse," while pounding the walls with his cane.

Mary Martha smiles at me and says, "You tell Charlie to come here this minute...Charlie, you get over here!" But her husband Charlie has been dead for ten years.

Mrs. Burdick, one of the charge nurses at the extended care facility at our regional medical center, is unperturbed by these outbursts. "Now, now, Margie, this is going to be another good day. Your daughter is coming to visit you this afternoon." Margery brightens visibly.

"Now Walter, you sit yourself down and eat your breakfast." "Yes, yes, Mary Martha, we'll tell Charlie you're waiting for him." Things begin to settle down.

Having just come over from the peace and quiet of the medical and surgical wings of the hospital, I'm amazed that these nurses can keep their cool in all this chaos. And why are they willing to work in an atmosphere so heavy with age and feebleness, confusion and anger?

One of the nurses at another elderly care facility gave me this simple explanation: "Oh, when we get to know these people we learn to love them, even when they're naughty. This is just the pediatric ward for these dear people."

In the book "Harvest Moon, Portrait of a Nursing Home," author and staff nurse Sallie Tisdale carries these comments a step farther. She writes that in nursing homes "patients are treated with understanding and compassion, something made of equal parts of love and disinterest." Her point is that nurses cannot allow themselves to become too emotionally involved. But rather than pure professional distancing, for Nurse Tisdale this amounts to a special kind of respect, "a recognition of another person, separate and complex, and not so very different."

The author wisely comments, as she observes her own clock of life tick on, "In this room are my past, my present, and my future. I am already old, and it is fine."

I highly recommend "Harvest Moon" for anyone considering placing a loved one in a a nursing home, now or in the future. It can bring comfort when these difficult decisions are being made.

A daughter or a son may have been caring for their parent in their own home, but now a change must be made. Mom or Pop has repeatedly soiled their bed, or they've fallen and broken a wrist or a hip. Or there was that frightening episode when dear Mom, hatless and coatless in

January, wandered away from home, finally to be found up by the police, talking to strangers in a gas station.

Jim Fluitt's plea to never be put in "a home" echoes a fear many of us have had, viewing being sent to a nursing home as the worst end to life's hard road. But now we know that the choice to keep frail or ill relatives at home is not always the kindest one. In most of these extended care facilities, patients are given love and compassion, along with professional care, and this knowledge should relieve the family's sense of guilt.

I recall the time when Margie's son thought that Mom had made sufficient progress so that he could bring her home. But Margie hadn't been back in the outside world for twenty-four hours before she was demanding that she be taken "back home — right now!" She wanted to return to the familiar place where she had old friends, where she was wiped and bathed, where she was comforted by the security of soft restraints.

Unfortunately, a long stay in such a facility can deplete Mom and Dad's reserve funds, and it is true that Medicare is very stingy when it comes to nursing home coverage. Medicaid is of help only when the personal funds are reduced to indigency levels. In "Harvest Moon," author Tisdale has included a wealth of facts and figures, including comparisons of for-profit and non-profit homes, as well as information on Medicare, Medicaid, and insurance.

My patient Jim surely isn't ready for any extended care facility, but he might be someday. If only I could persuade him to take the time to visit a relative or a friend or even a stranger in one of these homes, he might change his mind.

I'd like to say to him, "Jim, do this for me and for yourself. You go there and sit with a Margie or a Walter, hold a frail hand and say a few soft words. You do that, Jim, and even though they may not remember your words, they will remember your warmth and kindness. And as you walk away, your step will be lighter and your heart will beat more strongly."

*Pills and
Other Cures
For What
Ails You*

Introduction

IN MY YOUTH THE SOURCE from which all medications were dispensed was called a "drug store," and the person behind the counter — invariably a man — was "a druggist." Most medicines were "compounded" on the premises, each ingredient weighed on a delicate scale, then ground and mixed together by mortar and pestle. Prescriptions were then finally dispensed as "powders" wrapped in individual "papers," in hand-filled capsules, or as elixirs. The modern-day FDA would never allow that.

Today "drug" is a four-letter word, drug stores have become pharmacies, and today's druggists are skilled pharmacists. Medications no longer are compounded on the premises, but come pre-packaged, sealed and labeled in tamper-proof containers.

And today's doctor no longer writes his (or her) prescriptions in Latin, and the well-worn "doctor bag" gathers dust in the back of the closet, as "house calls" have become obsolete, largely replaced by hospital emergency rooms. And we MDs have been categorized (largely by the definitions of medical insurers) into primary physicians, specialists and sub-specialists.

Luckily, the patient remains the same. Though a bit more sophisticated and better informed, he or she remains a human being in need of help. And the pills and the potions we prescribe still need to have their effectiveness backed up by words of confidence from the physician.

1 A Cow, A Milkmaid and Your Good Health

HISTORIANS SIMPLIFY WHEN THEY TELL THE STORIES of scientific discoveries. Edward Jenner is given credit for the insights and observations which began our Golden Age of Immunology, but someone ought to erect a monument to a nameless milkmaid and her cow, both residents of Gloucester, England in 1773.

Around that time Dr. Jenner developed a special interest in the devastating plague of smallpox. He happened to have a probing scientific mind, coupled with an intense curiosity about the wonders of nature. Those parallel interests led him to delve into such diverse natural phenomena as hedgehogs and cuckoo eggs, and into the vexing similarity between smallpox and cowpox.

Jenner observed and wondered why milkmaids remained healthy during recurring smallpox epidemics, while so many other townspeople became sick and died. He conducted careful studies and concluded that cows which contracted cowpox had pox pustules on their udders, so that the girls who milked these cows developed pox pustules on their hands. When the milkmaids contracted a case of cowpox they were mildly ill for a few days, but this apparently made them immune to smallpox.

From that serendipitous discovery came the smallpox vaccination that has, for the most part, rid the world of that dread illness. (The cow, at least, is given some credit for this breakthrough: the term "vaccination" is derived from the Latin words for "cow" and "cowpox.") The only remaining traces of past battles against this disease is a small, round vaccination scar on the left upper arm of the members of the older generation.

Perfecting a safe and effective vaccine against polio was

another great victory in the immunological war on disease. Forty years ago the mere mention of poliomyelitis, "infantile paralysis," struck fear into the hearts of children and parents during the summer "polio season." Today, in the United States, Canada, Europe, Japan and many countries in Asia, polio has been effectively eliminated.

Doctors Sabin and Salk, working independently but with the same objective, produced a vaccine that is comparatively inexpensive and easy to administer. A few drops of the attenuated vaccine are given by mouth to infants at two months, and four months of age, and then again when the child is one and a half and four years.

Unfortunately, smallpox is still rampant in the tropics and sub-tropics — in India and the Philippines, for example, as well as in some countries in South America and Africa.

From the lowly beginnings in that dairy barn in England, a little more than two centuries later we have vaccines for a wide variety of diseases. Most mothers know about "DPT," the combination vaccine protecting children against diptheria, pertussis (whooping cough), and tetanus (lock-jaw). These immunizations are given on a schedule similar to polio vaccination. Also, today we routinely immunize children against the "childhood diseases," measles, mumps and rubella (German measles). This vaccine, referred to as MMR, is usually administered to children older than 16 months.

Vaccines also have been developed to protect you against adult diseases, such as pneumonia, and the various annually evolving strains of influenza, "the flu." And, if you're traveling abroad, you may need to be vaccinated against typhoid, typhus, yellow fever or cholera.

When some of these vaccines were comparatively new, those vaccinated sometimes suffered a strong, "positive" reaction — instead of just a touch of the disease they were being protected against, they came down with a serious case of it. Fortunately, today the newer vaccines have been carefully purified, making such reactions extremely rare.

So far I've been talking about immunity from a disease as though it were a simple, "either/or" situation. In fact, the process of immunization is extremely complex, involving lymphocytes, immunoglobulins, T-cells, immunosuppression, antigens and antibodies.

First, there are two types of immunity, "natural" and "acquired." As the first term suggests, each of us was born with a natural ability to resist certain diseases, or we received this defense mechanism in our mother's milk.

We acquire an immunity to certain diseases when our body responds to a "foreign" invader, called an "antigen." The offending substance which initiates the immunizing process may be bacteria, a virus, a protein or a vaccine, which our body recognizes as a kind of enemy, an intruder that must be resisted.

When this antigen is inhaled, ingested, injected or just rubbed onto the skin, it induces a foreign body "reaction," stimulating the production of substances called "antibodies." These tiny "anti-disease warriors" then will circulate in the fluid portion of the blood (the serum/plasma), vigilant for any future invasion by that specific antigen, ready to attack if the body's barriers are breached.

What remarkable advances we have seen in preventive medicine during the last two centuries! And the good news is that there's more to come. There's a high probability that researchers eventually will develop a vaccine to prevent certain types of cancer. Even now cancer specialists are able to control cancer by fortifying the body's immune system.

But that's another story....

2 The A-B-C's of Popping Vitamins

IN MEDICAL SCHOOL THEY DIDN'T TEACH US VERY MUCH about vitamins. We were told to advise our patients simply to eat a "well-rounded" diet of the basic food groups, protein, starch and a little fat, along with a daily quota of dairy products and plenty of fiber. Adults could more or less forget about supplemental vitamins, though we were admonished to be sure to give our kids vitamin pills and flouride pills until they were eight years of age, to harden their bones and their teeth.

Many doctors insist that we get all the vitamins we need simply by choosing a "sensible diet." Doctor Victor Herbert, a professor of Nutrition at the Mount Sinai Hospital in New York, wrote that, "taking vitamin supplements just gives you expensive urine."

In sharp contrast to this, in recent years various vitamins have enjoyed a faddish mystique and lore. For example, people gobbled huge doses of vitamin C after Nobel Prize laureate Linus Pauling extolled its cold-preventing virtues, though evidence of this particular efficacy is still lacking. Vitamin E enjoyed wild popularity because of its reputed power to prevent aging and to enhance sexual performance. Though hard evidence to support such claims is lacking, enthusiasts remain undeterred.

Health food advocates contend that "natural" vitamins such as rose hips and lysine will boost immunity and vitality. Or that vitamin B6 will reduce the monthly distress of PMS, and that vitamin A will smooth wrinkles and give you a rosy, youthful complexion.

Recent developments in the science of nutrition suggest that vitamins alone, in whatever dosages, are not magic. But that the judicious intake of vitamins, combined with a program of exercise, quitting smoking and moderating alcoholic intake, may indeed be the pass-key to good and enduring health.

We now are learning that certain vitamins may have the ability to fight disease, perhaps even to prevent or retard a number of ailments commonly associated with aging, though here the scientific support becomes a little shaky. However there is evidence that such vitamins as C and E and beta carotene accomplish this by taking on the role of "anti-oxidants." These are the substances that can de-toxify "bad molecules" that enter our bodies through inhaled tobacco smoke, exposure to sunlight, auto exhaust, and environmental pollutants.

That explains how foods containing these vitamins get credit for being able to prevent strokes and cataracts, to prevent or control heart disease and certain forms of cancer, and to help your immune system ward off infections.

Vitamin A/beta carotene occurs naturally in eggs and milk, as well as in many yellow, orange and dark green vegetables, such as spinach and broccoli. It may prevent night blindness and reduce your risk of contracting certain cancers. Medical researchers believe that adding zinc slows a gradual loss of vision, which occurs as part of the aging process.

Vitamin B, occurring in meat, eggs, fruits and some vegetables, is believed to have some value as a deterrent to cancer of the uterus. Vitamin B 12 is vital in the prevention of pernicious anemia, and now a growing body of research indicates that B 12 prevents or repairs nerve damage. Furthermore, B 12 taken during pregnancy may prevent nervous system defects such as anencephaly in the fetus.

Vitamin C, occurring in citrus fruits, strawberries, cabbage and leafy green vegetables, gives us healthy gums and teeth, and may help prevent cataracts.

Vitamin D, found in fish, eggs and milk, along with the help of sunlight, provides our youngsters with good bone growth, and may help prevent osteoporosis in oldsters.

Intake of Vitamin E may benefit your heart muscle, and also may boost the immune system of seniors. This vitamin occurs naturally in nuts, seeds, whole grains and vegetables.

Though we now are gaining new knowledge about the value of vitamins, which tends to widen their value to our health, nutrionists make a distinction between quality and quantity. The National Academy of Sciences counsels not to go beyond the Recommended Daily allowance (RDA) when taking vitamins. For example, gulping too much carrot juice can turn your skin yellow, and gorging on vitamin A can cause liver damage and hair loss. Scientific studies have determined that huge doses — megadoses — of vitamins or minerals are not beneficial, and in certain instances might even be harmful.

Today, when one of my patients asks about vitamins, I suggest they follow this formula: "Eat a well-rounded diet, search out the foods containing anti-oxidants, quit smoking, reduce and, if there is a need for vitamin supplements, read the labels and adhere to the RDA."

Simple as A-B-C.

3 Pills and More Pills for High Blood Pressure

NOT SO MANY YEARS AGO, treating high blood pressure was a simple and easy task for me. Simple because phenobarbital was the only hypertension medicine I could prescribe. Easy because the public was only mildly interested in the subject of high blood pressure.

But today we can select from a bewildering array of some 300 different medications to treat high blood pressure, the disease ominously nicknamed "the silent killer." My well-informed patients can recite the names of many of these drugs, and are quite concerned about hypertension, sometimes too much so.

Back in the days when it was "simple and easy" to treat high blood pressure, I'd begin with some fatherly advice. "Joe, you've just got to slow down. Take more time off. Get a little more exercise and lose some weight. Throw away that salt shaker. Then, after you've done all that, check back with me again in a month or so. If your pressure isn't coming down, we may start you on this little relaxing pill called phenobarbital."

Still very good advice: the primary and most effective way to treat high blood pressure is through a shift in lifestyle. Yet today we doctors and our patients are on a hypertension hype. Knowing your blood pressure reading is second only to knowing your social security number. Have we gone a little too far?

We in the medical profession are partly to blame for our patients attaching too much significance to blood pressure readings. Visit your doctor's office for just about any problem, and before you can even open your mouth to explain what's bothering you someone is taking your blood pressure. Worse, as they repeatedly pump up the pressure "cuff" on your arm, and watch the mercury fall in the gauge, the doctor or nurse may mention in an off-hand way that "your blood pressure is a little high today." A few minutes later you stumble out into the parking lot, mumbling to yourself "I've got hypertension — maybe I'm going to have a stroke!"

Around town you'll receive many other reminders about the dangers of high blood pressure. In the same category with bumper stickers wondering "Have you hugged your kids today?" or "Have you flossed your teeth today?" is the nagging query "Have you had your blood pressure checked today?" And you can have it checked weekly, although not always with the best accuracy, at your supermarket, your pharmacy, or your senior center.

Furthermore, because we physicians now have dozens of medications available to treat hypertension, with a new one coming along every week or so, it's natural that we prescribe them. Diuretics, beta-blockers, calcium channel blockers, ACE inhibitors. Our patients, in turn, expect to be given the benefit of these new miracle medicines they've read about in Reader's Digest or Time.

Even with all this attention now being paid to high blood pressure, many people aren't completely clear about what defines hypertension, and which of those two numbers is most important. There's a good chance my patient Joe will test his own blood pressure on the machine in the mall, then go home and tell his wife "My blood pressure was way up at 160 — I've got hypertension." But he'd be referring to the figure we express first, the systolic reading.

But it's the lower number, the diastolic reading, which is of far greater importance. The systolic reading can fluctuate widely as a result of stress, fatigue, anger and exertion. The lower, diastolic reading is more stable, and therefore a much more reliable measure of the pressure that pumps the blood cells through your arteries.

So as his physician I'd be glad to reassure Joe that he does not have hypertension, just because in that one instance at the mall his systolic reading was "160." His blood pressure reading of 160/82, taken on his way home after a hard day at the office, might well be 130/78 after he settled back in his easy chair at home.

Moreover, it is now accepted medical practice not to actively treat blood pressure with pills unless the diastolic pressure remains at around 95 or higher, in at least three readings on separate occasions.

However, if we do consistently get such elevated diastolic readings, we undertake medical management to prevent strokes or heart attacks. Yet the first step usually is to prescribe a change in lifestyle; intensive use of medications for patients with diastolic readings below the 95-100 level has not shown any advantage over the good old-fashioned remedies of weight loss, salt restriction and generally taking it easier.

In fact, studies done by the Veteran's Administration, the United States Public Health Service and at universities in the United Kingdom and in Europe, all indicate that using these medications in mild hypertension does not produce appreciable reductions in the numbers of people who become ill and die as a consequence of high blood pressure. Moreover, two well-designed research studies suggest that using medications to greatly reduce the diastolic pressure not only makes Joe feel lousy, but may actually increase his chances of suffering a heart attack.

In some ways it was easier for us years ago, with few medications to prescribe for hypertension. You might think, then, that today we are very fortunate to have so many choices. But in fact the multiple alternative medications have made life much more difficult for us. Now the physician must first decide whether the elevated pressure his patient exhibits really needs to be treated with medications and, if the use of drugs is indicated, which of the myriad antihypertensive drugs would best meet the patient's needs.

It would be nice if we could say "one size fits all," but while one type of medication may be best for the elderly hypertensive person, another will better suited for the youthful business executive.

The diabetic or the asthmatic patient may do well on a pill that is poorly tolerated by the person with kidney disease. And we know from experience that these new medications can have adverse side effects, carry certain contraindications, even occasionally have unfortunate interactions with other medications. Your doctor must take all these factors into consideration when he or she writes out that prescription.

Our pharmaceutical bible, The Physician's Desk Reference lists well over 300 antihypertension medications. Each reference is accompanied by paragraph after paragraph of fine print, important information about the effects of this particular medication, as revealed in the years of testing required by the Food and Drug Administration.

This is why your doctor sometimes may reach for that hefty book during your visit. And why he or she may heave a deep sigh of exasperation when a patient calls in and says "Hey, Doc, I just read about this new blood pressure pill — do ya suppose I should give it a try?"

4 Peg-Leg Pete and Chuck the Hook

PEG-LEG PETE AND CHUCK THE HOOK — those two fellows were childhood heroes of a sort for me, because they carried with them an aura of bravery and adventure.

Pete walked with a wooden leg because of what I mistakenly viewed as courage, but what really was sheer bravado. He had bet his playmates that he could race his bike across the tracks and beat the train. He lost the bet, along with his right lower leg.

We kids admired Pete not only for his bravery, but for what he could do with the leg that our local shoemaker had fashioned for him out of a broomstick and leather straps. Pete could run with us, he could dance a jig, and he was able to spin on his peg-leg like a whirling dervish.

Chuck, a millworker, also amazed us, as he carried his lunch bucket, drove a car, and flipped big boards around in the mill, all with the steel hook that took the place of his right hand. As I read Treasure Island I pictured Chuck acting the part of Captain Hook.

When we nosy kids queried Chuck on how he lost his hand he would say that as a child he had a bad habit of biting his fingernails, and that over time he had nibbled them down right back to his wrist. You can be sure that he cured a lot of youngsters of their nail-biting habit. We learned the real story much later, that his shirt sleeve had snagged on a board, and pulled his hand through the path of a cut-off saw.

Fortunately, such crude peg-legs and hand-hooks are a thing of the past. Today the specialized medical science of prosthetics and orthotics has perfected artificial limbs that function extremely well in place of lost arms and legs. "Prosthetics" is the branch of surgery or dentistry that deals with the replacement of missing parts with artificial structures, while "orthotics" is the practice of using braces to supply support to the body and to the limbs.

Creating and fitting artificial limbs is an extremely specialized skill, a combination of science and art. In our community Doug Potter is at once a designer, an architect, a mechanic and a carpenter. When a patient comes into Doug's office, usually on a referral from a physician, he or she brings along a medical history, along with a report of a physical examination. As a first step technician Potter visualizes the device his patient needs.

Following this, architect Doug takes painstakingly precise measurements, then goes to the drawing board to sketch out the curves and the contours of the limb he is to construct. As a third step this carpenter/mechanic builds a skeletal framework or armature, on which the limb will be formed. Then follows the tricky and complex design of the articulation — the way in which the artificial limb will move, whether from a ball-and-socket or the hinged joint. Also, figuring out the best way to attach the prosthesis to the patient, using cloth, leather, plastic and velcro, to give a secure and comfortable fit.

Finally this joint specialist must apply his extensive knowledge of body dynamics, especially the physics of stress and weight-bearing, to fit the device to the limb. As a final step, Doug patiently helps the patient learn to use this replacement for a lost body part. This can be a tedious and sometimes trying experience, and the patient may need to come back many times for fittings, adjustments and re-shaping.

Not surprisingly, such expertise can be expensive, up to $12,000 for a full leg prosthesis. But who would hesitate to pay that sum for the life-long ability to walk in comfort? Today's Peg-Leg Pete doesn't jig and twirl on a broomstick. Instead he can dance the light fantastic with the girl of his dreams, whirling on a leg of plastic, steel and velcro.

5   When Scratching That Itch Isn't Enough

> *There was a young belle of old Natchez*
> *Whose garments were always in patches*
>   *When comment arose*
>   *on the state of her clothes*
> *She drawled, "When I itches, I scratches!"*

"THIS ITCH IS DRIVING ME CRAZY — I wake up scratching myself until it bleeds!" Every doctor has heard that cry of anguish from patients, especially during hot summer months. The itching usually is caused by such simple irritations as insect bites, heat rashes, and itchy, scaling feet. We usually can relieve the itch, but still have difficulty explaining why and how a person itches.

You might think that this physical ailment, right out there on the skin where we can see it, would be easy to explain. There must be a simple answer to why we scratch, and why an itch can be worse than pain. But when patients ask I can't very well simply read them this definition from a dermatology textbook:

> *Sensory nerve impulses are integrated in primary central neuronal receptor pools, and from there secondary neurons are activated and conduct impulses along segregated specific fiber tracts to thalamic centers where tertiary neurons may be activated to send impulses to the sensory cortex.*

Got that? Scientific writers love to obfuscate. Translated this simply means that tiny, sensitive nerve endings (receptors) in the skin send messages to your brain, which identifies them as specific itch sensations.

That is, we "feel" the itching sensation in our mind, not in our skin. The same holds true, of course, for other sensations we perceive through the skin — heat and cold, pain and touch, wetness and tickle.

Some of the nastiest itching problems I see in my patients are caused by poison ivy. Characterized by pink, puffy welts or "hives" on the skin, the condition is given the clinical name allergic urticaria — from the Latin verb "to sting," and the noun for "nettle."

The mechanics of how poison ivy works are quite straightforward: toxic oils from the leaf of the ivy come in contact with the skin, causing an inflammatory reaction. Other forms of contact dermatitis can be caused by exposure to solvents, detergents and certain metals, such as the nickle in wristwatch bands, rings or earrings.

In contrast to these outer surface skin irritations, other and more complex dermtoses can come from within. Some people are allergic to shellfish, others to strawberries or to nuts. But they may not know it, making diagnosis difficult. In addition, some medications can induce an allergic reaction in a small minority of the population. These occasional offenders include penicillin, sulfa and phenobarbital.

Other common varieties of itchy skin inflammations are due to external, natural causes — but knowing this makes them no less tormenting. For example, fungal infections such as athlete's foot, jock itch and yeast vaginitis. Incidentally, "epidermophytosis" is a more genteel term for the athletes' irritation, and the scientific name for the lady's problem is candidiasis.

Any person afflicted with an itch is much less interested in the diagnosis than in getting rid of this pesky ailment. Fortunately, non-prescription medications usually can bring relief. Your physician can give you some brand names or, if your itching condition persists, can prescribe more powerful medications.

Obviously, the first step in treatment is to remove or avoid the irritant. If you have sensitive skin, remember to use rubber gloves when handling solvents or detergents. If you know you have food allergies, you'll of course avoid suspected foods. And if you know you are allergic to any medications, you should be sure that information is included in your medical records.

To fend off fungal itches, deny the little bugs that cause these problems the moist, warm home they love and flourish in. Dry, clean cotton socks are a must, and women should avoid tight-fitting nylon or rayon clothing, and wear cotton panties — perhaps the young belle from Natchez was allergic to synthetics! Before putting on rubber gloves, first slip on a pair of cotton "dermal" gloves, available in most pharmacies, to absorb perspiration.

To relieve mild, superficial itchiness, creams, lotions and moist compresses may suffice. Over-the-counter histamine tablets also sometimes help. But if these simple measures fail, see your doctor. He or she may attack your problem with more powerful topical medications, or even with cortisone, taken by mouth or injected. In extreme cases, hospitalization may be required.

Happily, most of the itches in our life are not that serious, and we certainly feel better when we scratch them. As the old Chinese proverb put it

> *Tis better than riches*
> *to scratch where it itches*

But there are limits to the pleasing relief, as the Russian saying reminds

> *Scratching is bad, because*
> *it begins with pleasure and ends with pain*

Finally, when it comes to itching skin inflammations, the best advice this physician can provide is

> *An ounce of prevention*
> *is worth a pound of cure*

6 Steroids, Good and Bad

"WOW, LOOK AT THAT HANDSOME HUNK! With those those muscles, he must be on steroids." This cause-and-effect evaluation came from my twelve-year-old granddaughter, as we watched male and female "body builders" on television. I had to agree she probably was right about the steroids, but I also had to wonder just how much she really knew about this particular group of hormones. And, for that matter, how much accurate information the average American adult has about steroids.

When I mention to a patient the possibility of treatment with steroids such as cortisone or prednisone, their usual response is something like "Don't give me any of that stuff, Doc, I'm afraid of it, I hear it's bad for you." Ironically, they're both right and wrong.

The particular steroids that have given this entire class of drugs a bad name are those in the anabolic/androgenic category. The term "anabolic" refers to constructive metabolism, a building-up process, "androgenic" to promoting masculine characteristics. Anabolic and androgenic steroids, AAS, are illegal drugs used by some few athletes, who hope to increase muscle mass and improve their athletic performance.

Production or sale of AAS may be punished by large fines and imprisonment. Most all anabolic/androgenic steroids are manufactured outside the United States, although the Federal Drug Administration believes there may be a few illicit, underground producers in this country. Whether imported or made in the USA, AAS pills command such exorbitant prices that traffic in them can be highly profitable.

Anyone using anabolic/androgenic steroids faces many serious dangers to his or her health. Long-term use can lead to high blood pressure, diabetes and premature hardening of the arteries, as well as possibly increasing a person's risk of developing cataracts and liver tumors.

These steroids confuse and disrupt the immune system, lowering the body's resistance to infection. AAS can cause greasiness of the skin, excess growth of body hair, and acne. Women taking anabolic/androgenic steroids may stop having menstrual periods and become sterile.

Knowing very well about the deleterious effects of AAS, I was relieved when I heard grand-daughter Sarah's comment as we watched those flat-chested women flex their bulging biceps: "How gross!" I would hope that someday this sentiment is echoed by the majority of young people.

Yet in spite of our awareness that the use of these drugs carries with it serious health dangers, androgenic steroids continue to be used by college and professional athletes, even by adolescents.

Government officials and physicians have passed laws and employed public information scare tactics to discourage the use of these illegal steroids, but I'm sorry to report that so far we seem to have achieved little success. It's difficult to get school children worrying about the risk of disease that may possibly strike them twenty years down the line. Young people have a vague feeling that, though they may not live forever, they'll be around for almost that long. And anyway, health problems happen to other people. And most young men strongly want to come off as strong, muscular and macho, and this desire outweighs fears about health in the far future.

On the plus side, recent studies have shown that an educational program directed toward young people, to inform them of the serious and substantial risks associated with the use of anabolic steroids, is far more successful than relying on scare tactics alone.

Part of this education can be to give some credit to the "good" steroid hormones, the corticosteroids. Produced by the adrenal glands, walnut-sized organs perched atop each kidney, these hormones can provide relief or cures for a wide range of human ailments.

Steroids reliably help the seasonal suffering of those with hay fever, and can help asthma patients breath easier. Exasperating itchy skin disorders that haven't responded to other medications often can be cleared up by corticosteroids. Inflammation and pain in bones and joints can be reduced or eliminated. Steroids may even be effective in treating certain rare growth disorders.

When used correctly and with care, corticosteroids are powerful agents toward better health. Anabolic and androgenic steroids can cause great harm, even death.

7 The Bald Truth About Hair Restorers

Ugly are hornless bulls,
A field without grass is an eyesore.
So is a tree without leaves,
So is a head without hair.

So spoke the Roman poet, Ovid, way back in 40 B.C. That baldness has been considered ugly for more than 2,000 years gives little comfort to those 55 million of us men whose faces extend over our brows to the top of our heads.

We valiantly try to put up a good front, not too convincingly asserting that we are proud of our shining pates. Perhaps to seek comfort from a support group, as well as to get their personal views on the bald state, I interviewed a few of my hairless friends and colleagues.

Happy Howard Lancaster laid the blame for his "chrome dome" deficiencies upon the strenuous studying he did in veterinarian school. Fellow physician Bill Wood made a similar claim, that his long years of medical training led to an early loss of hair. "And anyway," he added, "grass doesn't grow on a busy street."

Offering a similar defense, house-builder Stan Gustafson observed that "they don't put marble tops on cheap furniture." Dr. Harold Thysell snorted "Did you ever see a bald-headed bum?"

Yet in spite of these weakly positive protestations, more than a few who no longer have a full head of hair would be glad to have back what they've lost up there. They eagerly seek (and too often fall for) every new anti-baldness gimmick or magic hair restorer that comes along.

A few years ago a television promotion out of Reno, Nevada promised protection against further hair loss, as well as a hope of re-growth (money-back guarantee). I haven't heard anything recently about their "New Generation" products, so maybe their gamble didn't pay off.

Somewhat more authentic news has come with the announcement that a drug called minoxidil will grow hair. It has been approved by the FDA and is marketed under the name Rogaine.

Of course, that prospect has a seductive sound to those of us who really don't get our money's worth at the barber shop. But wait a minute, minoxidil has been around for quite a while, seeing limited use as a hypertension medication. It was only by accident that one of its side-effects was found to be the stimulation of hair-growth. This was well and good for us men, but the ladies rebelled when hair appeared on their foreheads, chins or backs.

And minoxidil had other drawbacks. For one thing, the stuff is quite expensive, about fifty bucks for a month's supply. Furthermore, the hair it stimulates is more in the nature of heavy peach fuzz, which gradually disappears when the drug is no longer used.

So, for my part at least, I'm not going to waste much time waiting around for a "cure" for my baldness. I know I "caught" this condition from the pattern baldness genes passed on to me from my father and grandfather. Instead, I'm just going to continue on through life, content with my lot as described by this ditty:

> *The Lord is just*
> *The Lord is fair*
> *He gave some folks brains*
> *The others, hair!*

8 How To Avoid Clogged Arteries

BY NOW MOST EVERYONE KNOWS THAT A MYSTERIOUS, fatty substance called cholesterol can be a killer, when bits of it get stuck to artery walls, impeding the flow of blood. The process is similar to how a buildup of rust and scale in a galvanized pipe slows the flow of the water coming out of the tap — but in your body the consequence of blocked arteries can be a stroke or a heart attack.

To prevent this we've long been warned to avoid fatty foods. But which fatty foods? And does "avoid" mean "give up altogether?" "C'mon, Doc," my patients are likely to say, especially around the holidays, "two or three butter cookies, or a couple of deviled eggs, aren't going to kill me!"

Probably not, especially in view of new findings on the accuracy of cholesterol testing, coupled with a much more comprehensive understanding to how cholesterol is handled by your body. First of all, just knowing your "cholesterol count" is not enough information for your physician to manage any incipient cholesterol problem you may have. It's a good start, but medical researchers now advise that we must begin to pay more attention to the different kinds of fat that are floating around in your blood.

As in the old cowboy movies, when it comes to fat in your blood there are good guys and bad guys. The ones wearing the white hats are the high density lipids, HDLs for short, who lubricate and prevent the hardening and narrowing of the heart's blood vessel. Very important for your health, there are life-saving and life-prolonging measures you can take to raise the level of your HDLs.

The bad guys responsible for the clogging of those coronary arteries are called low density lipids. They're the rascals who park in your arteries, steadily building up plaques which narrow these pipes, constricting the vital flow of blood to your heart and to your brain. Fortunately, researchers now are quite confident in recommending ways to keep your LDLs to a minimum.

Current thinking is that testing for the level of the third major cholesterol component, the triglycerides, is of lesser importance. However, the laboratory procedures used to measure triglycerides are also helpful in diagnosing and treating liver disease, alcoholism, and pancreatitis.

Here is a brief summary of what we now understand and can recommend about the state of your cholesterol, how to understand and manage those fatty good guys and bad guys racing around through your blood stream.

- A single "cholesterol count" is of some value as a screening test, but a measurement of the lipids and the triglycerides is also essential.

- A finger-stick cholesterol test done at a mall may be a useful starting point, but it also may be inaccurate. Furthermore, your risk of infection is increased in such mass screenings.

- To reduce the level of lipids in your blood, four specific steps are repeatedly recommended by researchers:

    1. Follow a low-fat diet

    2. Exercise regularly

    3. Lose some weight

    4. If you smoke, quit

- If you and your physician determine that additional measures are required to bring down your overall cholesterol count, and to drop your population of LDLs, you may begin taking small doses of Niacin, a constituent of the Vitamin B complex.

- Another natural substance that lowers the lipid levels is a component of your liver bile secretion known as "bile acid sequestrant." Questran is the brand name of a commonly used sequestrant. Available in powder form, it helps bring down the low density lipid level. Also, a psyllium seed product such as Metamucil or Citracel not only combats constipation, but further reduces the level of these "bad" lipids.

- If stronger measures are required to improve your cholesterol condition, your doctor may prescribe drugs such as Atromid-S, Lorelco or Mevacor. Each functions in different ways, and each has been formulated or a certain set of requirements.

At your next regular physical examination, talk over your cholesterol count with your doctor. And until then, here are five more important points about dealing with the fat globules floating around in your blood:

✓ Medication may not be necessary to treat elevated cholesterol levels; improvements in lifestyle may suffice, and diet regulation is still the first line of attack.

✓ Older patients can be given wider latitude on cholesterol levels.

✓ Younger members of families with a history of high cholesterol levels should be tested — the ability of a person's body to handle fats has a lot to do with heredity.

✓ Some of the medications you now are taking could be affecting your cholesterol level, either up or down.

✓ And, yet another good reason to quit, cigarette smokers have a higher level of LDLs, so they are more prone to coronary disease and heart attacks.

9 Prozac — Good News or Bad?

THE HANDSOME, GRAY-HAIRED ATTORNEY APPEARING on Larry King Live had fire (and dollar signs) in his eyes. He was on the show to lash out against the drug Prozac, its manufacturer Eli Lilly, and the hapless physician who had come to represent the drug company.

The heated controversy on this program centered around the suicides of two clinically depressed patients who had been under treatment with Prozac. The attorney talked about the million dollar product liability law suit he had filed, and suggested there might even be a class action suit in behalf of ten other plaintiffs — apparently all still alive, but who presumably had unfavorable experiences while taking Prozac (generic name, fluoxetine).

My heart went out to this research physician, who tried to logically present the facts as he perceived them, but who was repeatedly interrupted by this skillful and aggressive attorney, gruffly refuting each point. The doctor was flustered and defensive, not realizing that rudeness is an acceptable debating technique on television.

But beyond the fine points of vigorous discussion, more worrisome is that fact that, among the millions of people watching the show, thousands were taking Prozac for the treatment of their depression. Since its introduction in the late 1980s, it has continued to be widely used without serious adverse side effects.

As might be expected, many of the patients taking Prozac who had seen the show called their doctor right away to complain, along the lines of "Hey, Doc, what about this dangerous drug you put me on? After seeing Larry King Live last night, I'm more depressed!" The physician would heave a sigh, then launch into a half-hour explanation, to correct the wrong facts and impressions left by the television "discussion."

Since Larry King, Geraldo, Donahue, Oprah, 60 Minutes, Newsweek and Sally Jessy Raphael have entered the medical field, we physicians have had to spend significantly greater shares of our days supplying accurate information to our patients, to offset and correct the bad news and sensational health stories in the mass media. That approach attracts viewers and readers, but often can be counterproductive to American health.

Those doctors who were called by patients worried about Prozac probably began by pointing out that only after years of testing was this medication accepted by the Food and Drug Administration as an effective treatment for mild to moderate depression. They might have added that the very conservative publication Medical Letter, which each month supplies physicians with evaluations of new medications, pronounced Prozac to be "as effective as any other anti-depression medication."

Furthermore there are several reasons for the rapid and widespread acceptance of this medication to treat depression. First of all, Prozac does not cause lethargy and sleepiness as do some other anti-depressant drugs. In fact, most patients feel more alert, even wired, while being treated with Prozac. And some patients are able to lose weight, another way to relieve depression. Overall the medication can shift a patient's mood from a depressed "dysphoria" to an up-beat "euphoria."

The medical literature also contains some mildly positive reports of the successful use of Prozac to treat a number of psychological disorders, including bulimia, obesity, drug addictions, kleptomania and obsessive-compulsive neuroses. In addition, the drug has a wide margin of safety when carefully administered under medical supervision, and its usual once-a-day dosage makes it easy for patients to stay on their course of treatment.

It is true, however, as the lawyer contended, that some of the Prozac patients exhibited suicidal tendencies. It is also true that most depressed, despondent people, at one time or another, harbor suicidal thoughts. Paradoxically it is possible that, by converting dysphoria to euphoria, Prozac can infuse the patient with the aggressiveness and the motivation to take action on their suicidal thoughts.

The shrewd plaintiff's lawyer on Larry King Live, who seemed quite intent on reaching deeply into Eli Lilly's pockets, played heavily on this possibility. In doing so he probably confused many listeners, yet he carefully dodged these scientific facts:

- Carefully constructed retrospective studies have found no difference in suicidal tendencies in people using Prozac, compared with those on other anti-depression medications.

- Everything we eat or drink or take as a medication — from red wine to chicken chow mein, from aspirin to digitalis — can have unexpected adverse effects.

- Prozac continues to have the approval of the FDA as an effective treatment for depression.

The television "debate" about Prozac was but one example of how media hype can confuse and disturb the public. In the best of all worlds we could hope for more positive and truly informative health news on television. Unfortunately, for TV talk shows and news programs, bad health news is good news for their ratings.

10 Medications to Change Behavior

BY HIS OWN ADMISSION, movie star Sylvester Stallone was a wild and angry kid, a behavior problem on the street and in the schoolroom. "I used to beat up on cars, beat up on authority. I still sometimes do things for the shock value. That insecure little kid is still rattling around inside."

Sly Stallone was a hyperactive, hyperkinetic problem child. Born 20 years later he probably would have been given the benefit of behavior therapy, and possibly would have been put on Ritalin, a medication proven effective in calming kids who are "acting out."

Now as an adult he has sublimated his wildness, by shooting and bombing (only in the movies) his way to a multi-million-dollar annual income.

Reflecting on Mr. Stallone's angry childhood brought back memories of Paul Hawkes, a boy I first heard about from my son Dave, when they both were in the second grade. Paul behaved as though he were majoring in class disruption — every day he seemed to create some sort of anti-social mischief.

Comparatively minor infractions, but nonetheless irritating and frustrating to his teachers. Paul tripped Billy, sending him to the dentist with a chipped tooth. On the playground he snapped girls' heads by yanking on their braids, in the classroom he flipped soggy spitwads at anyone within range. Paul's disruptive activities continued into high school, where he was an increasingly frequent truant. Football was by far his best subject; on the gridiron he could vent his anger and his energy on hapless members of the opposing team.

Paul joined the Marines before he graduated — everyone agreed that tough military discipline might be able to productively channel his destructive energies. I don't know what happened to Paul after he joined the service, but I am sure that his drill sergeant and his other superiors were unimpressed by his wildness, and exerted their own draconian form of "behavior modification."

In retrospect I would diagnose Paul as having been suffering from hyperkinesis, uncontrollable hyperactivity. The condition is often given the name of Minimal Brain Dysfunction, MBD for short.

In addition to hyperactivity, the cardinal features of MBD include

1. **Distractability** — a short attention span, an inability to concentrate, also referred to as "Attention Deficit Disorder" or ADD

2. **Impulsivity** — for example, zipping across the street in front of traffic, seemingly unable to "stop, look and listen"

3. **Excitability** — temper tantrums, garrulousness, schoolroom disruption

4. **Antisocial activities** — such as clowning, acting out, reacting negatively to social constraints

Too often, but for good reason, the hyperactive child is avoided by other children, causing him or her to be reclusive, shy, depressed and resentful of authority figures. These are the children who may try to run away from home. This reaction is common in girls.

In the past teachers usually would happily give such hyperkinetic kids a "social" promotion to the next grade, so they wouldn't need to teach them two years in a row. But today, instead of putting up with Paul's (or Sly Stallone's) disruptive activities, the teacher and principal would have contacted the parents. Quite likely the hyperkinetic young person would be referred to a professional, with experience and training in treating such nervous disorders.

Before the start of any treatment, a detailed personal and

family medical history would be obtained. Then the child would be given a physical examination and a nervous system review, quite likely followed by tests of basic intelligence and achievement ability. In some isolated cases a brain wave tracing, an electroencephalography, might be ordered.

Then and only then, if the results of all these tests pointed to a diagnosis of pathologic hyperactivity — true hyperkinesis — would medical management with drugs be started, combined with a psychological program of behavior modification.

In medical management the drug Ritalin (generic name: methylphenidate) has proven most successful. A pediatrician colleague reports favorable reactions in 75% to 85% of the children he has put on a Ritalin program. Such combined medical and behavioral management requires close and continued cooperation among parents, physician, psychologist, social workers and educators.

Not so long ago, critics in the media were wondering if Ritalin was being used too frequently, and as a result creating a population of juvenile addicts. Some fair questions were raised, such as: How long must the medication be used? Do kids outgrow the need for this drug? What are the effects of long-term use of Ritalin?

There are no easy answers, but there is ample clinical evidence supporting the short-term use of Ritalin by a hyperactive child to increase his concentration, while decreasing his impulsivity and his distractibility. Ritalin calms him down and helps him learn.

Rest periods, during which the child stops taking Ritalin, reduces the possibility of addiction, while maintaining the medication's effectiveness. According to my pediatrician colleague, around 15% of this hyperkinetic population may require continued medical management as adults.

Some physicians and medical researchers contend that hyperactivity is actually a chemical and biological deficiency, a condition which justifies the use of the medication to offset the imbalance. They make the point that we use medications continuously to control hypertension, so why not do the same to control hyperactivity?

However, I must emphasize that this hyperkinesis is not a minor medical problem, to be easily solved with a quick cure. A parent cannot simply phone their physician to request a prescription for Ritalin.

Furthermore, some school psychologists prefer behavior modification programs, before drug therapy is attempted. The compromise is, of course, to use both.

We still have much to learn about this hyperactive syndrome. We are uncertain about the usual progression of this problem, and we cannot assume that it is precipitated by brain damage. At this point we believe it is a treatable dysfunction of the central nervous system.

It is, moreover, wrong to assume that all kids who occasionally are disruptive, have temper tantrums, beat up on cars, or threaten to run away from home are victims of hyperkinesia, and therefore have MBD. Most all normal children now and then exhibit such irritating behavior.

Medications work in complex ways. Ironically, it turns out that Ritalin not only quiets down the hyperactive child, it can brighten up the hypoactive, sluggish adult. In this connection, the medication also has been found to help those afflicted with a rare disorder, narcolepsy. These people abruptly drift off into short naps, sometimes while in a group, such as at the dinner table. In this case, the worst that might happen is that they drop their fork. Much more worrisome, and a strong reason to try Ritalin, is the prospect of this happening while they are driving!

11 Generic Drugs — Good or Bad?

Last week my patient Margaret Tunney reminded me to "Be sure to write that prescription so that I get generic drugs — that'll save me five or six dollars."

This week her friend Agnes, also a patient of mine, reported to me that "Those generic pills you prescribed just don't seem to do the job for me — I want to go back to the 'regular' tablets."

Two different opinions I and my fellow physicians hear all the time. Which is correct? Should your doctor prescribe "brand name" or "generic?"

One argument against generics is the commonly held assumption that they can vary in potency by as much as 20%. Doctor John Somberg, Professor of Pharmacology at the University of Chicago, explained this "20/20 rule," which states there can be no more than 20% plus or minus variation in the consistency and the "bioavailability" — the amount of medicine available to do what it's supposed to do — between the generic product and the brand name standard in the field.

This sounds as though generic drugs are allowed a wide range of potency, but the Food and Drug Administration responds that in most cases this variation doesn't really make that much difference. If that's true, you might ask why must brand name drugs stick to such strict standards?

Dr. Somberg and other specialists in pharmacology with whom I've checked believe that consistently strong potency is more important in some drugs than in others. For example in the case of heart medicines, epilepsy drugs and blood thinners such as Coumadin, the level of effectiveness might prove critical. Several of my local local cardiologist colleagues were of the same opinion. One prescribes only the brand name diuretic Lasix, instead of the generic furosemide, and the brand name Synthroid, rather than the generic thyroid extract.

I should emphasize that when generics first became available they sometimes were produced by unsupervised, less-than-dependable laboratories. The quality of generics has improved immensely, especially since several major pharmaceutical firms have entered the generic field.

Another concern some patients have is that pharmacists push generics because they are more profitable. In fact, the mark-up on some of the brand name medications may be higher, yielding the druggist a slightly higher profit.

The United States has some of the strictest pharmaceutical testing requirements in the world. Stemming from the Thalidomide scare some years ago, the long succession of animal and clinical trials can stretch from as little as five to as many as eight or nine years. This testing can cost pharmaceutical companies many millions of dollars, so you can understand how resentful they sometimes are when their branded product begins to receive competition from a generic formulation, immediately after its patent runs out.

So far I haven't presented you with a firm answer to the question, "Are generics good or bad?" When I talk this over with my patients, I offer the pros and cons on a range of points.

First of all, if the "20/20 rule" gives you concern, and if you wish to be certain as to absolute "bioavailability" of your medication, you will need to decide whether the added expense of the brand name drug is worth it.

Cost is, of course, also a factor. Let's assume that a hundred capsules or tablets of the brand name drug cost $20, whereas a hundred of the generic costs $15. If you take one pill a day the cost differential would be 5¢ a dose, or $18.25 a year.

In addition to the matter of money, you should rely on your doctor's advice when considering the necessity for high consistency and bioavailability. Put simply, which you buy depends on what it's supposed to do for you, and this is one of those cases where your doctor knows best. Day after day he or she reads through mountains of information about new and improved medications, including facts about the side effects, possible adverse reactions, comparative effectiveness and, of course, cost.

So, when it comes to deciding between brand name or generic drugs, the simple answer is that there is no simple answer...except that you and your physician should decide, weighing the pros and cons of each.

12 Laughter Is The Best Medicine — No Kidding!

> A Good Laugh and a Long Sleep
> Are The Best Cures in the Doctor's Book
> — Irish Proverb

THERE IS GROWING SCIENTIFIC SUPPORT for this happy proverb; clinical evidence indicates that laughter actually can discourage illness and help people to get well. To paraphrase the old saying, "he who laughs, lasts." Or, as the Bible puts it in Proverbs 17:22, "A merry heart doeth good, like medicine."

Older folks are well aware of the curative powers of humor, and those I know seem always to be on the lookout for a good belly laugh. Yet life is no laughing matter for teenagers and young adults. This contrast got me to wondering about how humor works, and why it seems to be so therapeutic.

More than 2,000 years ago a very wise Greek physician named Galen postulated that our minds and bodies were strongly influenced by the juices secreted by our various glands, secretions he called "humours." As these humours percolated through the mind and and body they produced "vapours" that brought good health and good humor.

Going all the way back to the start of cosmic history, it's obvious that God must have a delightful sense of humor. Why else would He, during those seven busy days, have created the platypus, the aardvark, or the ungainly skinny-necked ostrich. And the visually off-putting but actually delicious artichoke, or the avocado that's more pit than fruit?

Undoubtedly God created these creatures and foods quite late in the afternoon of the sixth day of His labors, when he needed a little good-natured relaxation. Today, in the same way, humor can be a refreshing restorative when we are tired or "stressed out."

Furthermore, medical researchers are finding that that laughter can be more than just a release, but can be provide a person with many of the same benefits as exercise. William Fry, a professor of psychiatry at the Stanford University School of Medicine, calls laughter "internal jogging." Dr. Fry admits that "It's not as vigorous as calisthenics or jogging, but you can exercise your laugh muscles at any time, at home, at the office, even while driving to and from work."

It is my contention that we doctors could learn to take ourselves a little less seriously, and do a better job of laughing. One of my medical school professors admonished us eager young students to "Take yourself lightly, but take what you do seriously."

The practice of medicine does have its very serious and sad moments, so perhaps physicians can be excused if they don't seem to be smiling all the time. Of course, this makes them a large target for those who would poke a little fun at them, and deflate their stuffy balloons:

> The new young physician had just moved to town, and didn't yet have a single patient. One morning when the doctor was sitting at his desk, doing the crossword puzzle, a

young man entered. Wanting to seem busy, the doctor immediately began talking into the telephone, apologizing to an imaginary patient that "things are pretty busy around here, I can't see you until next Tuesday afternoon." Then he put down the receiver and turned to his visitor, greeting him with "Good morning, how are you — that is, what's your trouble?" "Oh I feel fine," said the young man, "I came to hook up your telephone."

The positive effects of laughter are more than just mental. Laughter can actually stimulate your adrenal glands to produce catecholamines — adrenalin, norepinephrin and dopamine — all of which pump up your heart rate and increase your mental sharpness, just what we need in a time of psychological or physical stress or crisis.

> It had been a long morning for the surgeon. On his way down to the hospital cafeteria for lunch he dropped in to see one of his patients, the elderly Mrs. Jorgenson. As he listened patiently (no pun intended) to her enumeration of various aches and pains throughout her body (he secretly called it her "organ recital"), he spied a dish of nuts on her bedside table. Of course he had to try a few, and before he knew it he had eaten every last one of them.
>
> As he got up to leave he said "I'm so sorry, Mrs. Jorgenson, it looks like I ate your whole dish of nuts!" "Oh, that's all right, doctor," she replied, "since I lost my teeth I just suck off all the chocolate."

Laughter not only increases your heart rate and improves your circulation, it also can provide good muscular exercise. Doctor Fry has demonstrated that a half minute of hearty laughter can be equivalent to the exercise produced by three minutes of strenuous rowing.

Next time you go into a gut-busting, thigh-slapping spasm of laughter, observe how many different parts of your body are involved. Your abdominal muscles contract, your rib cage expands as your diaphragm pumps your lungs full of oxygen. You wave your arms, you clap your hands, and your lacrimal glands drip tears down your cheeks. Sometimes your uncontrolled laughter causes such intense muscular contractions around the intestines and the bladder that this leads a little loss of control in other departments.

Earlier in this collection of essays I related how author and psychologist Norman Cousins conquered a painful illness, ankylosing spondylitis, using a combination of humor therapy and modern medical therapeutics. He reports on his methodical application of happiness to cure himself in a very interesting book, "Anatomy of an Illness."

Humor and laughter can not only lighten the pain and anguish of disease, but that happiness can even increase the body's ability to heal, and to strengthen our immune systems. Every surgeon knows that the happy, optimistic patient has fewer post-operative complications, and so goes home sooner. Likewise, the pregnant woman who approaches her delivery with a smile and a positive attitude almost always has a speedier, easier birth. Medical researchers believe this is because laughter can produce endorphins, the body's natural morphine.

As Doctor Fry summarized, "Laughter is an activity that has both physiological and psychological energy — like sex and exercise and pleasureable eating."

So, have you heard any good ones lately? If you have, pass them around, because laughter is, indeed, the best medicine.

Sex, Babies and All That Stuff

Introduction

THEY DIDN'T TEACH US ABOUT HUMAN SEXUALITY in medical school, but they should have. Over fifty years of medical practice, with an emphasis on obstetrics and gynecology, have convinced me that sexuality can be a major factor influencing health and disease.

In my youth talking about S-E-X within our family circle never happened — sex was a four-letter word. Fortunately I had an older brother and sister who passed on some basic "facts of life," incomplete and inaccurate as they may have been. It wasn't until I got to Biology 101 that I acquired a little honest sex education.

In those days mothers often led their daughters to believe that sex was naughty, even "dirty," and that they should be wary of men's bestial instincts. Infecting daughter's with this suspicious attitude, well-meaning mothers may have laid the groundwork for future marital unhappiness.

How things have changed! No longer is information about sexuality delivered in a plain brown wrapper, it's on the newsstand. A Madonna mentality pervades movies and MTV. Pre-marital and extra-marital sex is accepted as the norm. Isn't it ironic that in this modern day the only deterrent to "sleeping around" is the fear of acquiring an incurable disease — AIDS?

As always, the pendulum will swing. We already are seeing a trend toward abstinence, and virginity is no longer derided.

Teaching the truth about the virtues and the wonders of human sexuality, as expressed by a couple's commitment to each other, is the foundation of enlightened sex education.

1 Can Kissing Be Dangerous To Your Health?

ROSEANNE'S TWO TV DAUGHTERS WERE WORRIED. One of their friends had come down with the "kissing disease," and these young women were wondering how kissing could possibly cause "mono." And was deep kissing particularly risky? (To one of the two it was undeniably disgusting: "I'd kill any guy who tried to stick his tongue in my mouth!")

I'm glad to report that ordinary osculatory activities (we doctors even have a clinical term for smooching) only very rarely lead to an infection. Yet your mouth is a menagerie of bacteria and viruses, some of which are harmless, others which definitely can cause disease.

That's why human bites often can lead to serious infection, caused by some of the nasty organisms swimming around in saliva. One of the occupational hazards faced by doctors and nurses, especially those working in emergency rooms, is the risk of being bitten by an intoxicated or otherwise irrational patient.

People bite other people more often than you'd suppose. In the emergency rooms of big-city hospitals, one in ten people with a bite to be stitched or bandaged were bitten by a fellow human. Many of these "bites" occurred when one person punched another in the teeth. Human bites can even be the result of child abuse, or over-enthusiastic sex play.

These are extreme examples of how mouth-borne bugs

can transmit disease to other people. Fortunately, much as they love the environment in your mouth, they don't live long in the outside world. The other day I noticed my secretary using an alcohol sponge to clean the mouthpieces of all our office telephones, to protect us from those nasty bugs hanging around during the flu and strep throat epidemic. I thanked her for her well-intentioned effort, but had to explain this probably wouldn't do much good.

To medical researchers those phone receivers are "fomites," no bad pun intended. A fomite is an object or material that might harbor or carry a source of infection, such as doorknobs, telephone mouthpieces, clothing, money and pillows. A great deal of research has been done on fomites, leading to the general conclusion that they are far less likely to be transmitters of diseases than sneezes, coughs and handshakes. Flu viruses and strep bugs, for example, can be spread by airborne droplets, launched by a sneeze.

Cupping your hand over your mouth or nose when you sneeze or a cough is an excellent way to protect those around you. This is a lesson most of us learned from our mothers at a very tender age, but the hands that covered the nose and mouth then may carry with them the droplet-born bacteria and viruses, and a little later contaminate someone else's hands or face. When that person puts his hands or fingers to his mouth or nose, this begins a new cycle of infection. That's why facial tissue and hand-washing are so important during the cold and flu season.

Your saliva is truly a buggy place! Some 200 different viruses have been identified in human saliva, including AIDS and hepatitis. While there is no proof that either of these diseases can be transmitted by a kiss, or even by a bite, this remains a theoretical hazard.

Patients with a cold often ask me, "How long will I be contagious?" My answer contains good news and bad. The bad news is that a person is most infectious early on, almost before he or she knows a cold is in the way. The good news is that once the illness is recognized and under treatment, infectiousness subsides rapidly.

A contemporary song talks of lovers sealing their vows with a kiss. This romantic notion had legal force in the Middle Ages when many people hadn't learned to write, and so would sign a legal document with an "X" and then kiss their mark. That kiss signified honesty and sincerity, and was accepted as a sacred oath to fulfill a promise.

In those days they weren't worried about paper acting as a fomite, harboring germs, as yet undiscovered. Neither do we need to worry now, as we all survive continual handling of Uncle Sam's biologically filthy folding green.

A few years ago on Valentine's day, our local paper ran two full pages imprinted with red lipsticked kisses. Roseanne's daughters could be sure those kisses from those lovely lips would be most unlikely to transmit any bad bugs, even though many hands had touched the newspaper.

In that same paper, a innocent but concerned reader asked Dear Abby if deep kissing can cause pregnancy. Abby's answer: "No, but it's a good start."

2   Birth Control, Today and Yesterday

NEARLY 80 YEARS AGO, MARGARET SANGER began her crusade for a woman's right to limit the size of her family. The Pill was made available to American women more than 30 years ago, giving them the power to control their reproductive lives, and at the same time beginning what many would term a "sexual revolution." Today another means of contraception, the "Norplant," has been added to a woman's birth control options.

Reviewing these twentieth century breakthroughs, we

might assume that birth control — more accurately called conception control — is a recent development, a result of modern social change and medical progress.

But an Egyptian papyrus from 1850 B.C. recommends preventing pregnancy by placing a small sea sponge, impregnated with honey and sodium bicarbonate, into the vagina before coitus. Another tip was the use of a vaginal suppository, whipped up from chicken fat and crocodile dung. And some of the wealthy favored inserting a gold ball into the vagina.

Back then and up into the nineteenth century, in addition to such "barrier" methods, women have taken various contraceptive potions by mouth. North African women were counselled to drink a mixture of gunpowder and the foam from a camel's mouth. Or to chew on a hunk of stale bread and a honeycomb containing dead bees.

Today, birth control using oral contraceptives and other methods is practiced worldwide by millions of sexually active men and women. Conception control is used by couples for three main reasons: To plan the timing of the birth of their children; a financial need to limit the size of their family; or for valid medical reasons. These are personal decisions arrived at voluntarily by the individuals involved.

On the other hand, in some countries the government has a hand in making decisions about conception control. In China, where over a billion people struggle to survive and prosper, authorities strongly encourage couples to have only one child. The government pays for prenatal care and the actual delivery in a first pregnancy, and the new mother is allowed a six week post-partum vacation with pay. But if she gets pregnant a second time the government withdraws all these benefits, and an official visits the parents to "strongly recommend" an abortion.

In the Philippines, also because of a rapidly expanding population, conception control is closely regulated by governmental agencies. When a couple marries, they must register with their residential district office. Within these districts a health officer keeps close tabs on their reproductive activities, making his rounds on a burro or a motorbike, providing educational material and contraceptives — I visualize him as a sort of contraceptive Good Humor man.

Though in the U.S. there has been no official effort to limit the size of our families, a "two-child" family is the norm. A hundred years ago, before contraceptives made family planning possible, families of a dozen children were not remarkable, especially on farms where there was so much work to do. Furthermore, infant mortality was high; it is not usual to find two or three infant headstones in family cemetery plots from the 1800s.

With the arrival of oral contraceptives in 1960, a woman no longer needed to depend on her male partner to prevent an unwanted pregnancy. The Pill at first won enthusiastic acceptance, and other means of contraception control — condoms, diaphragms, rhythm — were abandoned in favor of The Pill.

But before long, women began whispering to each other that the various oral contraceptives caused weight gain, blood clots, possibly even cancer. Blood clots and cancer happen only to other people, but weight gain — that was a worrisome prospect.

These rumors pushed medical researchers to belatedly discover that the 100 micrograms of the estrogen hormone contained in the original Pill was far more than needed to prevent conception. Without any loss of effectiveness, the dose has been reduced from 100 micrograms to 85, then to 50, and finally to 35 mcg. Today The Pill causes little, if any, permanent weight gain.

Moreover, studies conducted by the Center for Disease Control and the Fred Hutchinson Cancer Research Institute in Seattle have demonstrated, to our happy surprise, that the use of The Pill containing both female hormones, estrogen and progesterone, actually reduces by half the risk of cancer of the uterus or the ovary.

Not long ago, a media report by unidentified "experts" wondered if an increase in breast cancer could be blamed on birth control pills. So now we physicians have to deal with another scare headline.

The basic facts are these: (1) The increase in discovered breast cancer was in women over the age of 65, women who have been enjoying the benefits of increased life expectancy, and who probably never used the birth control pill. (2) The increase in the incidence of breast cancer (not of increased breast cancer deaths) is partly due to a greater awareness by women of the importance of self-examination, along with a willingness to get periodic, low-dose mammograms.

Furthermore, far too little emphasis has been placed on the allied benefits of oral contraceptives — and there are many. Research done by physicians at the University of Washington strongly suggests that OCs give protection against pelvic infection caused by chlamydia. The Pill may also protect against benign breast tumors and cysts. And oral contraceptives may reduce the risk of a woman developing rheumatoid arthritis.

Finally, any woman using The Pill will tell you that it's really nice not to suffer as badly from PMS symptoms, to no longer be painfully immobilized by menstrual cramps, and the pleasure of shorter and more predictable periods, with little blood loss.

3 Condoms, STDs and Morality

WHEN I WAS IN HIGH SCHOOL my friends and I talked about condoms, but only in hushed tones, when we were out of earshot of our parents. We passed around the information that "rubbers" would keep us "safe," though from what we weren't precisely sure. Referring to condoms as "prophylactics," a term as mysterious as it was unspellable, made us feel very grown up.

None of us had ever even seen a condom until Butch Krueger snitched a packet of them from his older brother's dresser. Brand-named "Trojans," their rather drab appearance gave no hint of the romantic sexual engagements we young fellows fantasized.

Butch told us that his brother had obtained the condoms up at "Doc" Woodcock's drug store, where many of our older brothers would buy them before they went out on a "hot date." After much rehearsal, they'd nonchalantly walk in and hand Doc fifty cents, praying no one they knew would enter while the kindly old druggist reached under the counter for that prized package of Trojans.

As a preacher's kid, I lived a rather sheltered life, acquiring most of my sex education in the schoolyard. It wasn't until I was in pre-medical studies in college that I learned condoms were termed "prophylactics" because they purportedly provided protection against venereal disease.

But at that stage in my life, syphilis and gonorrhea were nebulous afflictions that affected only skid row bums, or soldiers and sailors on lonely duty in far-away lands. My friends and I certainly didn't spend much time talking about VD.

But how times have changed! Today condoms are advertised on television, and women's magazines encourage readers to carry a packet of condoms in their purse, "just in case."

Is nothing sacred? Have we lost all modesty and constraint in dealing with these intimate sexual matters? A prime reason for this sharp change in our society's values can be expressed in three letters, "STD," standing for sexually-transmitted-disease.

By the 1960s, powerful new antibiotics enabled us to control venereal diseases. Yet now the public has been panicked by a trio of terrifying sexually transmitted diseases: herpes, chlamydia and the epidemic bombshell of incurable AIDS.

Genital herpes is an extremely painful and unpleasant ailment, rendering women physically and emotionally miserable. Furthermore, it is potentially fatal if contracted by a newborn infant.

Chlamydia is a less well-publicized malady, but in its advanced stage can seal the ovarian tubes of an unwary woman, causing sterility.

And the present horror of Acquired Immune Deficiency Syndrome has brought fear and trembling to people all over the world like no other disease in recent medical history. At this point, there is hope but no cure for AIDS.

All three of these diseases are mainly acquired through intimate sexual contact, and so the use during intercourse of some kind of a barrier, such as a condom, may afford protection against infection.

The threat of these three STDs has dramatically raised the status of the lowly rubber. Condoms now may be mentioned in polite conversation, as well as in the news media. No longer are condoms hidden beneath the druggist's counter; today in some convenience stores condom packets hang beside the cash register. Family planning clinics, health departments, even some schools, colleges and churches supply condoms for free or at minimal cost.

As a preacher's kid, I was taught that premarital or extra-marital sex was sinful, the work of the devil. I still find it difficult to accept a lifestyle that fails to equate moral commitment with sexual intercourse. I applaud the sentiment expressed in the story in which a young man asks his grandfather what he wore in his day to have safe sex, to which Grandad replied "A wedding ring, my boy."

And yet, as a physician, I'm very well aware that our Maker bestowed upon each succeeding generation an overpowering sex drive that sometimes can supersede moral convictions. The result is called "casual sex," the primary force in the spread of these sexually transmitted diseases.

It is indeed ironic that these three horseman of the sexual apocalypse — herpes, chlamydia, and AIDS — have revived a healthy social consciousness about sex. They herald the return of the wisdom of abstinence and the virtues of monogamy. Could it be that we must be faced with the threat of a serious disease to bring a renewal of old-fashioned morality?

4 Newer, Safer Intrauterine Devices

THE HISTORY OF CONTRACEPTION IS FASCINATING. We may think of birth control as a product of modern medical ingenuity, but a search of the literature, even including the Old Testament, reveals that down through the ages such matters were discussed quite frankly, usually related to the practice of the world's oldest profession.

Of the various non-hormonal means of conception control used over the years, the intrauterine device is the most recent, and certainly one of the most intriguing. Ancient records indicate camel drivers back in the day of the pharoahs gave us the first prototype intrauterine device. In order to forestall the inconvenience of a delay in the progress of the caravan across the Sahara, should a female camel go into heat, these ingenious fellows would insert a rock of the proper size and shape into the uteri of their lady camels. Those camel drivers were the gynecologists of their day!

The more recent use of IUDs goes back to the practitioners of fifty years ago who would use a device called a "gold stem pessary," a forerunner of the more modern "copper T." It was a device made of wire in the shape of a "Y," and at the lower end it had a small cap. Such stem pessaries, because of the perceived danger of infection, never received wide acceptance.

The more recent history of the IUD goes back to the early sixties, when the new plastic devices made their appearances and were accepted as dependable means of conception control and family planning. These devices came in various shapes, including the Lippes Loop, the Safety Coil and the copper wire wound Cu7. These devices functioned well, providing conception prevention rivaling that of the birth control pill.

Occasionally they did fail and an unplanned pregnancy ensued. There were apocryphal stories of babies being born with an IUD tightly clenched in their tiny fists. Occasionally, an IUD would drop out, perhaps during the cramping of a menstrual period, to be lost without the women being aware of it. That could lead to lawsuits, alleging "wrongful birth."

In response to these problems the A.H. Robins pharmaceutical company brought out out the Dalkon Shield, more specifically designed to stay in place and more certainly prevent pregnancy. Unfortunately the design and the string attached to it seemed to invite infections which, in a few cases, proved fatal. Multi-million dollar law suits followed, eventually causing the demise of this reputable pharmaceutical company.

The Dalkon Shield problems caused all IUDs to fall

from favor. It seemed the last chapter of the IUD story had been written. Because of the malpractice threat the only remaining producers of IUDs, Ortho Pharmaceutical and G.D. Searle, withdrew their devices from the market.

Not surprisingly there was an outcry from outraged women who had previously been perfectly satisfied with the safety and convenience of IUDs. Here is a sad commentary on how the public may be deprived of the use of medical advances through the gripping fear of malpractice liability.

However the age-old need for conception control will not long be denied. Women demand the fright to freedom of worry. Society respects the need for family planning. Already there are two new IUDs available, although so far they are seeing limited use. Additionally, the FDA has recently given the go-ahead to two conception control measures depending not on an intrauterine placement, but on hormonal prevention.

The history of a woman's right to control her own fertility carries on.

5 Norplant: The Ultimate Contraceptive?

FOR ITS EASE AND CERTAINTY IN PREVENTING CONCEPTION, Norplant is a major breakthrough. Consisting simply of six tiny silicone "bullets" inserted under the skin of a woman's upper arm, Norplant was 99.8% effective in preventing pregnancy for, believe it or not, over five years. Norplant is fully as effective as The Pill, and was approved by the Food and Drug Administration after tests on 55,000 women over a period of twenty years.

Sounds great, doesn't it? No more un-planned, un-wanted, out-of-wedlock pregnancies. Forget about taking pills, or using diaphragms or condoms. And no more need for abortions as a last-resort means of birth control.

The mechanics of the Norplant device are quite simple. Six silicone capsules, each the size of a small matchstick, gradually release carefully measured doses of Levonorgestrel, a female hormone similar to one component of birth control pills which suppresses ovulation. If a woman's ovaries release no eggs, she can't get pregnant.

The Norplant device is easily and quickly "installed" by a physician in his or her office, in a minor surgical procedure, using local anesthetic.

If all this sounds too good to be true, you're right. Unfortunately, as with so many other "miraculous scientific breakthroughs," Norplant is not the total and perfect answer to everyone's contraceptive, family-planning needs.

(1) The insertion and the removal of these "matchsticks" requires a surgical intervention by a physician. No surgery is completely "minor" — each procedure has its risks, costs, and possible complications.

(2) Some few women may suffer unpleasant side effects from the progesterone present in Norplant. These include weight gain, headaches, nausea, mood changes and acne. A woman contemplating the insertion of a Norplant device should review these risks with her physician.

(3) The most troublesome side effect of Norplant is its tendency to disrupt a woman's menstrual cycle. A significant portion of the women in the Norplant tests experienced irregular periods, inter-menstrual spotting, even total cessation of periods. These menstrual disruptions were severe and bothersome enough to prompt more than a quarter of the Norplant users to ask their doctors to remove the device.

(4) Norplant is not for everyone. The device is not recommended for women who weigh more than 150 pounds. Also, women who smoke are less favorable candidates. And high blood pressure, high cholesterol counts, diabetes

or a history of blood clots also may contraindicate a Norplant implant.

(5) Because of its comparatively high, one-time cost, $500 or more, Norplant may not be the suitable choice for the young single woman or the teenager — who, unfortunately, are at the greatest risk of an unwanted pregnancy. The women most likely to opt for this method of conception control are those who have completed their family but who are not yet ready for permanent sterilization.

(6) Finally, because the capsule outline is visible through the skin, some women may be reluctant to advertise their method of birth control.

Norplant is an excellent addition to our means of preventing pregnancy, but it does have its serious drawbacks. As a result it will see limited use until some of these problems are ironed out. Until then, couples will rely on past and proven means of family planning.

Of these, oral contraceptives will continue to be the most widely used. The Pill is 97% effective, and has few side effects in the low dosages now prescribed.

Intrauterine devices, with an effectiveness rating of around 95%, recently have fallen into disfavor because of infection and other complications. In the U.S. today, only two women in a hundred are using an IUD during their reproductive years.

Other means of temporary pregnancy prevention for women are waiting in the wings. A skin patch using the same ingredient contained in Norplant is under study.

In the spring of 1993 RU-486, the French abortion pill, is now undergoing clinical trials. Depending upon the outcome of these trials it is possible that the Food and Drug Administrations might approve this drug within two years.

Conception control in men, by means of a pill or a shot, lags far behind. We men seem quite content to allow the women to take the responsibility to prevent pregnancy.

Abstinence is, of course, the cheapest, safest, surest means of pregnancy prevention. But is there anyone out there who can boast of even a 50% rate of success in selling this concept to our teenage population?

6 *Virginity: New Teen Lifestyle?*

EARLIER THIS YEAR MARILYN came in for her pre-marital examination. During our conversation she proudly declared that she and Bob had decided early in their relationship that they would "wait."

I'm pleasantly surprised that I'm hearing this from more and more young couples these days, and to learn that "virginity" is a subject that can be talked about and is being talked about by couples, straight singles, and teenagers.

I can't deny that the fear of contracting AIDS and other sexually transmitted diseases (STDs) has focused our attention on the physical aspects of human sexuality. But beyond that there seems to be a renewed conviction among young women that it is acceptable and wise to "wait."

This is not to say that pre-marital sex is a thing of the past. Far from it. The natural sex drive is deeply programmed into the hearts and minds of men and women, especially young men and women. Indeed, teenagers have been described as "hormones with two legs." The wit who coined that term probably was a man: male hormone output peaks at 18, women's around age 30.

This inequity, combined with the age-old peer-pressure slogan "But everybody is doing it," are strong arguments against abstinence. On the other hand, we still can take every opportunity to refute the concept that because a young woman is still a virgin there's something wrong with her.

When a woman hears the tired line that everybody's

doing it, she has every right to say "This body isn't doing it!" That response often can bring her increased respect from her male friend, as well as from her female associates.

The medical facts favoring virginity and condemning promiscuity were well understood even before AIDS and other STDs forced a focus on the issue. Syphilis and gonorrhea were the sexually transmitted diseases a generation ago. Then penicillin came along as a cure-all and we relaxed, thinking we had the STD problem licked. Time proved us wrong.

AIDS continues to grab the headlines, but other sexually transmitted diseases, not immediately life-threatening, are serious problems as well. Herpes and genital warts are caused by sexually transmitted viruses, and not only are these ailments painful to the woman and dangerous for the pregnant woman's fetus, there now is reason to believe these viruses can cause cancer. Studies have found that a woman with multiple sex partners has a higher incidence of STD, as well as of cervical cancer.

Yet it seems wrong to rely on scare tactics to convince our daughters and grand-daughters to hang onto their virginity until they can hear the distant chiming of wedding bells. This conclusion must come from their own judgment and conviction. They can take heart from the fact that a recent survey found a majority of hot-blooded young swains wanted to marry virgins.

Some would contend that virginity is a "state of mind," that irrespective of the number of back seat skirmishes, a woman who at last comes to her beloved in total, intimate marital commitment comes as a virgin, just as Psyche came to Eros in Greek mythology.

Physiologically, virginity is both easier and more difficult to define. An intact hymen, the fold of mucous membrane partly covering the external orifice of the vagina, once was considered the mark of a virgin woman. Known familiarly as the "maidenhead," it's named for Hymen, the Greek god of marriage. But we know now that the use of tampons or vigorous sports activities, such as horseback riding and biking, can stretch out this fragile web of tissue. Only rarely does a physician need to dilate or snip this membrane, in order to facilitate intercourse.

The story of Megan, a 19-year-old student at a nearby university, is in sharp contrast to that of Marilyn, and underscores the value of virginity. Not long ago this poor young woman went through a horrible, terrifying experience, suffering through a long and bloody labor to deliver an unplanned and unwanted infant in the loneliness of her dormitory room. Her mind twisted by agony and anguish, she cast her lifeless infant into a dumpster.

Megan's life is forever scarred. Her first-born infant is gone. With her lingering sense of guilt, will this young woman ever be able to experience full and confident sexual happiness? We cannot help but wonder if she might have been spared this agonizing tragedy if during her early teenage years someone had been there to tell her that "Yes, it's all right to wait. Your body does not have to do it."

7 The Incredible Egg of Life

WHEN I WAS ABOUT SIX, I asked my mother about the red spot I'd discovered in one of the yolks of my breakfast eggs. She responded tersely, "That's from when the rooster got into the hen house." Her manner suggested that further questioning would yield no more or better information.

I didn't know it then, but this was my introduction to the mysteries of fertilization and reproduction. A dozen years later a chicken egg would again arouse my curiosity about the beginnings of life, when we pre-Med students in

Embryology 101 were given a fertilized egg to study through its entire hatching process.

Peering into our microscopes we watched the tiny "red spot" grow into a chick embryo, steadily developing a heart, lungs, limbs and sensory organs. That experience, still vivid in my memory more than fifty years later, laid the foundation for a life-long fascination with the process of reproduction.

What I learned from that chicken egg I later could apply to my understanding of how the human egg grew from an embryo to a fetus, and finally to a full-term baby. I recognized the similarities, and also was aware of the differences.

The chicken egg hatched in a matter of days outside the mother hen. The human embryo, on the other hand, broods for nine long months within the mother's body. Moreover, while the production of a fertilized chicken egg is easily achieved, the initiation of the human reproductive process can be chancy.

First of all, not all women in their reproductive years produce an egg each month. And when an egg is produced, the timing of the attempt at fertilization is critical.

Under the most favorable circumstances one egg (called an "ovum") pops out of a woman's ovary once a month, around the middle of the menstrual cycle, usually from the 13th to the 15th day. Then, attracted in the right direction by a wonderous process called "chemotropism," the egg floats over to one of the two fallopian tubes that lead down to the womb, the uterus.

Now timing is everything. The egg can be successfully fertilized only during its passage through the tube. That means a healthy sperm must have negotiated its way to that destination, valiantly swimming against the current, up through the uterus to the fallopian tube where the egg is passively waiting.

After this marathon swim the microscopic wiggler must

have sufficient strength remaining to crack the egg's outer membrane, to enter and complete the fertilization process.

Again, if the timing isn't just right, and all these events fail to take place within 48 to 72 hours after ovluation, hormonal changes re-set the menstrual clock. In the early part of the woman's menstrual cycle the lining of her uterus had been enriched into a lush nesting place for a fertilized egg. When none arrives she sheds this bed and has her period. Her uterus "weeps" at its failure to become pregnant.

On the other hand, if all goes well and fertilization is occurs, the "pregnant" time clock is turned on. The tiny egg soon splits into two, and then four, eight, sixteen, thirt-two cells, as it moves down the tube into the uterine cavity.

In the 10 to 14 days after fertilization, this pre-embryonic bit of protoplasm continues to divide by doubling, settling into its "nest" in the wall of the uterus. Even at this early stage, a doctor can detect a pregnancy by the use of hormone tests. Furthermore, something like two out of three embryos are spontaneously aborted in the first two weeks, usually because something isn't quite right.

In those pregnancies which continue, some of the newly-formed cells are converted into a placenta, called the "afterbirth" when expelled after the baby is born. This specialized organ burrows into the wall of the uterus to tap into the mother's blood supply, diverting nutrients, iron and oxygen to support the growth of the new intrauterine passenger. At the same time, the placenta dumps the embryo's waste products back into the mother's blood stream. And this busy organ also supplies the hormones essential to the continued growth of the pregnancy through nine months of gestation.

Early on, this pre-embryo has the appearance of a tadpole. By the fourth week — the sixth week since conception — a rudimentary embryonic heart begins to beat, and there is some reflex movement. By twenty weeks there may be sufficient brain development to provide the fetus with what the psychologists refer to as "sentience," an awareness and an ability to feel and respond to stimulus.

It is not until 25 to 28 weeks that the fetus is "viable," capable of existing outside the mother's womb, but only with the high-tech assistance of incubators and other sophisticated life support systems in hospital neonatal intensive care units.

Not too many decades ago, medical students were taught to recognize the time of viability by the onset of tangible movement, the biblical "quickening," when the mother could "feel the baby kicking." But now, obstetric science has created philosophic and legal confusion.

Today we can "look" at the size and shape of the floating fetus with ultrasonic probes, and listen to it with electronic fetal monitors. We can check the health of the developing human by analyzing the chemical content of the amniotic fluid. These technological advances have greatly increased pregnancy survival rates, but at the same time have confused the definition of the moment when human life — the life of the person — begins.

And furthermore, even with all our wonderful advances in obstetric science, there remains so much that we don't know or understand about the incredible egg, and the process which changes it into a living, active being. Why, for example, does the egg "know" to float into the tube to meet the eager sperm? What is that mysterious force that splits the single egg into the millions of cells that eventually constitute the amazing human body? No human brain has yet approached comprehending the development of the world's most awesome computer, the human brain.

In searching for the Reason, the Ultimate Force, the Cosmic Wisdom, there comes a time when Science and Theology must join hands.

8 Tough Abortion Choices for Lawmakers

A FEW YEARS AGO I felt obliged to ask my patients and friends to take pity on our Idaho state legislators, who had just had the very hot potato of abortion tossed into their laps. The majority of our representatives were baritones, none of whom had ever been pregnant, or felt the terror of a missed menstrual period

These conscientious if inexperienced legislators were asked to deliberate and decide on medical, moral and ethical aspects of the private lives of women such as Molly, Maggie and Martha.

Molly is a fifteen year-old teenager, in the early bloom of womanhood. At what was to be a happy, carefree weekend house party, in the company of a football hero, Molly was overwhelmed by a combination of the charms of her boyfriend, her own normal sexual urges, and a bit too much alcohol.

Six weeks later this tearful woman-child found herself at the family planning clinic with a positive pregnancy test.

Maggie, age 24, is a secretary whom I met when she was rushed to our hospital emergency room, bleeding profusely from slashed wrists. Deeply depressed over the break-up of a love affair with her boyfriend, who also happened to be her boss, she had attempted suicide when she learned she was carrying this man's unplanned, unwanted pregnancy.

Martha is a 43-year-old housewife, whose youngest child is nine. Her pregnancy with this baby had been traumatic, marked by hypertension, swelling and seizures, as well as by heart and kidney failure. For most of nine months it was touch and go for her, concluding with an emergency Cesarean section delivery. Martha's doctors strongly warned her not to become pregnant again.

As so often happens, at age 43, Martha considered herself beyond the age of fertility, and allowed herself to be a little careless. She was genuinely surprised to find that her middle-aged, poochy abdomen contained a 5-month-old fetus.

Stories such as these are poignant, real-life expressions of the abstract medical, moral and ethical dilemmas our legislators had to grapple with. Undoubtedly they wished the U.S. Supreme Court had left well enough alone, instead of tinkering with Rose vs. Wade. They knew that whichever way they voted, "pro-choice" or "pro-life," their political lives might be endangered.

Here were their broad options:

(1) Stay with the status quo. In spite of widespread public misunderstanding, the Supreme Court did not overturn the Roe vs. Wade decision of 1973. Abortion under certain defined circumstances is still held to be justifiable and legal.

(2) Go with the option presented by the Webster vs. Reproductive Services ruling, which said the state has a right to restrict the use of public facilities and funds for abortions. And, further, that if a fetus is "viable," a law prohibiting the abortion of that fetus can be considered constitutional.

(3) Or they could have gone back to the archaic Idaho statute that makes any abortion a crime. Although that law was never strictly enforced, it still held that whoever performed an abortion — a doctor, a midwife, or a backroom abortionist — that person would be guilty of a crime, punishable by a large fine and imprisonment. The woman undergoing that abortion also would be subject to fine and imprisonment.

More comfortable appropriating funds for buildings and budgets for state universities, most legislators strongly wished the Supreme Court justices had kept their hands off the Roe decision. Instead, the high court rubbed salt into the wound that had been gradually healing since 1973, widening again the rift between pro-life and pro-choice proponents. The lawmakers were faced with nothing less than trying to answer that question which can never be answered with firm certainty, "When does life really begin?"

Yet even in our comparatively conservative state, with a strict proscription against abortions, this question is implicitly answered every day. The Idaho State Department of Vital Statistics has informed me that if a fetus miscarries before 20 weeks, or weighs less than 350 grams, it need not be reported to the State for birth certification, apparently because it's not considered a person.

In all these legal considerations, "viability" is the key concept, the ability of a fetus to live outside the mother, albeit with the aid of life support systems. Here the water gets pretty muddy; the Supreme Court, in its Rose vs. Wade deliberations, couldn't conclude whether viability occurred at 20 or 24 or 28 weeks.

We doctors, with all our technical know-how — ultrasound imaging of the intrauterine fetus, enzyme analysis by amniocentesis — simply cannot say with certainty whether a 20-week or even a 28-week fetus would be able to live and breathe outside the womb.

The vast majority of physicians abhor the thought of abortion, and so we just don't do them. But we also abhor the amputation of a gangrenous leg, or the cutting off of life support systems of a terminal patient. Our training and experience has prepared us to accept the responsibility for those medical, moral, and ethical obligations.

Sometimes, of course, addressing the abortion question can get down to political tradeoffs. Idaho's neighbor state of Oregon not only allows abortions, Medicaid picks up the tab for those needed by indigent women. Apparently the legislators there reason that this approach is far cheaper than putting one more young life on the welfare rolls.

But that's a pragmatic, political choice. A much more

sensitive dilemma would have faced the legislators if they had faced the very personal problems that led Molly, Maggie, and Martha to consider the possibility of abortions.

For young Molly and Maggie the final decision had to be to have an abortion. This successfully accomplished, they picked up the threads of their lives, two wiser young ladies. For Martha, in her early 40s, the decision was much more difficult. At five months the termination of the pregnancy was considered hazardous. She went into labor at eight months and delivered a premature infant that barely survived.

Just three examples to show that, when it comes to human life, it's extremely difficult to legislate a single standard of what's right and wrong for everyone.

9 *Just Call Womb Service*

VIRGINIA, SEVEN MONTHS PREGNANT, is asking for advice on how to communicate with her baby right now, sixty days before she/he is due to arrive. She and her husband Alex have read entire books about the importance and value of early parental bonding, and so hope to get a prenatal head start. They have heard that parents can contact and influence their unborn progeny, even while their someday son/daughter is still floating in Mom's womb.

Virginia's friend Marcy regularly snuggled her pregnant abdomen up to a tape of Vivaldi's "Four Seasons" during the final three months of her pregnancy. And last year her cousin Sue bombarded her unborn baby with Bach and Beethoven. Both new mothers swear their babies' first cries had a special melodious quality.

Sound sort of silly? Sure it does, yet there is a growing body of evidence that the developing fetus is more than a blob of passive protoplasm, floating patiently in its womb room until the moment of birth, uninfluenced by the external world. On the contrary, we know the fetus is well aware of current events beyond mommy's navel, and is able to send as well as to receive messages.

A device called the Pregaphone was invented to help expectant parent communicate with their very little ones in utero. It's a simple, low-tech gadget, consisting of a length of flexible plastic tubing, with a mouthpiece at one end, an inverted funnel at the other. The entire contraption comes in tasteful "sunshine yellow," a color chosen by the inventor to be appropriate for either boy or girl babies.

The prototype Pregaphone was created by a marketing executive as a shower gift for her pregnant friend. Reaction at the party was so positive she refined and patented the product, and since has sold thousands.

In use, with the funnel resting on Mother's enlarging abdomen, she or the expectant father can dispense words of wisdom about life in general and how to succeed in it, or just offer a few happy words of welcome to the little pre-birth boarder.

Actually, this pre-birth communication is nothing new. For thousands of years mothers have been humming to their unborn babies, or have mumbled or grumbled to them, sometimes to be rewarded with a solid kick inside their lower abdomen.

Furthermore, mothers all over the world have long believed that external events can have a strong effect on the babies they are carrying. For example, Grandma was sure that it was her over-eating at the strawberry social when she was two months pregnant that produced a strawberry birthmark on Junior's leg.

Up until not so long ago, pregnant women easily accepted a variety of beliefs that certain physical, mental, or emotional shocks would "mark" their unborn baby. We now dismiss these notions as old wives tales, yet we know with greater confidence than ever that a pregnant woman's lifestyle can, indeed, have its effect upon the baby she is carrying.

- In the most extreme cases, the infant born to a drug addict can be trembly and jittery, experiencing a stormy course in the newborn nursery.
- The alcoholic mother may produce a baby with a shaky, unbalanced metabolism, and impaired liver function.
- The mother who is a heavy smoker may prematurely give birth to a puny baby.

These responses to external physical conditions emphasize the degree to which the unborn baby responds to external stimuli. And beyond these impinging physical conditions, you can appreciate that some sounds and even light register in the central nervous system of the fetus.

Sometimes these sensory stimuli set the baby to kicking when we disturb him. Mothers and doctors welcome these kicks as the baby's way of telling us that all is well within his cozy room, assuring us that his blood supply is adequate, and that the placental cafeteria is serving up good rations.

We can even "talk back" to junior using an "acoustical stimulator." Placing this hi-tech squawk box on the mother's abdomen, we send sound wave "messages" to baby, provoking a reassuring response.

So maybe the Pregaphone isn't so phony. Of course if you don't want to spend $12.95 for the real thing, you could send your words of love and guidance down the tube from a roll of paper towels. Or even through the hose attachment that comes with the vacuum sweeper. Just call womb service.

10 Having Babies, Naturally and the High-Tech Way

THE YOUNG WOMAN'S CRIES OF PAIN awakened me. I had dozed off, catching forty winks while waiting for Mary Prowaki to have her baby. I rubbed my eyes in the cold gray light of the Chicago winter dawn, abruptly remembering that I was about to deliver my first baby. To Mary I was a full-fledged doctor, coming to her apartment from the Chicago Lying-in Hospital, to help bring her first-born into the world. In fact I was an inexperienced medical student, and I was nervous.

Of course, I hadn't told her that this was to be my first hands-on obstetrical experience. That going out into the so-called "maternity district" to take part in a home delivery was part of my training in learning to be a doctor. Or that I probably was as scared as she was.

Late the evening before, the home-health nurse and I had been warmly welcomed into the modest home of John and Mary Prowaki, having climbed two flights of dingy stairs from a street that bordered on the stockyards. Mary's labor had begun and seemed to be going well, so we quickly made our preparations.

Instruments were laid out, water was put on the stove to boil, and near at hand was pile of newspapers to cover the birthing bed. By ten o'clock this young "doctor" and his nurse Mollie Fane were prepared to assist the baby's arrival.

Now it was early morning. Mary had gone through a long night of difficult labor, and was tired and worried. Her husband John was fretfully pacing the floor. "Can't you do something, Doc? Mary's sure hurtin' bad."

In clean, well-lighted University of Chicago classrooms, now far away on the other side of this town, medical school professors had taught us fledgling doctors all about the conduct of a normal labor, and the sequence of stages before the infant would arrive on the scene.

They forgot to tell us, however, what to say or do when the labor dragged on for hours, until the exhausted mother finally wailed in total desperation, "I just don't think I can do it, Doc!" Or when the expectant father's widening eyes seemed to suggest a panicked distrust of this hesitant young doctor.

To my rescue came Mollie, sturdy veteran of many such encounters. "You better do a pelvic, Doc, I thing the baby's hung up in there and it's trying to turn."

As my inexperienced fingers probed the birth canal, they touched the bulging bag of waters, and then the baby's head. Suddenly a gush of warm fluid whooshed out, drenching my shirtfront and trousers. I had inadvertently ruptured the amniotic sac, and now was a wet and embarrassed embryo doctor.

This time Nature came to my rescue. A moment later Mary shrieked "It's coming, it's coming!" Then suddenly a crown of brown hair appeared. With one last groan and grunt from Mary, a slippery baby boy emerged and was in my hands, kicking and screaming furiously.

Now there were happy smiles all around, husband John kissing the new mother, then congratulating me: "You did it, Doc, you did it!"

That was number one. Over the next fifty years I have "delivered" 4,434 more babies, and each time I've been reminded of the basic lessons I learned that early morning near the stockyards in Chicago.

The first lesson was one of humility. The realization that we physicians are truly only "attendants" at the birthing event. The mother, not the doctor, "delivers" the baby. We are present to offer the benefit of our training, our experience, and our technical tools, to make the process easier and safer for both the mother and the baby.

The next lesson I learned in that first delivery was an awareness, understanding and appreciation of the miracle of pregnancy and birth. The mystery of conception, the magnificence of the growth of the egg into an embryo, then to a fetus, and finally to the infant that bursts into this world, crying and kicking.

Being present at a birth is a wonderous experience, reaffirming my belief that there must be, indeed, a God in His heaven. One moment that bedroom was filled with pain and fear. In the next, pain forgotten, only with joy and tears of happiness.

The third lesson comes as a privilege of looking back over five decades of delivering babies. Early in my years as a physician, the increasingly apparent dangers of home delivery led to the creation of "maternity homes." Usually operated by a capable, experienced woman, a housewife and a mother, in the 1940s and early 1950s these institutions were a place for the mother-to-be to await delivery and then to have her baby.

In our north Idaho town, Bessie Oslund and Amanda Barnes each ran successful maternity homes, making up with on-the-job experience what they lacked in scientific training. They possessed a very personal understanding of "maternity," plus, they just loved babies.

But again, along came change in the name of progress, and soon the usual and expected practice was to have your baby in the hospital — more sterile, but also more impersonal.

Doctors and nurses were gloved and gowned, and husbands were excluded from the delivery suite, to fret with fellow expectant fathers in the waiting room. The newborn baby was promptly whisked away from its mother, into the sterility of the nursery, where Papa could view him or her through the window, sometimes wondering "Which one's mine?"

It wasn't long before the chilly, clinical atmosphere of hospital deliveries produced a movement in favor of a return to the warm intimacy of a "natural" home delivery. Hospital administrators responded by installing warm and bright "birthing rooms," with colorful wallpaper, an easy chair for Dad, and TV.

Gone were the masks and gowns and the swift and sterile separation of the newborn from its parents. Mom and Dad could cuddle their precious child minutes after the birth. If the proud father felt up to it, he could even tie off the umbilical cord.

In the next phase in the evolution of baby delivery, two powerful winds of change altered the basic nature of a doctor's obstetrical practice. First was the fresh, invigorating breeze of amazing advances in technology, including ultrasound imaging of the fetus, amniocentesis to determine the baby's condition and even its sex, and electronic monitoring during labor. Well in advance of a woman's due date, she might be given "stress tests," to check the health of the fetus, and its anticipated response to uterine contractions.

The second wind of change carried the dark clouds and squalls of law suits. Every pregnancy and delivery was expected to produce a "perfect" baby. As a result, the physician was forced to simultaneously practice good medicine in behalf of the mother and infant, as well as "defensive" medicine to fend off possible malpractice suits.

These changes combined to dramatically increase the cost of delivering a baby, causing couples to think twice before entering upon a pregnancy.

And physicians, who might otherwise "let nature take its course," may cover their exposure to possible litigation by intervening in the course of the delivery process, even to the extent of taking the baby by Cesarean section. Many fine obstetricians, frustrated by the parents' expectations of a "perfect baby" with every pregnancy, and by the prospect of parents eager (with the help of attorneys hovering nearby) to sue when everything isn't perfect, are throwing in the sponge — and the birthing forceps.

Looking back into that dingy bedroom near the stockyards in Chicago where I delivered a healthy baby onto newspapers, I can only conclude that that young doctor lucked out. His exhilarating experience there inspired a life-long wonder of the natural beginning of new life.

It's too bad that the embryo doctors of today, with a roomful of high-tech machines and the threat of litigation just outside the birthing room door, are denied a similar inspiration.

10 Cesarean Section: A Better Alternative Today

JULIUS CAESAR IS SUPPOSED TO HAVE ENTERED this world by way of a cut in his mommy's abdomen, and this is why the surgical delivery of a baby by this abdominal route is called a "Cesarean section." Yet it is highly unlikely that a women could have survived this operation around 100 B.C., and Caesar's mother lived for many years after his birth. Furthermore, history books make no mention of this operation being performed before the 16th century. Perhaps Ceasar's birth was given a kind of mythological cast because he was so gifted and versatile.

There is precedent for such flights of mythologic fantasy. It excited our schoolboy imaginations to read the story of how Prometheus split open the head of Zeus with an Olympian ax, allowing Athena to spring out, fully armed, ready to act as protectress of the ancient Greek cities.

Biblical scholars have long pondered the symbolism of Eve's birth as related in Genesis: "And the Lord God caused a deep sleep to fall upon Adam, and he slept, and He took one of his ribs, and closed up the flesh instead thereof."

Many theologians accept this story of the very first surgical birth as allegory, meant to demonstrate the oneness of Man and Woman, husband and wife, as they bring into life a newborn person, "bone of our bones, flesh of our flesh."

The first recorded abdominal delivery in which the women survived was performed by a German pig gelder, named Jacob Nufer, in the year 1500. This fellow, presumably distraught by his wife's cries of anguish during labor, used his gelding instruments to make an abdominal cut, and "snatched the infant from his wife's loins." By some miracle she survived, and went on to give birth to two more infants, via the normal vaginal route.

Five hundred years later, we have the surgical skills and the technological support systems to perform "C-sections" with a high percentage of success. In the past twenty years, the proportion of babies delivered this way has risen to around one in five.

Sometimes, in extreme cases, the procedure is used to attempt to deliver a living child from a dead or dying mother. Though the aims are noble, the procedure often is not successful, because time is such a critical factor. For example, not long ago a pregnant woman killed in an automobile accident was rushed to our hospital in an attempt to save the baby, due in a few weeks. But the best efforts of a skilled team of doctors and nurses was unable to perform a post-mortem Cesarean section in time to deliver a living baby.

Only a generation ago, a C-section was resorted to only after all other efforts at vaginal delivery had failed. The most common indication was "cephalopelvic disproportion," meaning the baby's head is just too large to pass through the birth canal. The other common reason was hemorrhage, resulting from premature separation of the afterbirth.

The general limitation of Cesarean sections to such emergencies resulted in the surgical procedure being used only about 5% of the time. Today, in most hospitals, the figure has risen to around 20%.

There are several reasons for this increase. The most frequent reason for a C-section these days is "failure to progress," an apparent and worrisome delay in the rate at which the birth passage opens to allow the downward progress of the baby trying to be born. The rate of dilatation and descent is charted by the nurse on what is called the Friedman Curve, and deviation from a "normal" curve is considered cause for concern.

Not so many years ago, if at this point we had noted a lack of progress in the rate of delivery, we very well might have sedated the mother and turned her on her side, allowing her a few hours of sleep to regain her strength. In most cases when she awakened, she would go into active labor and deliver a lusty baby.

Another cause for the increased use of Cesarean sections is the greatly improved technological monitoring systems. In labor and delivery rooms today an Electronic Fetal Monitor sends out a constant "lub-dub, lub-dub," recording the baby's heartbeat on a strip of paper. The frequency of this lub-dub slows with each uterine contraction — called "decceleration" — but promptly returns to a steady normal beat as the contraction subsides.

Now then, if this re-acceleration doesn't occur as promptly as it apparently should, that fact is duly recorded on the tape — and on the awareness of the patient, the husband, the natural childbirth Lamaze coach, and of course on the nurse and the doctor.

Flashing before the eyes of the poor physician is a vision of the attorney for his patient — now a plaintiff — waving the tape in front of a jury and screaming, "Why, doctor, when you saw that decceleration, why didn't you immediately perform this simple little operation, a C-section?"

So, faced with this prospect, the doctor naturally doesn't elect to allow nature to take its course. He or she opts for the safest course (for the doctor), and leads a team in a major — by no means a "little" — surgical procedure. Often the baby lifted from the mother's abdomen is pink and crying lustily, showing no negative effects from "decceleration." In most instances the mother now must have all future babies delivered by this abdominal route.

Happily, modern surgical techniques and the availability of antibiotics enable rapid healing, and have made Cesarean sections relatively safe. Advances in anesthesia also have increased our willingness to resort to an operative delivery. No longer is it necessary to hastily "snatch the baby from the womb" in three our four minutes. Now the procedure can be carried out deliberately and methodically.

Here, then, are the obvious reasons why the delivery of babies by C-section has become much more common. On the one hand we have become very confident in the comparative safety of the operation, while on the other there is the ever-present fear of malpractice litigation, if the physician courageously persists in assisting the mother in a difficult vaginal delivery, rather than giving in to the surgical procedure.

As we reflect upon the changes that have taken place so rapidly during the past two decades, we cannot help but wonder what the year 2000 will bring. Will we continue to depersonalize this business of having babies? Will pregnancy and delivery become mechanical and painless? Will surgical delivery eventually take precedence over vaginal delivery?

Can we conjecture that genetic engineers will take over the reproductive duties? Will artificially inseminated test tube fetuses grow not only in the wombs of surrogate mothers, but in plastic uteri in the reproductive laboratories? Will baby X then bond to it incubator, rather than to its human mother?

Heaven forbid! Even though God said "In sorrow thou shalt bring forth children," the Eves of tomorrow will continue to conceive babies, and willingly bear that pain. Mothers-to-be somehow know that, when they hear that first cry of their newborn infant, the pains of childbirth miraculously disappear.

Come what may in the 21st century, my forecast is that future Adams and Eves will stay with good old-fashioned way of making babies, and that in the strong majority of the cases their children will be delivered in the natural, normal way...just like Julius Caesar.

11 Twins!

"OH NO, DOCTOR, IT CAN'T BE — there aren't any twins in our family. Are you sure?"

I was confident in my diagnosis that Janice was carrying two fetuses in her uterus, and showed her the ultra-sound "picture" which confirmed this.

Once her surprise had given way to acceptance, excitement took over. The expectant mother happily phoned family and friends to announce "We're going to have twins!" Husband Jim went around busting his buttons, bragging about his virility to the folks down at his office, and to anyone else who would listen.

But as the prenatal months dragged on, and Janice's abdomen swelled to enormous proportions, she began to worry. Will the labor be twice as difficult? Will I be able to nurse two babies? Will my tummy ever go back to its normal size? Will I die?

Jim also has had to face some sobering consequences of having twins. There will be twice as many sleep interruptions with babies to feed and diapers to change. There will be twice as many shoes and everything else to buy. College tuition will be doubled.

Fortunately these fears disappeared at the moment of delivery, when six pound, two ounce Johnny came into the world kicking and screaming. Ten minutes later out came Jason, five pounds twelve ounces, crying a little less lustily, but also perfectly healthy.

Now Janice could shed a tear of joy and relief as those prenatal nightmares vanished. And Jim could give the good news to grandma and grandpa, and then head out to buy two dozen roses and two boxes of cigars.

The delivering physician, now almost forgotten as the babies were rushed to the hospital nursery, wiped his brow and gave thanks that all had gone well.

Through the last months of Janice's pregnancy he had quietly reflected on a doctor's special concerns about a woman carrying a multiple pregnancy. There was an increased chance of elevated blood pressure as well as a condition called toxemia of pregnancy, characterized by hypertension, fluid retention, edema and protein in the urine. Extra bed rest might be required during the last weeks of the pregnancy. The possibility of a complicated delivery would be much greater with twins, and the chance of hemorrhaging would be increased.

Because twins were involved there was an increased risk that one of the fetuses might not make it — sometimes the weaker of the two dies while still inside the uterus.

Once Janet knew she was carrying twins, on every prenatal checkup visit she would have a list of questions about dual births. For example, her first and most basic, how and why do twins happen? My reply could only be that multiple pregnancies are an accident of nature. With all our scientific know-how, we still can't explain why a fertilized egg will split in half to produce two fetuses that will develop into identical twins. It just happens.

We also know that a woman may sometimes produce

two eggs during a single monthly cycle, and that in rare instances both these eggs can be fertilized by two different sperm cells. The result is two fetuses with two entirely different sets of genes. Called fraternal twins, the two are twins only in the sense that they shared an intrauterine life, and because they were born at approximately the same time. Genetically they are just ordinary siblings, often not of the same sex, two different people.

We think twins are cute, and encourage that cuteness by clothing them in identical shirts and dresses. Their hair ribbons and their tennis shoes must look alike, and their hair is trimmed and parted in the same way. Doublemint chewing gum exploits our fascination with twins by using identical twin boys and girls in their TV ads.

Aside from the obvious physical similarities, from time to time we hear about mysterious extrasensory perception experienced by some twin pairs. How even though the two may be miles apart they have the same thoughts, the same dreams, even the same attacks of appendicitis. Female twins may experience their first menstruation simultaneously.

Twins often will date the same type of person, often with similar names, even if they have been separated from each other, living in different cities.

Born with the same complement of genes, some twins seem to become more similar as they grow older. Literature abounds with examples of twin-induced confusion, sometimes embarrassing or humorous cases of mistaken identity.

On the other hand, in terms of behavior, twins are not strictly "slaves to their genes." A study at the University of Minnesota examined the lives of 350 identical twins who had been raised in different families. They concluded that identical twins are not necessarily identical in behavior.

Personality traits such as leadership, imaginativeness and vulnerability to stress seemed genetically linked. On the other hand, assertiveness, agressiveness and social consciousness can be influenced by upbringing.

Some believe it's not such a good idea to strongly stress the similarities between identical twins. One is Ann Landers, the twin sister of "Dear Abby," who contends that parents use this accident of nature to attract attention. She believes that twins should be allowed to be strictly on their own, so that they can become self-dependent and self-confident.

Just which course Janice and Jim will take in rearing their new twins remains to be seen. At least they have avoided that cutesy trap some parents fall into of naming their twins Pete and RePete, or Kate and Dupli-Kate.

Yet now that they are gradually recovering from the shock of having twins, I'm guessing they agree with the 19th century humorist Josh Billings:

"There is two things in this life for which we ain't never really prepared, and that is twins!"

12 *Circumspect Circumcision*

ONCE CIRCUMCISION WAS LOOKED UPON as standard procedure. Because parents simply assumed their baby boy would be circumcised, we physicians would almost routinely remove the penis foreskin soon after birth. In our small north Idaho town no surgical consent form needed to be signed by the parents, and I would be surprised on those rare occasions when parents asked us not to circumcise. Why would parents resist such a normal, acceptable procedure?

During the past ten years or so, attitudes toward circumcision have changed, in response to a number of studies which have raised questions about the value of routine circumcisions. Now the parents of the newborn boy are provided information for and against the procedure, and the hospital requires a written authorization.

Generalized public feelings questioning routine circumcision have been focused into a movement by a half dozen organizations. Foremost among these is NO CIRC, an acronym for the National Organization for Consumer Information Research Centers, a group consisting of nurses, pediatricians, and lay people.

The people of NO CIRC will gladly supply you with a sheaf of informational literature. Among their anti-circumcision arguments...

- The foreskin has a protective role, protecting the penis against venereal disease
- As with any surgery, there are risks in performing a circumcision
- Great pain is inflicted by this surgery
- Circumcision can be a mutilating operation, leading to sexual dysfunction and suicide
- Circumcision is an "unnecessary" surgery, performed on a non-consenting infant.

If you agree with these five arguments you must imagine I feel extremely guilty, as I reflect on the phallic indignities I have inflicted upon more than two thousand baby boys I've delivered over the years. Good heavens, I even allowed my two sons to be circumcised!

As a surgical resident at Chicago's Presbyterian-St. Lukes Hospital, I introduced interns to the basics of surgery techniques, using the simple steps of circumcision. As residents we also were privileged to watch Jewish ritual circumcisions, celebrated with wine and cake by the assembled family. One rabbi reminded me that he was following the orders stated in Chapter 17 of the Book of Genesis: "Every male child among you shall be circumcised as a covenant between God and Man." Moreover, in the Book of Samuel it is recorded that David slew 200 of those heathen Philistines and brought their foreskins to the king as a dowry for the hand in marriage of his daughter Merab. Not too different from collecting scalps as trophies of war.

Recalling these Bible injunctions, I felt less guilty. Then I turned to the current scientific literature and found that...

- A study at Walter Reed Hospital in Washington determined that uncircumcised men had ten times as many genital infections as those who had been circumcised.
- Clinical statistics indicate that circumcision using modern techniques and specially designed instruments carries with it only very small risks.
- As for "great pain," neurologists believe that, in the newborn, the sensory nerves which conduct pain messages to the brain are not yet developed.
- The statement that "circumcision leads to sexual dysfunction and suicide" simply does not stand up to careful, unbiased scrutiny.
- Various courts of law have held, sensibly enough, that parents can consent to surgical procedures in behalf of their infants.

Aside from such specific rebuttals, there are a number of reasons why circumcision is so widely accepted in the United States. Among them...

- It is easier to keep the circumcised penis clean and free of odor.
- Cancer of the penis is extremely rare in the circumcised male
- The incidence of cancer of the uterus is significantly higher in the wives of uncircumcised men.
- With the majority of males already circumcised, a boy with an intact foreskin may suffer locker room embarrassment.

- Circumcision forestalls the development of phimosis, a stricture of the foreskin which prevent easy retraction.

Yet the current controversy surrounding circumcision is a good thing, serving as a reminder that the decision to do this or any surgical procedure should be based on good reason. And it emphasizes the point that, before any surgery is contemplated, the patient or those responsible for the patient have a right to know the advantages and the disadvantages of the procedure, so that they can give informed consent.

13 Dramatic Changes in Adoption

MOST ADULTS AND MANY CHILDREN know that babies aren't delivered by Mr. Stork. But now specialists in reproductive science have devised techniques to make it possible for a human being to be conceived in a laboratory test-tube, rather than in the bedroom.

That amazing triumph has opened a large can of worms, releasing all sorts of slippery social, medical, ethical and legal problems. Babies can be bought, wombs rented. And they don't come cheap.

Before obstetrics became so entangled with technology, we physicians were dealing mainly with "blessed events." Dollars then didn't seem to matter, and many babies were never paid for. To me and to many physicians this wasn't of great concern, because there was something really rewarding and satisfying in helping bring a new life into the world.

Moreover, a couple's infertility was generally accepted as an act of God, endured for a time and then finally resolved through the happiness of a simple and relatively inexpensive adoption. In my early days of practice in northern

Idaho, in the 1940s and 1950s, there always seemed to be plenty of "unwanted" babies. In fact, I occasionally would have to scout around to find adoptive parents.

One reason was that safe and sure contraception, such as provided by the birth control pill, wasn't available. Furthermore, youthful unwed pregnancies were probably inevitable, given the sketchy and not so reliable schoolyard sex education program.

Also, abortions had not yet become legal, and certainly were not as socially acceptable as they are today. When a doctor determined a pregnancy should be terminated, to protect the mental or emotional health of the woman, he had to refer her to the local abortionist, who many gentle folks knew about but no one talked about. Or she could drive about thirty miles to a little rundown motel over near the Spokane airport, where abortions were performed while the authorities looked the other way.

It followed, naturally, that most of the unwanted, unplanned pregnancies went to term. The young woman would drop out of school, deliver, then put her baby up for adoption. Not infrequently the mother of nine children would in desperation offer up her tenth offspring for adoption.

Adoption procedures were simple, and carried out with complete confidentiality. In today's litigious climate it may be hard to believe that there was no signed contractual agreement — the young mother's word and that of the family were sufficient.

It was the custom then, also, to immediately whisk the baby to be adopted out of the delivery room and into the hospital nursery, to avoid any post-partum anguish the mother might suffer — and to make sure she wouldn't change her mind. The only charges to the adopting parents were the hospital and doctor's fees.

To make the baby a legal child of the adoptive parents,

attorney Ward Arney usually would handle the details. His fee was $25 — or nothing, if that seemed proper.

Today, even though sex education is a part of our school programs, and condoms are easily available, teenage pregnancy is extremely common. Also common are abortions, as well as unwed mothers. No longer do pregnant teenagers drop out of high school in total disgrace. And as a consequence, no longer are there enough babies for adoption: 90% of those unwed teens who go through with their pregnancies will keep their babies as a badge of adulthood.

This situation helps explain the desperation felt by those couples who yearn to have a baby, to be parents, but haven't been successful. Scarcely a week goes by that I don't receive at least one letter from a man and wife pleading for information on adoption. They usually list their excellent qualifications and their ability to pay. Usually they enclose a glossy color photo of the handsome couple.

Given such a shortage of babies to adopt, no wonder some couples are willing to spend $25,000 to $30,000 to obtain a baby through surrogate motherhood. It's a sad state of affairs.

With discoveries such as The Pill and Norplant, family planning has become easier and more reliable. In this overpopulated world, beset with disease and famine, this is all for the good.

But some of you may wonder if medical scientists have not gone too far, unnaturally invading the uterus to artificially produce human life.

There are a few rays of sunshine breaking through these black clouds of controversy over surrogate parenthood. For one thing, given the much-publicized shortage of babies to adopt, those parents who in the past few years have been lucky enough to adopt a child have been reminded of their great good fortune.

And any woman who at one time in her life made that

heart-rending decision to give her baby up for adoption, can now know for certain that the choice she made was the right one. She unselfishly made a precious gift of a lifetime of happiness, not only to the adopting parents, but to her child.

14 *Happy Ending to Teen Pregnancy*

THIS IS THE TRUE STORY OF TWO YOUNG WOMEN, Diana and Sarah, whose lives crossed without their knowing it. It's a sad story, with a happy ending.

Diana was a the 17-year-old daughter of a broken marriage. At 16 she fell in love with Tom, the captain of the high school basketball team and, as so often happens, her search for a loving, caring relationship resulted in a teenage pregnancy.

For Diana and her family, because of their religious beliefs, abortion was out of the question. Fortunately, she came under the care of an understanding family physician, who listened to her worries and dispensed a fair amount of fatherly advice. Even though marriage was not contemplated, the doctor urged Tom to remain loyal to Diana. Surprisingly, he came with her on prenatal office visits, and stayed at her side during the entire labor and delivery.

A week before Diana was due to deliver she confided to her doctor, her eyes brimming with tears, that she had decided to give up the baby for adoption. In spite of pressure from her peers urging her to keep her "baby doll," and in spite of her unhappy family background (or could it have been because of it?), she had the maturity of judgment to come to this difficult decision.

The day of delivery produced strong tugs on the heart

strings of everyone involved. When the chubby, lusty baby boy was delivered, the young mother and father choked back tears, refusing to look at the infant or even to ask its sex, probably fearing they might not be able to hold to their decision to give the baby away. There were tears on the cheeks of the nurse who carried the baby to the nursery. The doctor was glad he could hide his own emotions behind a surgical mask.

Then came the time to pick out the proper adopting parents. In this day of The Pill and easy abortions, every doctor who delivers babies has a long list of prospective adopting parents: there are far more who couples who want to adopt than there are babies available. When one does come along, the physician must select which husband and wife will be rewarded for their patience. Will the new parents provide a good home, filled with loving care? He or she must also consider the age of the parents, their religion, and even their complexions. Fortunately, in this case the decision was easy — Sarah, the other woman in our story — just had to have this baby.

Sarah was a very pretty, 22-year-old woman, a patient of the same family physician since she was in kindergarten. Two weeks before her wedding she visited her doctor for her premarital consultations. To his utter dismay, and of course to hers, his pelvic examination revealed a large tumor on one ovary. The physician had to decide whether to advise Sarah and Bob, her husband-to-be, that immediate surgery was indicated? Or to proceed with the wedding as planned, and have the surgery when they returned from their honeymoon?

After he carefully stated the options, along with the risks of postponing surgery, this young couple decided, without a moment's hesitation, to go ahead with the marriage.

Two weeks after the honeymoon, the physician operated to remove the tumor. A biopsy specimen was whisked over to the hospital laboratory, but the pathologist was unable to make a definitive diagnosis at that time. So the surgical team closed the incision, hoping the tumor would prove to be benign.

Unfortunately, upon further study the pathologist concluded that the tumor was a rare type of cancer, yet fortunately one with a high rate of cure. But it would be necessary to operate again, to remove Sarah's uterus and her other ovary, to prevent future spread of the cancer. This was done and, to make the cure all the more certain, she was given a course of cobalt treatment. Of course, Sarah now could never have children.

Through this entire traumatic newlywed experience, Sarah and her husband were cooperative and uncomplaining. Hospital and radiation therapy costs were high, but they drew on their meager savings and managaed to make regular monthly payments. All the health care people who dealt with this young couple — doctors, nurses, therapists — were touched and inspired by their courage and their loyalty to each other. "I have no trouble, whatsoever," said the physician to a colleague, "in deciding that Sarah and Bob just have to be the adopting parents of this newborn baby."

Good things aren't always easily accomplished. Because the natural mother was a minor, the court was unwilling to accept her consent to the adoption. Diana's parents were divorced and remarried, and were living in other cities, so they had to be tracked down and their signatures obtained. To add to the delay, the hospital administrator was reluctant to allow the baby to be discharged without a court order. Getting all this done took another two and a half days.

But finally we came to the happy endings. A beautiful baby boy was placed in the arms of Sarah. There were more tears, but they were tears of joy. Her young husband has taken on extra jobs, and her mother went back to waiting on tables to help with all those bills. No question about it,

Sarah's new baby would be well loved!

Diana's happy ending has been less dramatic, slower in coming. After her release from the hospital, she fell into a deep depression. Counseling from her physician and from her minister helped, and gradually she came out of her understandable post-partum blues. She returned to high school, and hopes to go on to nurse's training. Tom is studying auto mechanics at our community college, and is assured a job when he graduates. Then he and Diana will make plans for a church wedding.

Diana will begin a new life with Tom, and they will start a family. She and her new husband will take comfort in knowing that because of her courageous decision, somewhere in this world her first-born baby is in a good and loving home. Her emotional sacrifice brought a lifetime of happiness to two people who were denied the privilege of having a child of their own.

15 Women Are More Than Just Equal Already

I'm all for woman's lib
Make women equal to men, somehow
Instead of being so darn superior
The way they are now
           — *Nipsy Russell*

LET'S FACE IT, OUR WIVES AND MOTHERS have out-smarted us men down through the ages, letting us think we are their superiors, and that they are the weaker sex. Hogwash! They've known all along they are our better halves, the stronger sex. And there is plenty scientific evidence to prove it.

Peering through a microscope, you can see this female superiority even before life begins. Sperm carrying the Y chromosome to make boys may swim a bit faster and may be a little more aggressive, but in the long run the X-type female sperm outlasts the male, being more durable and more patient in achieving its goal and destiny.

The male sperm, because it's speedier and more aggressive, does manage to impregnate a higher percentage of ova. But that's an empty victory: more males are spontaneously aborted in early pregnancy, and more males are stillborn.

At the time of delivery the female fetus seems more able to withstand the rigors of the passage through the birth canal. Brain damage secondary to birth trauma is more common and more serious in boy babies.

Come to think of it, how many of us men could go through nine months of pregnancy, and then survive the delivery?

The female child matures physiologically, psychologically and emotionally much sooner than boys. And girls go through the socialization process much earlier, enabling them to be "social beings" throughout their lifetimes.

When a headline shouts that "Heart Disease is Mankind's Public Enemy Number One," the writer is, in fact, referring to men. Rarely do premenopausal women suffer heart attacks, and the female hormone, estrogen, may protect women against coronary disease.

This explains, in part, why women have a greater average life expectancy. A baby boy born today can look forward to 72 years of life on this planet; a baby girl has a life expectancy of 80 years. Now that ain't "equal!"

There is growing evidence that the female brain is anatomically different from that of the male, and in some ways physiologically superior. For example, neurologists believe skill in speaking is governed primarily by the left side of the brain. Because the female of our species appears to make better use of the left hemisphere, she is more communicative, more sensitive, more interested in people — again, a more social being.

There are a few compensating factors, of course. Males seem to make better use of the right side of their brains, and so are more adept at visual-spatial tasks, excel at manipulating things, and at jobs that require manual dexterity. Men are the aggressive hunters, the bruising football players. The male brain seems to more easily handle mathematical and analytical problems.

Yet as the 20th century comes to a close, the gender gap begins to narrow. More women are seen in the ranks of architecture, engineering, medicine. Women are flexing their political muscles.

The most recent census found that not only is our nation's population growing older, it's growing more female. Will we in the next century see an evolutionary shift to female predominance? Let's face up to it, men, it looks like we are in a losing cause.

Yet there is one last vestige of macho male superiority left for us, and we must struggle to preserve it. So far we men do not wear one single thing that zips up the back!

16 *When You're Having Trouble Having Children*

UNWANTED PREGNANCIES AND WORLD OVERPOPULATION are serious global problems. But on a local and personal level, the problem facing my friends John and Jane Archer was just the reverse: they were eager to have a baby, but hadn't been able to conceive.

During their first year of marriage, they used contraceptives, then decided they were ready to start a family. But after eighteen months of trying without success, Jane went to her physician for an explanation.

Most newly married couples simply assume that, when they are ready to have a baby, "her" egg and "his" sperm will come together in a loving embrace. In most cases they're correct.

But for John and Jane it wasn't that simple. They came face to face with what's called "comparative infertility." Yet as they learned more about the mysteries of reproduction, they began to have hope.

First, their doctor dispelled the common misconception (no pun intended) that "it's always the woman's fault." In at least a third of the cases in which couples are having difficulty conceiving, the male partner shares responsibility.

He also told them that the timing of coitus can be critical. Most women ovulate in the mid-portion of their monthly cycle, around the 14th day. And during that time the egg has a 12-hour period of peak fertility, when a single sperm can penetrate and induce fertilization.

Some women sense they are ovulating, and some experience mild cramping or spotting. To more accurately determine her time of ovulation, Jane's doctor suggested she keep track of her "basal" morning body temperature. This is your basic temperature after your body has been at rest all night — at ovulation time a woman's temperature may rise 1/2 to 3/4 of a degree.

Jane also was advised to remain lying down for 30 minutes after coitus, to reduce the challenge for the sperm swimming upstream.

If John's sperm count turned out to be low, a more thorough physical examination could indicate problems for which there are remedies, some which are quite simple. When some animals are "in heat," the male's testicles drop down into the scrotum to allow the cooler temperatures to enhance sperm production. This suggests that prospective fathers should change from tight-fitting jockey shorts to cooler boxers. Long hot tub baths also won't help matters.

Some men may have a "varicocele" — a bunch of varicose veins in the cord that supplies the testicles. This impediment can be easily repaired with minor surgery.

John was happy to learn from his wife that the doctor prescribed a little relaxation for him, to improve their chances of conceiving a baby. Romance and the pleasure of loveplay apparently generates a full supply of sperm in the ultimate ejaculate.

If the couple had continued to have no success, Jane's physician would have ordered tests to make sure her two fallopian tubes were not blocked or obstructed. And if he suspected that her ovaries were failing to pop out an egg each month, he might prescribe a pill called Clomid, to stimulate ovulation. Using this particular medication slightly increases the chance of having twins, but isn't a "fertility shot" that may lead to multiple pregnancies.

As is so often the case, medical intervention wasn't necessary. A few months after going home and following the doctor's advice, Jane and John received the happy news that her pregnancy test was positive. Today their son Todd is nearly two, and his brother or sister will be born soon!

17 PMS Blues...And Worse

ARE SOME WOMEN NOT TOTALLY MENTALLY COMPETENT, just before their period? A few years ago a Virginia judge went along with this defense, when he dismissed drunk driving charges against a 42-year-old woman.

The state trooper who made the arrest testified that he

pulled the defendant over when he observed her zig-zagging across the center line. After being ordered out of her car she refused to take a sobriety test, showered the officer with obscene expletives, and tried to kick him in the groin.

Expert witnesses stated that a woman suffering from PMS can indeed involuntarily commit criminal acts, because they are temporarily bereft of their full mental capacities. Often these women are unable to control their emotions, and therefore cannot distinguish right from wrong.

Premenstrual syndrome has been described by medical textbooks and journals for more than a half century, and in recent years law enforcement agencies have found a direct correlation between PMS and child abuse, wife-beating, and other forms of domestic violence. In 1981 the potential power of PMS over a woman's psyche received worldwide attention when a high court in Great Britain accepted premenstrual syndrome as a defense for manslaughter.

In the case of "The Crown vs. Mrs. English," the facts revealed that the defendant, in a jealous frenzy and propelled by what her barrister called "an uncontrollable disruptive explosive disorder," drove up behind her husband as he walked home from work and speared the surprised fellow on the car's bumper, then impaled him on a nearby fence post. A medic at a nearby infirmary pronounced the hapless chap DOA.

The day after this sensational incident, Mrs. English began her menstrual period. Almost immediately she became calm and contrite, once again a sensible lady.

Noting this extreme contrast, the judge ruled that the defendant has committed involuntary manslaughter under wholly exceptional circumstances, totally beyond her control, and for that reason she should be held blameless. Mrs. English was, however, prohibited for a period of one year from getting behind the wheel of her instrument of death.

Such bizarre and extreme manifestations aside, PMS is

now widely accepted as a proven clinical entity. Nonetheless, many boyfriends and husbands can recall how frustrated and befuddled they felt the first time they experienced their best-beloved's erratic and capricious PMS mood swings. Most concluded either that "it's all in her head," or "she's going bonkers."

Even some physicians (obviously of the male gender) consider PMS to be an imaginary illness, a purely psychosomatic disorder. But if this were true, why does the condition recur cyclicly, always just prior to the onset of the menses? And why do the symptoms so quickly evaporate when the menstrual flow begins?

As many as 50% of all women experience PMS sometime in their lives, though fortunately only about 5% of these women are severely incapacitated. When the PMS symptoms are at their hottest peak, marital quarrels flare and divorce may be threatened.

To assist in diagnosing PMS, a physician may ask the patient to fill out a questionnaire or to begin a daily diary of physical and emotional symptoms. Psychologists might administer standardized tests such as the Minnesota Multiphasic Personality Inventory, the Dyadic Adjustment Scale, the Beck Depression Evaluation, or the Locke-Wallace Personality Scale.

Solid, scientific stuff. But any woman who has been afflicted with PMS doesn't need questionnaires or diaries to make her own personal diagnosis.

PMS typically makes its appearance during the week prior to menses. Among the physical symptoms are swollen, tender breasts, bloating, fluid retention, weight gain, headaches and backaches, lower abdominal distress. Women suffering from PMS sum it all up by saying "I just feel rotten all over."

The physio-chemical changes which anticipate menstruation induce psychological changes as well. Medical textbooks use terms such as dysphoria, dysthymia and compulsive-obsessive neuroses. Translated into plain language these terms mean the blues, the blahs, a feeling that life isn't worth living. Husband or boyfriend doesn't love me anymore; everybody is picking on me.

Women suffering from PMS often have an intense urge to snack, to smoke or drink, or to indulge in salty foods, ice cream or chocolate.

A woman in the grip of premenstrual syndrome may even have uncharacteristic thoughts of suicide or homocide — remember Mrs. English. And she may insist her soul-mate sleep in the back bedroom...or she may demand ardent love-making, to the point of near exhaustion!

Some psychologists would have us believe that PMS is an unhappy symptom complex that is handed down from mother to daughter. They contend that a mother conditions her daughter to think of her menses as the curse of being female, and that the PMS symptoms are an expression of the anxiety felt in anticipation of the onset of her hated period.

This seems a little far-fetched in this day of enlightenment regarding the naturalness of the menstrual cycle. In my experience, most modern mothers teach their daughters to look forward to menstruation as the first step toward womanhood.

Neurologists and physiologists blame PMS on "neurotransmitter dysfunction," resulting from a menstrual mix-up in the production of dopamine, endorphins and catecholamines.

This theory, though quite difficult to prove, would give justification to the use of tranquilizers, anti-depressants, even lithium. These can help offset mood swings, but have their negative side effects, making careful supervision mandatory.

Just why women are afflicted with this monthly period of unhappiness is not fully understood. Certainly there is no single cause but, because PMS is closely correlated with a woman's menstrual cycle, hormonal imbalances are suspected. A few years ago British researchers postulated that the downswing of progesterone in the days just before the menstrual period was responsible for the PMS miseries.

Acting on this hypothesis, suppositories containing progesterone were inserted into either the vagina or the rectum of women who regularly suffered from PMS, in an effort to prevent the onset of these symptoms. Some women were helped, others were not, and at $20 to $25 a month this treatment could put large holes in a working girl's pocketbook. Birth control pills, which also contain progesterone, are a simpler, more economical and often successful approach, perhaps because they suppress ovulation.

The sports enthusiasts insist that exercise — tennis, aerobics, swimming, fast walking — bring relief from PMS. There is no question that such activities relieve menstrual cramps by the production of endorphins, and it may be that this carries over into relief of the PMS symptoms.

Water retention is a frequent component of PMS. A woman finds her rings are tight on her fingers, that she's gained a pound or two, and that her breasts are tender — all reminders to cut down on salt in the week before the start of her period.

PMS sufferers often report severe headaches, and it is entirely conceivable that a puffy brain pressing against the skull could be expressed in a huge headache. In some cases doctors have prescribed the temporary use of a diuretic such as spirononlactone, when water retention seems to be a particularly severe aspect of a woman's PMS symptoms.

Arthritis pills (prostaglandin inhibitors) can reduce the aching and slow the menstrual flow. Anti-depression medications help some women, and an anti-panic pill, Xanax, has met with mixed success.

Dietary management as a way to control PMS has many true believers. Eliminating salt, sugar, coffee, tea and chocolate might make sense. Pyridoxine, vitamin B6, has its advocates. Alcoholic beverages are to be avoided during these PMS days: a single drink can unleash an aggressive, destructive outburst.

It seems grossly unfair that womanhood has had to bear the burden of these cyclic hormonal rages. Who knows how this monthly female malady may have shaped world history? Indeed, I wonder where Eve was in her hormonal cycle, when she offered Adam a bite of the apple.

18 Hysterectomies: Too Many? Unnecessary?

THE SUPERMARKET TABLOID SHOUTS "Doctors Doing Too Many Hysterectomies!" A TV report cites a study which concludes that 22% of the hysterectomies done in the Chicago hospitals were "unnecessary."

Unfortunately, this kind of sensational information may raise doubts in the mind of a woman who has been told by her physician that she may need a hysterectomy. Quite naturally, such scare stories might lead her to doubt her physician's clinical judgment.

One good that can come from such sensationalism is that surgeons will go to even greater lengths to make certain their patients are fully informed about the pros and cons of the hysterectomy procedure, and why it appears to be the optimum treatment under the present circumstances.

The doctor's first step will be to make certain that the woman understands the anatomy and physiology of the female reproductive system. She will be told that the uterus is simply a muscular organ, a superbly designed pre-natal baby carriage. At a time in life when the need for more pregnancies is over, the organ's primary function is at an end.

Not all women will readily accept this explanation. Some believe the uterus is the center of femininity, and that a woman's sexuality will be diminished if that organ is removed.

Today we know this isn't so, but Socrates believed it. He taught that the "hystera" — the Greek word for "womb" — was the regulator of a woman's emotions by virtue of the "humours" that exuded from it. This is the source of the word "hysteria," a condition characterized by uncontrollable outbursts of fear, weeping and irrationality.

Women in their reproductive years, as well as their husbands and boyfriends, will relate to this description of one aspect of PMS. But many of them know that it's the ovaries, not the uterus, which control the switchboard of emotions and the thermostat of a woman's heating and cooling system.

The uterus is one of the most remarkable bodily organs we physicians deal with, pervading a major share of a woman's physical and emotional life. From the time a girl enters womanhood at the onset of her menses, to the end of her reproductive life at menopause, a woman is acutely aware of the state of her uterus.

Moreover, I can think of no organ that can manifest such a wide variety of medical conditions. To act as a site for the creation and nurturing of a new life is the most visible and most wonderful. Less wonderful are the uterine-based cramps, bleeding, miscarriages, tumors, cancers, pelvic pain, and urinary incontinence — what other organ has so many potential problems?

"Too many unnecessary hysterectomies?" Most people in our town probably don't know that at our hospital we have a committee that reviews all the hysterectomies, to make certain that the diagnoses are correct and that the operation would benefit the woman's health and well-being. I can assure you that doctors are extremely sensitive to criticism by fellow physicians in such a "peer review."

There are many justifiable indications for hysterectomy. Early cancer of either the uterus or the ovaries has a high rate of cure. Fibroid tumors that cause bleeding, pressure or pain need to be removed. Infection and painful endometriosis certainly justify surgical treatment.

There are, however, female conditions that have no such demonstrable "pathology," but which to be corrected may require a hysterectomy. These include dropping down of the female organs, loss of urinary control, and abnormal bleeding which fails to respond to conservative hormonal management.

Physicians are concerned that some women believe "hysterectomy" is a dirty word, and that the fear engendered by this misleading publicity might cause a woman to shy away from a vitally necessary surgical procedure.

Over the years, I have conducted my own clinical study of women who have had hysterectomies. My modest survey consists of a single question: "Mrs. Jones, now that you have had a hysterectomy, and no longer have a uterus, have you any regrets?"

The response invariably is along the lines of "With no more cramps, nor more bleeding, and no worries about pregnancy — Doctor, that's the best thing I ever did!"

19 Three Paths to Menopausal Happiness

HOT FLASHES AND NIGHT SWEATS, the so-called "vasomotor" symptoms of the menopause, used to be primary reasons for taking female hormones. For some women these medications also brought relief from moodiness and depression, the general personality shifts that some husbands uncharitably refer to as "midlife bitchiness."

In the past when physicians prescribed hormone therapy for women in menopause, they were treating symptoms, for the most part successfully. Ordinarily, hormone pills or shots were used as a stop-gap measure, to tide the woman over this trying time, as she made her transition from her reproductive years.

Recently, however, we've shifted our focus on helping women get through menopause. We continue to strive to relieve the symptoms, but now are also taking a closer look at the physiology of female aging. Rather than simply trying to ameliorate the symptoms, we now place greater emphasis on improving a woman's total quality of life. And when we prescribe female hormones to relieve the sweats and the flashes, we know we're giving our patients two additional benefits: reducing their risk of osteoporosis and of heart attacks.

This change in the treatment of menopause came about as a result of two discoveries: one that estrogen can prevent, or at least deter, the loss of calcium from the bones; the second that this female hormone can have a favorable effect on a woman's cholesterol level.

These new findings have led doctors to more frequently prescribe estrogen, which has led women to ask more questions:

What dose of the hormone is proper?

Do hormones cause cancer?

What are the disadvantages?

What is the best way to take these hormones?

Shall I use the brand name or generic?

How long should I take these medications?

The proper dose is, of course, the amount that will control the vasomotor symptoms. In most cases, a dosage level of

.625mg. of conjugated estrogen, the pill most commonly used, is the amount needed to adequately control the loss of calcium. We used to believe that taking calcium was all-important in the prevention of osteoporosis, but now we know that it's really the estrogen that prevents the broken hips and wrists, the "widow's hump," and the compression fractures of the spine.

At least statistically, brittle bones are a larger threat to the lives of older women than is cancer. This year around 15,000 women will die as a direct result of hip bone fractures, while fewer than 3,000 will die of cancer of the uterus. In this same year 700,000 women in their mid-fifties, who still have a third of their life expectancy ahead of them, will begin to lose their bone mass unless treatment is begun.

In fact, whether female hormones can cause cancer is still unresolved. Most authorities will answer "absolutely not," but we do know that some female cancers are "hormone-dependent." They contain "hormone receptors," and will grow if stimulated by the administration of hormones.

Of course if a woman has had a hysterectomy she doesn't need to worry about cancer of the uterus. On the other hand, women who have had their first pregnancy very late in their reproductive life, or who have never had any pregnancies, may be at increased risk. And because some cancers may "run in the family," a woman whose mother or sister has had breast cancer should remember to do her self-examinations, and to have mammograms at specified intervals.

The disadvantage of taking hormones are few, especially when compared with the proven advantages. It's true that large doses of estrogen may cause breast enlargement and tenderness, similar to the discomfort noted at period time. And it's true that this hormone may cause a little water retention. Estrogen medications may in some rare cases cause a mild nausea, which can be overcome by taking them at bed time.

But in adding up the disadvantages of estrogen therapy, we now need to factor in another important advantage to be gained from moderate dosages of the female hormone. We all know that men can have heart attacks in their 40s, 30s, even in their 20s. Women, on the other hand, rarely have heart attacks until they are well beyond menopause, after their ovaries have stopped producing estrogen. Now that an American woman's life expectancy is approaching eighty, heart attacks have become the number one cause of death in older women.

Doctor Frank Sacks, working at Harvard Medical School, found that as women pass the menopause and their estrogen levels fall, their cholesterol counts increase. In addition, their high density lipids (HDLs) decrease — these are the "good" lipo-proteins that are thought to clean out some of the fatty plaques that may have accumulated inside the blood vessels, in a process somewhat like flushing the sediment out of a car radiator. It follows that by supplying estrogen to these post-menopausal women we can raise their HDL level, thereby reducing the incidence of atherosclerosis, which can precipitate heart attacks.

As for the best way for a woman to take estrogen, she needs to work that out with her physician. The majority of women use the pill form, and the one most commonly used is the "natural" conjugated estrogen, Premarin. Don't be turned off by the fact that this medication is derived from the urine of pregnant mares; the ingredients are carefully purified, and then formulated to exact dosages. Another estrogen medication is estradiol (brand name Estrace), produced from the lowly yam.

Your doctor may suggest you take a progesterone pill with the estrogen, to reduce your chance of cancer of the uterus. If you combine the two, you'll need to decide on a dosage schedule. The cyclic use of these two hormones will cause your menstrual periods to continue, at least for awhile.

Moreover, the use of progesterone may reduce some of the benefit that estrogen provides in reducing the cholesterol level. Once again you are faced with choosing your priorities.

Estrogen can be taken by injection by women who cannot take (or who have trouble remembering to take) oral medications. Taking estrogen shots may reduce some of the cholesterol-reducing benefits, because the hormone goes directly into the blood stream, bypassing the liver.

Estrogen now also can be administered through a skin patch, and there is vaginal cream containing estrogen. Hormone pellets placed under the skin are not as yet widely used in the U.S.

When should you start taking estrogen and how long should you continue:? Menopause doesn't happen overnight, and so the lowering of estrogen production is a gradual process. Likewise, calcium loss and the decrease in HDLs occurs over many months. Whether to begin supplementing your female hormone production before you experience any symptoms of menopause, or to wait until your change of life begins or your menses cease, is something you and your doctor need to talk over.

How long should you take estrogen? Some physicians recommend taking the hormones for at least five years, while others believe you are justified in taking estrogen until you are 85 or 90. In any case, you are entitled to and should cooperate in taking advantage of regular follow-up examinations while you are taking hormones, simply because our knowledge about these matters is changing and growing each year.

We doctors have a number of medications we can prescribe that serve double purposes, but rarely are we fortunate to have a pill with triple benefits. Amazing estrogen is not the "feminine forever" pill, yet it does bring blessed relief from many of the menopausal symptoms, while at the same time postponing those penalties of the aging process

— osteoporosis and atherosclerosis — broken bones and brittle blood vessels.

20 Androgen vs. Estrogen: Man/Woman Stuff

LET'S TALK ABOUT TESTOSTERONE. Just what is this magic elixir of virility? The basic ingredient of macho? If semantics is your thing you'll find roots of that term for the male hormone name in "testicle" and "steroids." And if you think back to high school biology, you'll remember that the lifelong traits of maleness are developed by this endocrine secretion. Included are a hairy chest, a deep voice, acne, swollen prostates, wet dreams and snoring...the last few being things a lot of us guys could do without.

This endocrine essence also is what causes men to be aggressive, competitive, dominating and boorish. Too much of this high-test hormone can lead to violence, crime, anti-social sexual behavior, wife abuse, extra-marital affairs and, ultimately, divorce. Pretty potent stuff!

But beyond all these negatives, testosterone is responsible for broad shoulders and strong muscles, as well as for speed and endurance in athletes. And in addition to these physical influences, for the basic urge to acquire and protect a mate and to form a family.

All of us, both male and female, have testosterone and estrogen circulating in our bodies. It is the proportion of each that determines the sexual characteristics that will be ours throughout our lifetime. At the moment of conception the whirling wheel of fortune deals out the X and Y chromosomes, which stamp "boy" or "girl" upon the just-conceived embryo.

Androgen Vs. Estrogen • 329

All of a woman's ova, her eggs, contain only X chromosomes, female chromosomes. About half of a man's sperm cells contain X chromosomes, the other half possessing the Y or male chromosomes. If a sperm cell containing the X chromosome is the first to penetrate the X-marked ovum, the two X's combine to create a female embryo. On the other hand, if a Y sperm gets there first the XY chromosome combination produces a male embryo.

As intrauterine growth progresses, the female embryo develops the internal female sexual organs — vagina, uterus, fallopian tubes and ovaries. In contrast, the male embryo develops the external genitalia, the penis and the testicles, and the internal prostate.

At birth, a boy baby's testosterone level is low, and the phallus exists mainly for male identification (and possibly to be subjected to circumcision). As childhood moves toward puberty, the organ gradually enlarges; it may at times stiffen and, much to the boy's surprise, emit a spurt of fluid.

As puberty arrives, for reasons no one knows, a male's testosterone level increases tenfold, complicating life accordingly. The boy/man is plagued by a voice that cracks, clothes no longer fit him, hair grows in places it has no business growing, and his armpits smell. Girls begin to look interesting, maybe even worth talking to. Now and again he notices a troublesome bulging in his crotch.

Then a miracle of love, courtship, marriage and family set the stage for the reproductive period of his life. He becomes aware of how another life cycle is begun, as his external genitalia unite with the internal organs of his mate to produce a new being, to recapitulate Nature's magnificent plan.

Endrocrinologists have determined that man's hormonal sex drive is highest at age 19, whereas a woman peaks in her early thirties. Yet actually men experience daily and seasonal fluctuations. Towards the end of the day a man's testosterone level is at its lowest, having been depleted by work-a-day struggles. During the night his hormonal reserve is abundantly repleted, and often he will awake with an erection.

There is a seasonal variation, as well, the highest levels being attained in the fall, perhaps explaining the abundance of spring babies. Allan Mazur, a sociologist at Syracuse University, found an elevation of the testosterone level in tennis players after winning a close, hard-fought match.

Synthetic testosterone is available and can, in certain instances, be used to remedy hormonal deficiencies. A word of caution, however, especially for those Schwarzenegger wannabes who have lofty ambitions of building bulging biceps. Small, carefully regulated doses of this hormone may be good; large doses of steroids can do harm.

21 The Myth of Male Menopause

THIRTY YEARS AGO physicians believed that men, like women, underwent a "change of life," brought on by a diminished output of testosterone, the male hormone. But men don't experience the same set of symptoms of the change in hormonal status — the hot flashes, night sweats and mood swings — as women do.

Furthermore, men haven't been menstruating for 35 years or more, a sometimes bothersome and painful monthly cycle for women, which now comes to an end with menopause, literally "a cessation of the menses." In the members of the stronger sex, God in His (or Her) wisdom turned off the ovaries at around age 45 to 52, and with it a woman's reproductive ability.

Men do not ordinarily experience this same age-linked

conclusion; their testicles continue to produce sperm indefinitely. The Bible relates how one-hundred-year-old Abraham begat a son with his wife Sarah, and often today we read of "December-May" marriages in which a man in his 70s sires a child.

Though a man may continue to be potentially sexually vigorous through and beyond his middle years, the fifties for many men is not a happy decade. Yes, there is a gradual reduction in the secretion of testosterone, but external psychological pressures play a larger role in what has been wrongly called "male menopause."

At this time a man's present can become his future. Rarely does a man attempt any major career changes after the big five-oh. At this time a man perceives a decline in his stamina, often experienced as a gradual diminution in his hard and steadfast capacity for physical and mental work. Many men closely link their identity and self-esteem to their jobs, their position and status in a larger organization, so this downward shift also can cause a decline in a man's perception of his youthful attractiveness.

Also in these middle years, just when many men would like to slow down and take life a little easier, along come significant increases in financial pressures, notably the horrendous cost of educating his children.

Moreover, from time to time the poor fellow reflects on the fact that Einstein sketched out The Theory of Relativity before he was 25, while here he is at the advanced age of 50, losing 100,000 brain cells a day to cosmic bombardment, with little of enduring merit accomplished in his half century as a resident of the earth. Not much time left; life isn't fair.

Also at this time in his life, many a man discovers monogamy equals monotony. His need for marital sex may diminish in frequency and ecstacy; he frets and wonders about his lessened libido. Scientific studies suggest that stress and fatigue may be key contributing factors. In one survey researchers found that fireman (perhaps because they have plenty of time between fires for rest and relaxation, including hours in the firehouse library to read Playboy) have the highest sexual frequency, while high-powered executives and hard-working doctors have the lowest.

To a man these bedroom blahs can be upsetting. He may secretly respond to a slight reduction in his sexual stamina with irritation that it is the man who must perform in sexual arousal, while the receiving female can feign ardor.

Outside the bedroom this can be a tough time with kids. The mid-life man's first-born son may have grown tall, strong and independent, and now is covertly or even overtly challenging his parents, especially his dad. The father's teenage daughter may feel an uneasy but exciting rustling of hormones within her bosom, bringing mood swings and urgings toward independence — her strong and solo love for her father may now extend to a younger man...who surely (Dad thinks) isn't good enough for her!

This mid-life malaise, brought on by a slightly diminished stamina or a dwindling sexual prowess, can be hard on dear old Dad. For the first time in his life he begins to reflect upon his own mortality, often out loud. His wife may suggest a physical check-up and, if he reluctantly consents, he may complain to his physician that "I'm falling apart, I must be getting old."

His doctor can help. First, this man in his fifties must be assured that these problems are primarily psychological, caused by events outside his body. Furthermore, he should realize that any decline in sexual interest or performance isn't his fault, and that there are a lot of other husbands out there with the same problems.

Third, his physician will strongly advise against seeking romance outside the marriage. Too often such foraging attempts to regain a self-perception of attractiveness and sexiness turn out to be dismal failures. Also, his doctor will caution against excesses of work and exercise as being self-defeating. If the patient has experienced a few episodes of impotence, he will be reminded that stress and fatigue can be main contributors. With those pressures relieved, the mid-life man's former prowess likely will return.

If absolutely necessary the doctor may prescribe testosterone shots or tablets, but he will continue to emphasize the importance of the mind in matters of the heart. And he will share with this man in his middle years the wise counsel that wives first cherish loving tenderness and intimacy, with or without the physical act. A little romance, a bit of fantasy in a relaxed weekend hideaway, may marvelously stimulate the flow of the natural male hormone.

22 Widows and Widowers Aren't Fourth Class Citizens

HERE IN THESE GREAT UNITED STATES OF AMERICA we like to say that "all men are created equal," and that we are without class distinction or prejudice. Yet if we are honest, many of us must admit we are guilty of some biases based on age and sex.

First of all, we worship at the altar of youth and youthfulness. We pamper our kids, forgiving them their iniquities, giving them special privileges. Even the courts have a category called "youthful offenders."

Their parents work hard, striving always toward tomorrow. Then, sooner than they might have expected, tomorrow is today, and they find themselves in another class called senior citizen, an artificial, government-created stratification beginning at age 65. That group also is pampered to some extent, as they are rewarded for staying alive with Social Security and Medicare.

Largely within this latter group is a fourth class, the widows and widowers. A group of societal orphans whom we sometimes see fit to ignore, people who still are very much alive, but who in our culture are all too often relegated to a life of isolation and loneliness.

Try to picture yourself as a temporary member of the Fourth Class who has just lost a spouse. In this scenario you will for the first few weeks after his or her death be showered with attention by family and friends. You will have little time to reflect on your recent loss, because you'll be too busy answering the flood of telephone calls, and trying to eat your way through the gifts of food, enough to feed a small army. There'll offers of help in sorting clothes and personal belongings to give to the Salvation Army. The couples you formerly saw socially will dutifully give you solo invitations to dinner parties.

Then, ever so gradually, this attentiveness will begin to evaporate. Invitations will dwindle, and you may deliberately back away, feeling uncomfortable as a "fifth wheel." And anyway, out in public at these social gatherings you miss your spouse more than ever, because it was he or she who always led the conversation at a sprightly pace.

This is the time of danger when depression may set in. You may resort to alcohol to relieve the blues and the blahs, only to find that alcohol actually worsens the depression. At worst you may consider suicide.

Then, too, from time to time there will be a stirring in your heart to remind you that you're still a sexual being. You will recall that old song lyric that "it's so nice to have a man (woman) around the house." Perhaps your only need is to have a friend or a companion, like the woman who inserted this want ad in the Singles Connection section of the Hemet, California News: "Lonely widow misses husband. Needs tight-fisted, ornery old coot for companionship."

On the other hand, you may be tormented by deeper needs. In the dark of night you may dream of days years before, of romance and love making with your spouse who now is gone. Some of these dreams will be so vivid that you are panicked awake, emotionally spent, your pillow wringing wet.

Fortunately, in our present culture an elderly man who gives in to his sexual drive is no longer thought of as lecherous, and the sexual woman is not considered a tramp. Cohabitation by unmarried but committed senior couples is acceptable — Uncle Sam even encourages such living arrangement, by penalizing those who remarry by reducing their Social Security payments.

It is encouraging to see that we are ridding ourselves of these myths and misconceptions about healthy sexuality among mature men and women. Now it is normal for widows and widowers to affirm that the fires of sexuality still burn brightly, and that physical and emotional expressions of love can be immensely satisfying in their golden years. No longer are these widows and widowers relegated to being Fourth Class Citizens.

23 *The Quest For An Aphrodisiac*

I'D JUST GIVEN PAUL RICHARDS HIS ANNUAL PHYSICAL, and we were chatting in the examination room. He's been my patient for nearly twenty years, and over that time I've gotten to know him pretty well. Plus, I've purchased three Buicks from his dealership. As he was knotting his tie he said, with an attempt at off-handed casualness, "By the way, there's this other problem my wife wanted me to mention. You see, I'm having a little trouble getting it up."

Paul used the standard code for an inability to obtain and maintain an erection, and his feigned casualness masked a terrible fear that he was "losing his manhood." Along with that there was a deep concern that his marriage was in danger — his wife had intimated that maybe he was "giving at the office" and so was unable to give at home.

Men will pretend to pass off their concern with a "ha-ha" and a half-hearted smile, but doctors know that this is most certainly not a laughing matter. The joking is a cover-up for the shame this genital dysfuction causes.

Over the centuries man has been searching for a cure for this troubling sexual problem — a quest for a magic potion. Unfortunately most aphrodisiacs, named after Aphrodite, the goddess of love in Greek mythology, have only mythical powers of sexual stimulation. Yet both Western and Oriental cultures continue the search.

On an African safari our Kenyan guide told us how ground-up rhinoceros horn is sold for hundreds of dollars an ounce, to be snuffed into the nostrils as an aphrodisiac.

In China herb doctors were happy to tell us how dried sea horse, *hai ma*, is crushed and slowly simmered in a wine concoction. They use it to "warm the kidney" and cure impotence.

One of the most notorious aphrodisiacs is Spanish fly, made from powdered beetles. The active ingredient is cantharidin, which can in fact cause swelling and tumescence of the bladder and the penis. Unfortunately this tumescence can be painful, and the erection may persist into a pathological condition called priapism, which may require emergency medical intervention and has been known to end in death.

A more modern medication is yohimbine, a chemical compound obtained from the West African yohimbe tree. This drug is listed in our Physician's Desk Reference as "possibly having aphrodisiac properties," but has no guarantees.

In men who have an actual glandular deficiency, the male hormone testosterone may have benefit. This form of therapy is not without hazard, and of course should be administered only under a doctor's direction. Among possible contraindications is a remote chance of liver damage, or of accelerating the growth of an existing prostate tumor.

A wide variety of prosthetic devices are available for the treatment of impotence, which illustrates how frantic this quest for erection can be. Among these are plastic rods implanted in the penis, miniature balloons which can be pumped up when the need arises, and a negative pressure pump which traps blood in the organ, producing a temporary tumescence.

Unfortunately, many of these prostheses ultimately fail, simply because they are artificial or mechanical devices, and love-making should be neither artificial nor mechanical. Moreover, well over two-thirds of the cases of impotence arise from psychogenic rather than organic causes — originating in the head, rather than in the pelvis.

Nonetheless, organic causes need to be considered and eliminated in the process of arriving at a diagnosis. Diabetes, hypothyroidism, or true glandular dysfunction must be ruled out. Also, sometimes certain medications can be the cause of impotence. But mental and emotional causes are by far the most common.

Psychogenic sexual dysfunction can be described as the four A's: Anxiety, Anger, Apathy and Angst.

- A person who is anxious or depressed invariably has a low libido level.
- Anger at one's partner, or interpersonal conflicts, block the production of love-making hormones.
- Apathy and fatigue simply are not conducive to conjugal happiness.
- Angst — the fear of failure — can perpetuate the problem. A one-time inability to perform, for whatever reason, may engender apprehension in a man, who

frets "What if I can't get it up the next time?" Stewing over this prospect can lead to a self-fulfilling prophecy.

Such psychogenic impotence is curable, and relaxation techniques are the key: "Don't worry about performing, just relax and enjoy it." In Masters and Johnson's method of sexual counselling, such relaxation is given the fancy name of "non-genital sensate focussing." This emphasizes aspects of love-making that are entirely apart from the physical act of penile intromission. They give it the name of "love play" rather than fore-play.

Women are better at this than are men. Again and again wives tell me that, above all else, they cherish the warmth and tenderness of the coital togetherness. The snuggling and the cuddling and the feeling of security. The lack of haste while experiencing the consciousness of giving as well as receiving pleasure. It's the wise husband who learns this early on in marriage.

Human sexuality is a function of the mind, and that separates us from the animal kingdom. Animals copulate, propelled by an instinctive reproductive drive. Humans experience coitus, from the Latin for a "coming together," mentally, emotionally and spiritually.

Good and Bad, Right and Wrong

Introduction

When I began to practice medicine, in the late 1930s, it was both easier and more difficult to care for patients than it is today.

It was easier because patients expected less of their doctor — they knew the limits of medical science, and didn't expect man-made miracles. We had far fewer medications in our doctor bags, though we were at the edge of an era of wonder drugs, capable of curing potentially killing diseases such as pneumonia and peritonitis.

Furthermore, in those days people weren't in such a rush to sue each other, so we physicians had much less fear of being caught up in a malpractice suit. Back then the good doctor was revered, the patient-doctor relationship was secure, and we never felt the need to practice "defensive medicine."

Babies were welcomed into the family with their minor or major imperfections. Doctors helped the delivery along, and did all they could for the mother and the child, but weren't implicitly held responsible for delivering a perfect baby every time, irrespective of what variations nature had dealt each infant.

Medical decisions made by physicians were accepted without question, and no second opinions were required. Doctors knew what was right and wrong, so there was no need for ethics committees to oversee the standards of medical practice.

How things have changed!

Technology has given doctors amazing new diagnostic capabilities, and near-magical (and very expensive) medicines, tests and procedures. Today we can save tiny babies, born many months prematurely, or with tragic birth defects. And, at the other end of the spectrum, we can extend the terminal patient's life for many months, depriving them of "a natural death."

In some ways such amazing advances of biotechnology make the practice of medicine much easier. Yet at the same time they have made a doctor's life more difficult. Such high-tech healing and life support is exceedingly expensive. A physician may, at times against his better judgement, put a tiny "preemie" on a life support system that will cost society hundreds of thousands of dollars. Or a doctor may place a terminal patient in a $1,000-a-day intensive care unit to prolong their life — or, more accurately, to postpone their inevitable death. Yet after ordering such "heroic measures" we all too often are taken to task by the government, the insurance companies and perhaps even the hospital ethics committee.

The doctors of today face a dilemma. We can cure more diseases and save more lives than we could fifty years ago. Yet societal pressures and costly technology have produced a radical change in the practice of medicine. Our Hippocratic Oath has been bent and broken. But the Golden Rule still works.

1 Ethical Preparation By The Next Generation

SEVERAL TIMES A YEAR I lead a seminar on ethics at our local college. Each time I do I'm encouraged at how thoughtful and sensitive these young people are when discussing the big issues of right and wrong. If they are to be the politicians, the legislators, the community leaders of tomorrow, then our future is in good hands.

We usually begin by talking about much of what we read in the newspaper every day, questionable ethics in government and the banking industry, including the savings and loan mess, and the public's lack of respect for Wall Street financiers. But we soon move on to consider the ethical dilemmas now facing the health care industry.

We talk about living and dying, AIDS and abortion, the proper and appropriate application of medical technology. These students are impressively swift at understanding the issues as, using actual case presentations, I share with them some of the daunting ethical decisions we physicians must make almost every day.

For example, the need to arrive at a fair and unbiased conclusion about treatment for an AIDS patient who had been admitted to the hospital with what undoubtedly was terminal pneumonia. Was it right to give this man an antibiotic that might prolong his life, or would it have been ethical (and perhaps even merciful) to withhold that medication, to let the natural dying process take place?

Should abortion on demand be condoned or rejected? Is abortion justified in situations where the life of the mother or of the baby is threatened? Should the decision whether or not to have an abortion be left to the woman's conscience and the wisdom of her physician, or should legal restrictions enter into the picture?

Was that grandma correct in going through a pregnancy for her daughter, who had been born without a uterus? And what about the couple who decided to have another baby, simply to provide a source for a bone marrow transplant for an older sibling afflicted with leukemia?

We discuss the pros and cons of "passive euthanasia," at issue in the widely-publicized cases of Karen Ann Quinlan and Nancy Cruzan: under what circumstances is a physician ethically justified and legally protected in withholding intravenous food and fluid, to hasten the dying of a terminally ill patient?

I even challenge these bright young men and women to consider whether it ever would be ethically acceptable for a doctor or any health care worker to perform "active euthanasia," drifting a terminally ill patient off into a permanent sleep with a lethal dose of a "hemlock elixir," such as Dr. Jack Kervorkian has been doing with his "suicide machine."

In the brief fifty minutes I spend with these college students, my faith in our future is always strengthened. Most of them are old enough to vote, and are ready and willing to tackle these crucial life-and-death decisions that now face their generation.

I wish I'd had the opportunity when I was their age to have been so thoughtfully challenged. Contrary to what some of us Seniors might think, these Juniors are acquiring and sharpening the ethical judgmental skills they'll need to keep this wobbly world of ours on an even keel.

2 Doing What Was Right Seemed Much Easier Then

THE DELIVERY WAS OVER, and baby Deborah Kay was placed in her mother's arms. It had been a long wait for this baby's 40-year-old mother, nine months filled with mixed emotions.

Nor had it been an easy time for the father. Well into middle life, with three teen-agers in the household, this couple had put aside any thoughts of possible pregnancy. Contraception had been hit-or-miss. But they had missed. The pregnancy test was positive.

At first there was anger, then panic. Husband accused wife, wife harangued husband. What would friends and relatives say? What will our kids think? Because this was 1957, in a small own in northern Idaho, an abortion was out of the question.

Slowly frustration gave way to resignation, and then even to guarded happiness. Maybe it would be a special thrill to have one more "bundle of joy." When Mom and Dad finally told their teen-aged boys they yelled "Hey, that's cool." Their 13-year old sister happily promised to be the baby sitter.

Now, at long last, the baby had arrived. With the mother cared for, I turned my attention to the infant girl. She was chubby, a little puffy, with a hint of a different look about her. But newborn babies, with their molded heads and squeezed faces, are anything but pretty. Anyway, I was relieved she was here, alive and well.

I glanced up at the large clock on the wall of the delivery room; it was just after two AM. I'd give Deborah Kay a more thorough examination on my morning rounds, but now I wanted to catch a few winks.

"There's something peculiar about this little one you delivered this morning, Doctor." Nurse Joan McDonald had brought Deborah Kay to me to examine. Sure enough, the baby's face was still puffy and her eyes were slanted and almond-shaped. The nose was flat and the legs lax. Surely we had to give consideration to a diagnosis of Down's syndrome.

Joan's response was natural: "Oh, no, what will we tell the mother?" "First of all," I said, "let's be sure of the diagnosis. And, if it's confirmed, we'll be sure to use the proper name, 'Down's syndrome,' not 'Mongolism.'"

As we expected, all the tests confirmed the diagnosis. Now I would have to face Mom and Dad with the bad news.

It wasn't easy. After I had finished telling them that Debbie would have these defects, that she would be mentally retarded and would live a life of utter dependency, there was only tearful silence. Then... "You're very sure, are you, doctor?" I explained all of the exhaustive tests that had been used to arrive at a final diagnosis. Hurrying on, I suggested that parents often decide to place these little ones in institutions, and this was a choice they would be entitled to make.

Mom and Dad looked at me in bewilderment. "Doctor, do you know what you are saying? This is our baby. No way will we give her up."

So it was that Deborah Kay went home into the loving arms of a family welded together by the need to cherish and care for and protect this little person, who would live her life in perpetual childhood, never attaining true mental maturity.

Bringing up Debbie was not always easy; her mental and physical inadequacies called for special effort and lots of patience on the part of every family member. Teaching Deborah to eat with a fork and a spoon went slowly; fingers seemed to work so well.

On the one hand, matters such as toilet training and personal hygiene were treated with exasperating indifference by this young lady, while, on the other hand, her first menstruation was a terrifying experience: "Mommy, am I going to die?"

Because Debbie was so slow and awkward, other children would laugh at her, taunt her and run away from her. As a result, brothers and sister and Mom and Dad would set aside time to be her surrogate playmates. In return, over the years she showered them all with her smiles and hugs, and lots of love. And with that the family was given a sense of fulfillment at having accepted the responsibility for the complete care of another human being.

A few weeks ago Debbie and her now 43-year-old sister came in for their routine physical examinations. At last year's checkup I had noted an enlarged uterus and, because her extremely heavy periods had caused anemia, we had given some consideration to a hysterectomy. Today's examination showed her uterus to be much smaller, and her sister reported that Debbie's periods had stopped completely. Obviously, Debbie was passing through menopause.

How ironic it has been, I thought, as I then examined her older sister, that here is the teen-ager who at age 13 happily promised to be the new baby's "baby-sitter," and who for the past 35 years had been just that, even after she had married and reared her own family.

And here was Debbie, whose body I had examined as she grew up physically, through infancy, puberty, her middle years and now menopause, in the span of three and a half decades. Yet here was a person whose entire being had been imprisoned in a fruitless childhood. But during those years what blessings of togetherness she had brought to this fine family as they nurtured her and protected her! How fortunate it was that 35 years ago Mom and Dad had made the wise decision to take her home.

Having finished my afternoon appointments I reflected on how much had changed since Deborah Kay came into the world in 1957. I thought about how I might have reacted differently if that 40-year-old pregnant woman had come into my office today.

An intelligent and well-informed woman would now know that at age 40 there was a slightly increased chance her baby might be born with congenital defects. She might very well expect to have a special test — an amniocentesis — done to check this possibility, while the fetus was still in her womb. If the results raised some questions, she would know that she would have the option of an abortion.

Occasionally the test can prove inaccurate, only to add to the dilemma. Rarely, it can cause a miscarriage, resulting in the loss of a normal pregnancy.

With all these misgivings, what decision would we make today? As a physician I would have to bear in mind my legal liabilities. These days parents expect — indeed, demand — a perfect baby be delivered to them.

Finally, would these two people — this husband and wife — who were beginning to feel great joy at the prospect of having a treasured "late-in-life" baby, now have to suffer the anguish of having to make a decision, one that may plague them every day of their lives, whichever course they chose?

Right now it was easy for me to say that the choice they made back in 1957 definitely was the correct one, having been privileged to watch Debbie's life unfold in the tender embrace of devoted family members.

Moreover, 35 years ago the choices were not that hard to make; Debbie's parent knew there was just one way to go.

Today the way is strewn with hard stumbling blocks. Now Debbie's embryo would be the concern not only of the parents and the doctor, but possibly the courts, the legislature and the hospital bioethics committee.

3 "Above All, Do No Harm"

WHEN I RECEIVED MY MD DEGREE from the University of Chicago I took the Hippocratic oath, a symbolic promise to "do unto others as I would want to be done by," and always to be guided by the Latin dictum *primum non nocere*, "above all, do no harm."

If somehow or other the patient didn't get well, or if we didn't have the right medicine for the problem, or if the baby wasn't "perfect" — all this was accepted as "God's will," and the physician would be given credit for "having tried."

But in the past few decades several extraneous factors have diluted the purity of purpose expressed in this oath — I think of them as "the three M's" — Money, Malpractice and Medical Technology.

Money - In years past we physicians didn't worry so much when a patient couldn't pay a bill. But the advent of widespread private health insurance, plus the federal Medicaid and Medicare programs, weakened the bond between the patient and the physician, because someone else was paying the bill.

At the same time, the doctor feels less ethical concern about controlling medical costs, as long as the patient has "good" health insurance. He or she became less reluctant to order all manner of medical diagnostic goodies — lab tests, x-rays, CT scans at $500 each, MRI scans at $700. While this explains how this problem occurred, it does smack just a bit of dishonesty, or at least of poor medical ethics.

Malpractice - Until not so long ago the quality of my practice of medicine was scrutinized mainly by my peers and by the hospitals. But in recent years the courts and lawyers have intensified their surveillance. Once physicians relied upon their eyes and ears, their hands and their stethoscopes. But now this increased and too often adversarial surveillance means we are far more likely to order more diagnostic testing, and possibly to engage in more intensive forms of treatment. This sense of vulnerability has contributed to increased health care expenses in the United States, the practice of what has been called "defensive medicine."

When I began my practice of medicine in northern Idaho in the late 1930s my annual professional liability insurance premium was around $100. Now a physician in our area who delivers babies or does major surgery will pay around $20,000 for insurance coverage. Doctors in major metropolitan areas, where malpractice suits are more likely, pay much higher premiums.

Medical Technology - Medical ethics is now a vital issue in the beginning of human life, the end of life, and everything in between.

High tech has changed the simple and natural process of having a baby into a complicated, almost mechanical procedure. We can look into the womb and see the fetus move, and sometimes even determine whether the baby will be a boy or a girl.

We can stick needles into the uterine cavity and draw out amniotic fluid, to assess whether the fetus appears to have any congenital abnormalities. If there seem to be problems, termination of the pregnancy must be considered — a tough ethical decision to make.

When labor begins we hook the mother up to an electronic monitoring device, to provide us with a constant readout on the infant's progress, and the strength of the mother's contractions. A significant change in the baby's condition may support a decision by the doctor to go directly to an operative delivery of the baby, a Cesarean section, rather than to take any chance of having a difficult delivery, or to reduce the risk of losing the baby.

Early in my training at the Chicago Lying-In Hospital the Cesarean section rate was 5% — only one in twenty deliveries might be done by C-section. Today, at our regional health center in north Idaho, a fifth to a quarter of babies are delivered by surgical Cesarean section. Though in the past half century we've made tremendous advances in the safety and certainty of deliveries though the natural birth canal, to protect themselves doctors often opt for surgery, which happens also to involve more people and equipment and so is more expensive. Can that really be ethical?

Modern technology also enables us to extend a person's life far beyond the normal expectancy, often beyond what our patients may desire. Too often they become prisoners in a life artificially prolonged by intravenous feeding, massive doses of antibiotics, and breathing ventilators. Hospital ethics committees now must wrestle with deciding "when to pull the plug."

Ethics committees usually are composed of physicians, hospital administrators, laypeople, and sometimes members of the clergy. To help them make their difficult decisions, anyone entering our hospital for treatment is required by law to comply with the requirements of the government's Personal Self Determination Act. When they are being admitted each patient is asked if they have a signed Advance Directive, or a Living Will. Also, if they have designated a person to have their Durable Power of Attorney, to act in their behalf in case their mental powers should be incapacitated, and they no longer are able to make their own life and death decisions. You can just imagine how these kinds of major mortal questions can be disturbing to a person entering the hospital for an appendectomy or a hernia operation.

One of the newest challenges to medical ethics is the wide scope of problems brought about by the exciting opportunities enabled by genetic engineering. Since the discovery of deoxyribonucleic acid (DNA) as the force within our body cells that determines what we are to be as human beings, scientists have been tempted to manipulate these genes to prevent or cure certain diseases.

One of the first attempts to put genetic engineering to good use was an effort a few years ago to change the DNA structure of a little girl with cystic fibrosis. Blood was drawn from her body, taken to the laboratory where the genes were altered, and then transfused back into her blood stream. It is possible that in the future similar efforts will be made to deal with inherited diseases such as sickle cell anemia in Blacks, or Tay-Sachs disease in Jews. At some point in the not-too-distant future a couple planning to be married might be checked for genetically-transmitted diseases, and if they tested positive they could have their genes "engineered" before having children.

Even more ethically befuddling, some day not so long from now it might also be possible for parents to "customize" their children by genetic tinkering with their DNA, to "order" such characteristics as their height, color of their hair, their mental capacity, even their longevity. Would that be ethical?

Only a few decades ago we scoffed at the idea of being able to produce a baby in a test-tube. Now that's not only technologically possible, for a large portion of our society it is ethically acceptable. Every so often we read about a grandmother who was successfully impregnated with a test-tube embryo, produced from her daughter's egg, fertilized with her son-in-law's sperm. Which, if nothing else, should put an end to all those mother-in-law jokes!

But it won't put an end to serious and substantial questions of medical ethics. Issues ranging from sperm banks to euthanasia expand and become more complex each day, paralleling technological advances. Wise health care specialists will come to good decisions, but only with the advice and guidance of a well-informed public.

4 A Case of Life or Death

This was our dilemma: should we, as Sam's physicians, allow him to take his dream trip to Australia, or should we tell him the truth and urge him to stay home and start treatment, to begin his battle against a life-threatening illness?

As we mulled the matter over, we once again concluded that though medical schools equipped us with all the tools we needed to diagnose and successfully treat thousands of diseases, they failed to teach us how to make swift and correct ethical decisions. This we had to learn out in the real world of medical practice.

Sam's primary care physician and I knew that he and his wife Martha, happily married for nearly forty years, had long planned to return to her native Australia. As a 12-year-old girl Martha had been torn from her playmates, her school, and her childhood memories when her parents emigrated to the United States, in search of financial advancement. Although she grew up to be a proud American citizen, throughout her married life she longed for a return visit to her homeland.

With this in mind , Sam and Martha planned and saved toward what was to be a memorable month-long vacation Down Under. Their son and daughter joined in their enthusiasm, regularly sending Christmas and birthday checks to swell the dream trip fund. Finally dates were set, tickets were purchased, reservations were made. In just four months, Sam and Martha would be on their way.

Then disaster struck: Martha suffered a massive cerebral hemorrhage and died.

Sam was distraught and deeply depressed. Without Martha his future seemed empty, life no longer seemed worth living. The dream of a trip to Australia had ended in an ugly nightmare.

Weeks passed, and the deadline for cancellations approached. But when Sam announced to his children that he planned to give it all up, they disagreed, saying "Mom would have wanted you to go, you should do this in memory of our mother."

For the next two days Sam thought of little else, as he struggled to decide what to do. He finally was able to agree that he could serve as Martha's surrogate, by making this pilgrimage to the land of her birth. For a time during his depression Sam had doubted that life was worth living, and even harbored thoughts of suicide. Now his enthusiasm gradually returned, as he once again had a purpose in life.

His children suggested that he should have his annual physical examination before he left for Australia, and it was during this exam that the doctor discovered a cancer in his prostate — a serious type of cancer, but amenable to treatment. As my colleague reviewed the pathologist's report he was distressed and angry that this could happen to his friend and patient at such a critical time, just when it seemed that a few rays of sunshine were coming back into Sam's life.

And why should he, as Sam's physician, be forced to decide whether to risk throwing his patient back into a deep depression by telling him he had cancer, and that he must give up his trip in order to undergo treatment?

Now my fellow physician was asking for my advice. Should I advise Sam's doctor to tell him a white lie, to inform him of the diagnosis and need for treatment only after he returned from Australia? Perhaps he could tell only Sam's son and daughter, letting them share our burden.

Or should we carry the whole burden ourselves, saying nothing to anyone at this time, hoping the cancer would remain dormant until Sam's return? On the other hand, what if this cancer were the fulminating, fast-growing type?

Thinking only of ethical issues, putting aside all legal

considerations, how could we two troubled doctors arrive at the one right answer? Our hospital's medical staff has hard and fast protocols for almost every clinical contingency, but none for such complex ethical puzzles.

Where could we turn? Our ethics committee might be able to help, but there was no time for their objective deliberations: Sam was scheduled to leave in three days. Moreover, that committee, like most committees, often provides as many answers as there are members.

No, the ethical decision was ours to make, even though the courts might one day prove us wrong. It was up to us to answer these tough questions: Shall we remain silent and allow Sam to take his long-waited trip? Or shall we make the cool and calculated (and legally correct) decision to fully inform our patient?

So we searched our hearts and finally arrived at a decision. We hope it was the right one. Only time will tell.

5 Is the Genetic Genie Out of the Bottle?

IN THE NOT TOO DISTANT FUTURE, genetic engineering and molecular biology may bring us cures we didn't dare dream of only a decade ago. Research scientists manipulating genes are zeroing in on how to prevent or reverse the ravages of such terrible wasting illnesses as AIDS, Alzheimer's and cancer.

But there is a dark side to this story of molecular manipulation. At the same time we are unlocking the secrets of the most basic chemical composition of our our bodies, are we also letting a monstrous genetic genie out of the bottle?

Today's high-tech, big-budget genetic engineering began

very modestly in the mid-nineteen-hundreds. An Austrian monk named Gregor Mendel, an enthusiastic gardener, found that he could breed and cross-breed pea plants to obtain different colors of the blossoms, as well as to increase the size and the quality of the peas and their pods.

The methodical Mendel kept careful records of his experiments, and after several years was able to set forth some principles of heredity. What came to be called the Mendelian Law states that the ratio of the dominant and recessive traits determines the exact character of the genetic end product.

In the middle of the twentieth century, American scientists were able to isolate the essential life substance which contains the genetic information to create these highly predictable hereditary outcomes, deoxyribonucleic acid, DNA. Consisting of twisted strings of protein, whirling around in the 46 chromosomes that are found in each and every human cell, these tiny strands of DNA have been called "the immortal coil of inheritance."

After these important discoveries it didn't take long for the genetic scientists to realize that if they could somehow effect a change in the DNA, they might be able to alter the development and functioning of all the organs and systems of the body.

Partly by scientific tinkering, partly by serendipity, researchers working with a youthful patient suffering from cystic fibrosis found that by exposing the CF patient's blood cells to an enzymatic action they could fracture the cell's gene structure, changing the faulty configuration to a normal one. That done, they then added a special bacterium, Escherichia coli. Ordinarily a bad guy, this bug started creating new normal cells by "cloning," which then could be re-injected into the patient.

This knowledge gives us hope that genetic engineering may lead to cures for other such inherited afflictions, such as Tay-Sachs syndrome, sickle cell anemia, hemophilia and color-blindness, in addition to cystic fibrosis.

Animal experimentation using frogs and mice also has shown some promise in the cure or prevention of Alzheimer's disease, AIDS, arthritis and diabetes. Researchers have been able to protect mice from the development of cardiovascular disease by giving them high density lipid (HDL) genes that will protect them against strokes and heart attacks. Just think, if we all could have those new genes we could gorge on eggs, cheese and ice cream!

Since the discovery of "oncogenes," mutant genes that can under certain circumstances produce cancer, there is hope that manipulation of the DNA in these oncogenes might prevent some cancers.

Yet despite all of these magnificent discoveries, many members of the scientific community have a feeling of uneasiness about the implications and responsibilities of such tinkering. Now that we know DNA carries the inherited traits of height, hair and eye color, intelligence, even resistance to disease, what is to stop a parent from paying a genetic engineer to insert those special attributes into the genes of their offspring?

Of more immediate concern is the possibility that health insurers, employers and the government could gain access to your genetic "fingerprints," and use this information to discriminate against you. Even worse is the frightening scenario of a nation deciding to create a superior human race.

Fortunately, groups of scientists are setting up safeguards to control this genetic genie, as he struggles to emerge from his magic bottle. A concerned and well-informed public is necessary to help them make the right decisions.

6 Research Using Fetal Tissue Can Be Very Pro-Life

A FEW YEARS AGO A DRAMATIC MEDICAL SITUATION, the case of Baby Theresa, underscored and amplified the opposing points of view in the Pro-Life versus Pro-Choice controversy. The parents of a child sadly born without a major portion of her brain were blocked by a Florida court from allowing her organs to be transplanted as a living gift to another endangered baby.

The court held that Theresa's organs could not be removed until all nerve system activity had ceased, including her breathing and her heartbeat. Baby Theresa died at the young age of 10 days, but her parents' hopes that their baby might give a flickering spark of life to some other needful human had expired several days before.

The case of Baby Theresa focused public attention on another organ transplant issue, the use of aborted fetal tissue in the experimental treatment of such chronic diseases as Parkinsonism, diabetes, cancer and Alzheimer's. Considerable success already has been attained in the treatment of chronic and genetic diseases. In a widely-reported breakthrough, a Denver man so badly afflicted with Parkinson's disease that he was forced to crawl on the floor found he could walk again, even without a cane, after being injected with normal fetal cells.

Each side in this debate has good and strong points, but where you stand can be influenced by personal experience. Once a staunch Pro-Lifer, the Reverend Rev. Guy Walden changed his views when his son Nathan was successfully treated with a fetal tissue transplant for a life-threatening and genetically-transmitted condition called Hurler's syndrome. Commenting on his shift he said "We're not talking about whether a person has a right to have an abortion....If we can save a life, shouldn't we?"

Pro-Choice supporters argue that cases such as these demonstrate the value of research using fetal tissue from abortions. Pro-Lifers contend that social acceptance of fetal tissue transplantation would only increase abortions, by tilting vulnerable women toward going ahead with the procedure.

Both sides in this debate agree that abortion on demand is a poor method of conception control. But we know that research on genetic and degenerative disease must go on. Perhaps the time come for us all to take a searching look at our moral, medical and ethical beliefs.

7 It's Getting Difficult To Die With Dignity

IT'S GETTING HARDER TO DIE. In years past when hope was dim for a patient's recovery, the physician would make his pronouncement, the clergy would give solace and communion, and then the patient and the family would do the rest. God's will would be done.

Today, all too often, it takes a committee to arrange this natural transition. Now the dying process may involve not only the doctor and the clergy, but attorneys, hospital authorities, social workers and ethicists, even the courts and state legislators.

Magnificent medical technology is the main reason for this shift. Today we not only can prolong life, using what are sometimes called "heroic measures," we sometimes can even bring back to life a person who by some technical definitions is dead.

This can make deathbed decision-making very complicated. Shall we prolong life with intravenous fluids, antibiotics, ventilators, resuscitators and other high tech — and very high cost — equipment? Just because we can do it, should we do it? Who will have the courage and the wisdom to make the decisions?

Attorneys, when asked for an opinion, must answer cautiously, always protecting the legal and financial interests of the terminal patient, as well as those of the survivors.

Hospital authorities are on the horns of a dilemma. They know that as the costs of care for the terminal patient mount, many of the bills will go unpaid, whether by the family, the insurers, or the government. And they all harbor a lingering fear of becoming involved in a legal action charging "wrongful death."

Decision-making also has become harder for the family, torn between saying "Spare no cost, give Grandma all of the very best care available," and "Keep her comfortable, but let her die with dignity."

And amidst all this bedside confusion, physicians are likewise caught in a bind. Almost without exception my older patients have said to me, "Please, please, when my time comes, make them let me go!"

But physicians have taken an oath to do everything possible to preserve life. Even in those instances when we know that death is inevitable, and we would desperately wish to hasten the end, we are confronted with that nasty word "euthanasia."

Sometimes loving relatives of a dying patient take matters into their own hands. When a man shoots his invalid wife, to put her out of her suffering, he receives a suspended sentence. Doctors and hospital administrators probably were relieved when a distraught young father disconnected his dying son's life support systems, while he kept them at bay with a gun.

In addition to such isolated, individual instances of "mercy killing," "suicide doctor" Jack Kervorkian has relentlessly focused public attention on the right to die and who is justified in assisting individuals to make their "final exit."

Clearly technology has raced ahead of our society's legal and moral standards. Are mercy killings such as this ever justifiable? Mr. and Mrs. John Q. Public are asking for an answer. The United States Supreme Court has agreed to enter into this dispute, considering the now famous Cruzan case, passing judgment on whether physicians have a legal right to discontinue giving food and water to a terminally ill patient. Their decision is discussed in chapter nine.

8 Suicide

IN THE SPACE OF ONE MONTH two of my friends, kind and gentle Arthur and thoughtful and caring John, died violent deaths by their own hand. Their suicides left me with a deep hurting inside.

When someone we know commits suicide, this can fill us with despair and guilt, as we wonder where we went wrong. What more could I have done for Arthur and John, as a friend and as a physician?

Arthur had been my patient for many years, and always had enjoyed good health. He recently had retired from his job in the business office of a local lumber mill, and was eagerly looking forward to spending many more days out on the golf course.

One warm and muggy August afternoon, while lining up his putt on the tenth green, he felt a sudden wave of weakness, as if he were about to black out. Because his strength didn't return, and his speech seemed confused, his golfing partners hurried him to the hospital emergency room.

After an extensive battery of tests a tentative diagnosis of transient ischemic attack (TIA) was made. Arthur was sent home after being reassured by the doctors that this was, indeed, a "transient," temporary episode. A neighbor remarked, "Oh, you must have had a small stroke" — a well-intended comment, but we learned later that this lodged the term "stroke" firmly in Arthur's mind.

Surprisingly, the effects of this "transient" attack seemed to persist; my patient just didn't make the expected return to good health. He put away his golf clubs, and continued to complain of fatigue and extreme weakness.

Further laboratory testing revealed no abnormalities. A brain scan showed nothing out of line. A consultation with a nerve specialist gave no indication of any organic neurologic defects. I prescribed a mild anti-anxiety/depression medication, and scheduled weekly office appointments for him.

He came in a few times, and seemed to be making some headway. Then one day kind-hearted, soft-spoken Arthur ended it all with a bullet.

John, a practicing psychologist, was a friend and colleague, a well-liked member of our medical community. I knew him best by the positive feedback I got from the patients I had referred to him for counselling. They would gratefully tell me of Dr. John's kindness and compassion, of his gentleness and understanding as he patiently listened to them pour out their worries and sorrows.

It seemed to me that John worked very hard, and took his responsibilities very seriously. So often as I talked with him, at the hospital or at our weekly Rotary club luncheons, I was impressed by his reserve and his infrequent smiles. At times he would seem distracted and lost in thought. I assumed this to be normal for an overworked counselor, carrying the heavy burden of his patients' problems on his shoulders.

Then one day our community was shocked and grieved to learn that John had ended it all with a rope.

Again, where had we gone wrong? Don't we doctors have the vision and foresight to prevent this horrible hurt of suicide?

Unfortunately, even with all of our training, experience, and high technology, we must confess that we are not always able to foretell and forestall such tragic incidents. For all of us physicians who work with anxious and depressed patients, suicide is not only a worry but a continuing enigma. Which of our unhappy, despondent patients might be considering suicide, who might be the next to exit with pills, a bullet, or a rope?

The fact remains that not even the most experienced practitioner, no more than a friend or relative, can unerringly predict an impending suicide. But we do have some guidelines to to assist us.

"Have you ever thought of suicide?" In the past we may have been reluctant to pose that question, but now we know this can be exactly the query a person with suicidal tendencies wants to hear. They may have been sending out cries for help for months, cries that went unrecognized. These are the people who murmur about their worthlessness, or give subtle suggestions that life is no longer worth living. Or who even send out a warning message by way of a small overdose pills, or who scratch their wrist with a razor blade.

It's reassuring to know that fewer than one or two out of a thousand patients who make such threats actually go on to successfully commit suicide. Yet all such cries for help must be heeded and answered.

Scientists exploring the psychodynamics of suicide have

concluded that this is truly an illness, a disease caused by an organic brain disorder. They theorize that an imbalance in the biochemistry of the limbic system of the brain, the vital areas where our emotions are stored and regulated, can lead to suicidal thoughts. Soon we may be able to measure the limbic system's chemicals — the norepinephrins, the serotonins, and the dopamines — much as we today measure our serum cholesterol and our blood sugar.

But until that day we suicide survivors — doctors, friends, family — are to a degree absolved of the responsibility of recognizing this biochemical disorder. We can be forgiven our failure to prescribe what might have been the appropriate anti- depressant chemicals.

Until then we professionals can say to the other survivors, those who were so close to the victims, that the Arthurs and the Johns were suffering unbearable anguish from a perplexing illness that was not of our doing, and for which we do not as yet have a simple cure.

Until then we must learn again that life goes on, and that life is for the living.

9 Pulling the Plug

ON JANUARY 11TH, 1983, Nancy Cruzan was accidentally thrown from her car on an icy road just out of Carthage, Missouri. For twenty long minutes her brain cells were dying, as they were deprived of oxygen. But her body lived for seven more years as this young woman, comatose and paralyzed, was kept alive by oxygen, antibiotics and tube feeding. This in spite of repeated pleas by her mother and father that she be allowed a natural death.

Through these seven years Nancy' Cruzan's life and

death struggles were dragged through the courts, finally to the Missouri Supreme Court and on up to the United States Supreme Court. The State of Missouri contended that the treatment of this brain-damaged woman should be continued, because it was unclear what her wishes would have been under this set of circumstances.

Ultimately, in a split 4-3 decision, the U.S. Supreme court ruled that the Missouri court was within its rights to compel continued life support, in spite of the wishes of Nancy's surrogates, her parents. But of great added significance was the court's additional ruling that an individual does, indeed, have the right to refuse life-sustaining treatment.

Then, ironically, as the hospital bills continued to mount, the State of Missouri decided it was time to withdraw from the case, abruptly dropping the legal action it had begun.

In response a courageous county probate court judge ruled that the doctors could accede to the surrogate's request to have the artificial support withdrawn. This was immediately done, and a few days later Nancy Beth Cruzan passed away, quietly and painlessly, with Mom and Dad at her bedside.

The Nancy Cruzan story was dramatic and received national focus. But similar stories are being played out in big cities and small towns throughout the United States. Here are two from our north Idaho area which illustrate the ethical dilemma, and emphasize the need to make your wishes known in advance of an emergency.

"John" and "Jane" each were involved in auto accidents that resulted in severe brain damage. Both became comatose and both were paralyzed. Both were being kept alive by artificial life support systems. Neither had living wills.

A year and half ago John had failed to negotiate a curve

with his motorcycle, and plunged over a steep embankment. He survived, but suffered a fractured skull and fractured neck bones. Eventually, after his condition stabilized, he was transferred to a nursing home. There he was sustained with tube feeding, continual urinary bladder drainage, and around-the-clock-nursing care. John could not talk, walk or swallow, and had to be assisted with his bowel functions. To prevent pressure sores, his position was changed regularly. To enable him to sit up for short periods, he was lifted into a straight chair and supported with soft restraints.

As the months passed, John's condition deteriorated, while the cost of his care steadily mounted. His attending physicians called on the hospital's ethical support committee to review the case, and make recommendations as to the future care of this patient. John's wife told the committee that she no longer held out any hope, and asked that artificial life support be withdrawn. But several members of the family pleaded, "Isn't there anything more that could be done?"

Giving in to these wishes, the doctors ordered another brain scan. This test did reveal a mild hydrocephalus, "water on the brain." Going the extra mile, an attempt was made to relieve this pressure through brain surgery.

Unfortunately, there was no apparent improvement — the brain damage was far too extensive. So, as John's condition continued to worsen, the family finally came together to request that all support be withdrawn, to allow the natural course of events to transpire. With the tubes removed, death came easily.

Jane was a 70-year-old housewife from our town, who was involved in an auto accident in Texas where she was visiting friends. A fractured skull and a broken spine left Jane in a vegetative state. Like Nancy Cruzan she was comatose, quadriplegic, her life artificially maintained.

Jane developed lung and kidney complications and was transferred to the intensive care unit in her Texas hospital, where she was attended by heart, lung and kidney specialists. She was placed on a respirator, given large doses of antibiotics, and fed intravenously. As you can imagine, this all was extremely expensive, and medicare and her private insurance were paying only part of the bill.

As weeks passed into months her family decided to bring Jane home to be with them. This was accomplished through the use of an "air ambulance" — for $9,000.

Now it was decision-making time for Jane's husband, her three daughters, her minister, her attending physicians, and the members of the hospital ethical support committee. After long and often heart-rending deliberations, the consensus was reached to allow Jane to pass away naturally. Thirty-six hours after her tubes were removed she died peacefully. There were many tears, but everyone in that hospital room knew the right decision had been made.

Throughout our nation mothers and fathers, sons and daughters, physicians and ethics committees are struggling with these same life and death decisions. The Supreme Court's specific ruling that the individual does have the right to refuse life-sustaining treatment is a real breakthrough, but it only has value to an individual if these wishes are put into writing.

Fortunately, a good share of the public seems to have recognized the need and taken action: in the six months after the court decision, in New York City alone, health agencies were deluged with 800,000 requests for living will forms. Nancy Cruzan's father was able to see this brighter side of his daughter's tragic young death, observing that "Hundreds of thousands of people can now rest free, knowing that when death beckons they can meet it face-to-face with dignity."

10 Living Wills

NORA HAD LIVED 84 YEARS, enjoying a full and fruitful life. She loved children, her own and everyone else's, playing their games with them throughout her fourscore years. Her son called her the "oldest teenager on the block." And now we three attending physicians were sitting across the conference table from Nora's son, trying to answer the questions he threw at us: "What good is my mother's living will if you doctors won't honor it? Why can't you abide by Mom's wishes and let her die?"

His sturdy Scandinavian mother had been in robust health until the evening nearly a month ago when she was rushed to the hospital emergency room, laid low by a perforated gastric ulcer. Now Nora was hanging onto life by a slim thread, in the grip of what seemed to be unsurmountable postoperative complications. She had been semi-comatose for over three weeks, and was now supported by a ventilator, oxygen, IV fluids, and an ensemble of exotic antibiotics.

A member of the family had located a living will that Nora had signed nine years ago, and now we two surgeons and an internist were being asked to abide by the wishes she had expressed almost a decade before. But we were hesitating, remembering that such a will had to be renewed every five years. Technically and legally our hands were tied, because the will was outdated. We also recalled that a living will was defined as a directive made by a patient who was suffering from a "terminal" condition, such as cancer. But our patient was dying of cardio-renal failure, secondary to peritonitis, and therefore did not fall into the proper "terminal" category. We were on the horns of a legal dilemma; it seemed easiest to procrastinate.

Finally, under family pressure, we cautiously withdrew part of the artificial life support — the ventilator, the tube feeding, the antibiotic medications. But we just could not bring ourselves to go all the way, to turn off the oxygen, to "pull the plug."

And so Nora, gasping and struggling for every breath, clung to that thin thread of life.

At last a sister, the eldest member of the family, no longer able to watch this suffering, drew on her stalwart Swedish courage and demanded that all artificial life support be removed. After an hour-long conference with our ethics committee, and another meeting with the entire family, we gave in to their wishes and discontinued the oxygen.

Three and a half hours later Nora stopped struggling for breath, and quietly slipped from this earthly life.

In retrospect we doctors realized that our timidity had caused needless anguish. And what a waste of time and money! Yet we could plead for forgiveness on two counts: first, because we physicians by training and tradition are compelled to preserve life at all costs; and, second, because the contemporary litigious climate saps us of our courage.

We physicians will continue to be besieged by requests for a quicker ending when a loved one's life is ended, for allowing God's will to be done. Perhaps in the future we will be more responsive, when we reflect on the experience of those of us who have regularly worked with terminally ill patients, a clear understanding that most people are not so much afraid of death as they are of dying.

Pardon me, doctor, but may I die?

I know your oath requires you to try to keep me alive
  so long as the body is warm and there is a breath of life,
  but listen, Doc, I've buried my wife.

My children are grown and on their own,
  my friends are all gone, and I want to go, too.

No mortal man should keep me here,

when the call from Him is unmistakably clear.

I deserve the right to slip away
  — my work is done and I am tired.

Your motives are noble but now I pray
  you can read in my eyes what my lips can't say.

Listen to my heart and you'll hear it cry:
  pardon me, Doc, but may I die?

— Anonymous

Doctoring

Doctoring is fun. Doctoring is rewarding.

Family doctoring brings with it the privilege of welcoming a new life into this world, of working with children, adolescents, adults — real people of all ages — as a friend and counselor throughout a lifetime. And then possibly being at their bedside when they finally go on to glory. Without a doubt this personal involvement with the patient and the family is the key to what makes doctoring so rewarding and fun for me.

After a long career in medical practice I am repeatedly grateful that the course of events in my younger days guided me toward doctoring. But did I deliberately choose to be a physician? Of course not. Like most young people I arrived at my career decision by happenstance, through trial and error.

As youngsters we have vague ideas about what we want to do when we grow up, partly because we don't know about many of the options. Today little boys want to be firemen or astronauts; little girls may hope to be nurses, actresses or veterinarians — or astronauts. My father wanted me to become a minister, to follow in his footsteps. In high school I secretly wanted to be an architect because Mr. Lamereau, my mechanical arts teacher, showed me how much fun it was to plan and draw houses.

It wasn't until my sophomore year at Crane Junior College, on Chicago's West Side, that a "life and death experience" first pointed me toward medicine. I'll have to admit that, up until that time, I hadn't given much thought to living and dying.

It began when Mr. Zig Carlson, my zoology teacher, taught me how take a life by thrusting a probe into a designated spot between the eyes of a little green frog. Mr. Carlson called it "pithing" but, when that little fellow gave his last quivering struggle, I called it "dying."

As I performed my first "operation," dissecting my frog, I rebelled at the grisly task. But as the weeks passed I found I was increasingly interested in anatomy, the study of the body's structure. And all the while I kept thinking about the fragile balance between life and death.

A second similar learning experience clinched my decision to go into medicine. Toward the end of that semester I learned that to get an "A" from Mr. Carlson I'd need to dissect a cat. The catch was that I would need to obtain the cat myself.

In those days stray cats were plentiful in the back alleys of Chicago, and reducing their population was not only condoned, it was encouraged. Yet I still cringe when I think back to the day I caught my cat and doused it with a can of ether, quickly ending its life. That skinny alley cat gave up its nine lives to further my knowledge of anatomy.

After that, the die was cast. I switched my major from liberal arts to pre-medical studies, and embarked on the long and grueling course that would lead to an M.D. degree. How ironic that the death of two animals could instill in this embryo doctor a compassion for life, and imbue him with a respect for the art of healing!

And ultimately, during my first year of medical school, as I spent hours dissecting the human cadaver I'd been assigned, I couldn't help but wonder if the soul of the little green frog, of my skinny tomcat, and of the cadaverous woman now under my knife, had flown to their appropriate heavens. I surely hoped so...then maybe my minister father would forgive me for what I was doing!

One of the privileges that has come through a long career in doctoring is having been able to witness the amazing changes that have taken place in the practice of medicine. Most of these changes have been good, bringing us all better health through preventative medicine, improved hygiene, changed life style, and of course through advanced medical technology.

Yet I have seen how the march of medical technology is at least partly to blame for the strong calls today for health care "reform," in what is no longer simply the practice of medicine but instead is called "the health care industry."

Many of the essays in this final section reflect on those changes. The "good doctor" is a different person than he was a half century ago. No longer does an "M.D." title confer the right to practice the art and the science of medicine for a lifetime. Now the family practice physician must keep abreast of medical advances by enrolling in continuing medical education courses, and periodically undergoing "re-certification."

Most of the evolutionary changes in the way we practice medicine today are commendable. We now save the lives of heart attack victims that in yesteryear we surely would have lost. Doctors now salvage the lives of one-pound premature babies, sustaining their tiny bodies in fabulous neonatal intensive care units. Advanced medical technology now enables surgeons to transplant hearts, lungs, kidneys and eyeballs, and to replace worn out joints with steel and plastic substitutes.

Through "genetic engineering" scientists can modify the DNA of a plant or animal — even the human animal. Through what are sometimes called "heroic measures" we can prolong the life of the aging patient, or the terminal cancer patient, far beyond what was previously thought of as a "natural death."

Such amazing medical developments have brought along two unhappy side effects. One is the extremely high cost of high-tech diagnostic techniques and procedures, and the other is the need for physicians to seriously weigh the ethical aspects of their medical practices — including grappling with an issue which greatly pains doctors even to think about, the rationing of health care. While doctors are willing to work first and foremost for the benefit of their patients' well being, paid or unpaid, the vast expansion of medical technology soon will make it necessary to decide who will or will not benefit from these costly medical miracles.

Over the years it has been my good fortune to visit a number of countries, to study their health care systems and to exchange views with fellow doctors there. Wherever I went, I found family practices flourishing at every level, including the comparatively uneducated but capable "barefoot doctor" in China, and the "middle-educated" doctors in the former Soviet Union.

In America we are fortunate that our family doctors are highly educated specialists in their own right, possessing a wide range of knowledge and understanding of the basics of health care. At the same time we are blessed with an amazing array of sub-specialists, technically proficient in one particular area of practice. We are lucky to be served so well by both.

1 Diminished Image of the Doctor

PEOPLE DON'T THINK AS HIGHLY OF DOCTORS as they used to. A recent survey found the first five "Most Admirable Occupations" were fireman, paramedic, farmer, pharmacist and grade school teacher, in that order. In past polls physicians regularly were first or second, but this time they didn't even make it into the top ten.

Doctors once were idolized (as in "My son, the doctor"), but today often are the target of angry sarcasm. On television the kindly and caring Marcus Welby MD has been replaced by the far less flattering depiction of Dr. Doogie Howser, and the often disgruntled New York doctor Joel, out of place in the Alaska of "Northern Exposure."

In a movie of a few years ago, "The Doctor" is a cruel and uncaring heart surgeon. Only when the physician himself fell victim to a serious, life-threatening disease did he learn humility. Another film, "Doc Hollywood," ridiculed big city MDs while attempting to glorify small town doctors. To make its points, the movie frequently dispensed with real world truthfulness, and ladled out large dollops of Hollywood hyperbole.

A young doctor, played by Michael J. Fox, just out of his training and still not quite dry behind his ears, is by sheer accident transformed into a revered, caring family physician. In the short span of 72 hours, he saves the life of an elderly doctor who is having a heart attack; heroically and

and of course successfully performs an extremely difficult delivery; hurriedly sees a host of sick and needy patients in the little clinic; and still finds time to fall in love with a beautiful young lady who drives the rickety old ambulance.

Please, dear reader, that just ain't how it happens out in the real world!

If you believe TV and Hollywood, the doctors of today have hearts of stone and feet of clay. Even the usually upbeat Erma Bombeck took off on us in a recent column, noting that the audience, filing out after seeing The Doctor, "had smiles on their faces. They had seen good triumph over evil. They had seen arrogance rewarded with revenge."

"Evil" and "arrogant" may be a little too strong, but the fact remains, we physicians aren't admired and respected as we were when I began practicing medicine. I think there are at least five reasons for this shift. Our patients complain that...

☛ We docs are often too busy, making patients wait too long, forgetting that their time is just as valuable as ours.

☛ We sometimes don't listen, and don't take the complaints of our patients seriously, when they come in worrying about heart attacks or brain tumors.

☛ We can be insensitive, not taking the time to go into the deep-down causes of what's really troubling our patients.

A second group of reasons for doctors' dip in popularity are caused by circumstances largely beyond our control...

☛ First of all, money, a consideration mostly ignored by physicians of yesteryear, who were notoriously poor businessmen, often not knowing who did and didn't pay their bills. Many times their pay for a baby or an appendectomy was a hind quarter of beef or a two-cord stack of firewood.

Now Medicare, Medicaid and largely universal private health insurance have forced doctors to become very aware of the practice of medicine as a business. Big Brother in Washington, at Blue Cross, or deep inside some other claims handler has come between the patient and his or her physician. "Somebody else" now pays the bills, and this means at least some of the patient's gratitude is directed toward someone other than his doctor: "You know, Doc, I didn't have pay one cent!"

And, in the same way, we physicians are aware that we are working not only for the patient, but for a third party payor, especially when there is a misunderstanding, perhaps about a bill. Then the blame falls on the shoulders of the doctor and the hospital, rather than where it belongs, in the lap of the Health Care Financing Administration.

ಌ Modern technology also has diverted admiration and respect from the doctor, as amazing scientific machinery has replaced some of the diagnostic acumen and therapeutic wizardry which used to be totally attributed to the physician. Now the knowledgeable patient will come in or call and ask, "Doc, I've got this hip problem, so don't you agree that I should have a CAT scan or an MRI?"

These five causes are all aspects of a decline in the personal relationship between the patient and her or his physician. This tendency has been accelerated by the increase over the past few decades in the number of specialist doctors, physicians who a person may see only a few times, and only for very specific problems.

However, there are signs of a new trend among new MDs to "specialize" in family practice. This may be why another recent survey, done by the Gallup organization, found the public's favorable opinion of their personal physician had increased to 87%, up from 80% a few years before.

2 Men Medics/Hen Medics

WE MALE MEDICAL STUDENTS called our very few female classmates "hen medics," and looked upon them as rare birds not likely to fly very very high over the medical practice horizons. When I was doing my training in the 1930s, we viewed these young women studying to be physicians with at least some degree of condescension. We were sure they would end up in a government or public health job, or taking care of heathens in Papua, or at best in a teaching position.

Moreover, these female medical students were rarely looked upon as dating material. As interns and residents we dated nurses. There were a lot more of them, we worked side by side with them, and shared our tiredness and our strained emotions with them. Many of us married a nurse, as I did, and lived happily ever after.

Once out into the real world, the practice of medicine was, for the most part, considered to be a man's job. That was certainly the case when I arrived in north Idaho in 1939. Our medical fraternity was, without apology, a "good 'ole boy's club."

Then one day Doctors Don and Jane Gumprecht came to town, and soon the barrier was broken. These two young graduates of the University of Minnesota were our community's first husband and wife medical team. From the very start, their practices were marked with professional capability and success.

Doctor Jane wasted no time in setting us straight about "hen medics." With her quiet and unassuming manner, she quickly became known as a capable, caring family physician. Doctor Don won many friends as a hard-working general practitioner, the kind of a doctor who could do everything. This included setting broken bones, delivering babies, snipping out gall bladders, or treating your sniffly, runny nose or your aching and flu-ridden body.

In their spare time, the Doctors Gumprecht brought four fine children into this world, including three sons who have become doctors.

If Drs. Don and Jane broke the ice, the arrival of Anita Robinson and Chris Kutteruf quickly melted away any remaining icy chunks of prejudice about female doctors and husband/wife practices.

Doctor Robinson can hook you up to a remarkable device that produces a special heart tracing, called an echocardiogram, that gives us a reading on the condition of the heart valves and the heart muscle, and an estimate of how the old pump is functioning.

Doctor Kutteruf, a gastroenterologist, can look at your insides from top to bottom (literally), using a gastroscope for the stomach and a colonoscope for the bowels. These flexible little tubes can wiggle around the corners of the colon or stomach, searching for polyps, tumors, ulcers and cancers. A tiny light on the end shows the way, and a miniature clipper can snip off a bit of tissue for further study.

Soon the men medic/hen medic melt turned to a flood, as three more doctor-couples came to town, perhaps attracted by north Idaho as a good place to raise a family, as well as to practice medicine.

Doctor Patti Moran and Doctor Eugene Kresbach arrived via the round-about route of the University of Minnesota medical school and public health work in Alaska. Patti is in family practice, Eugene works as an emergency room physician.

Then came Doctors Mary Jo and Robin Shaw, she a pediatrician, he an E.R. physician at our regional hospital. Incidentally, these two handsome young doctors met in medical school anatomy class at the University of Arizona — love at first sight over a very stiff cadaver!

The most recently arrived husband and wife doctor couple, Steve Malek MD and Leann Rosseau MD, met at Carroll College during their pre-med years. Doctor Malek is an emergency room physician, his wife Doctor Rosseau a family practitioner.

This positive evolution of the place of women in our local medical community reflects a national trend. "Hen medic" is no longer a derogatory term among medical students — it hardly could be when medical schools boast that nearly half their students are women.

Though each member of our local husband/wife doctor teams has chosen different areas of practice, they all share a common bond of love for their family, their community and their patients. Furthermore, they understand and accept telephone interruptions at the dinner table, and broken hours of sleep.

3 Angels of Mercy

I ARRIVED AT OPERATING ROOM Five a little early, there to assist in a total hip replacement for one of my patients. I took this opportunity to observe nurses Carol and Darcy move confidently and swiftly around the room, making everything ready for this complicated team operation.

Across the room our "scrub" assistant Jerry was laying out thousands of dollars worth of gleaming surgical instruments, which during the operation he would place into the waiting hands of the surgeons, in the precise sequence and at the precise moment they are needed.

At the head of the operating table, behind the surgical drapes, stood nurse-anesthetist Rich, ready to deftly adjust dials and valves, buttons and switches on his $30,000 anesthetic machine. Throughout the operation, this sophisticated apparatus would provide him with a steady readout of the patient's pulse, blood-pressure, oxygen level and heart tracing.

After the surgery is completed, and the patient's condition pronounced stable, he'll be moved to the intensive care unit across the corridor where Sarah, Larry and the other specially trained ICU nurses will watch over this patient until there he's completely returned to consciousness, and his "vital signs" — blood pressure, pulse, heart action and so forth — are considered satisfactory.

That done this newly-hipped gentleman will be moved back to his room on the surgical wing, where Doris and Ione and their nursing staffs will continue to monitor and care for him, providing pain medicine, sedatives, intravenous fluids, and possibly antibiotics.

In just a few days, the fellow will be up and about, gently jigging around on his brand-new hip, thanks to the efforts of smooth-working teams of doctors and nurses.

The notion of doctor-nurse teamwork is comparatively new. Down through history, the nurse was often viewed in a far more subservient role. Although there is mention of "the nurse" in the Talmud and in the Bible, and even in Egyptian papyri, the true beginning of modern nursing history dates back to Florence Nightingale.

At a time when nursing was thought to be an "unsuitable occupation for a woman of high birth," this second daughter of a wealthy English family resolutely set out to be a nurse. After visiting hospitals and studying nursing in Germany, in 1854 she organized a group of 38 woman nurses to attend to the wounded in the Crimean War.

This effort brought her much positive public acclaim, and she spent the rest of her years writing and speaking about the need for education as well as "training" for nursing students. Called "The Lady With the Lamp," because she believed a nurse's duties were required both night and day, in 1860 Florence Nightingale was instrumental in creating a nursing school in London.

Notwithstanding the high esteem in which the public held Nurse Nightingale, for many decades female nurses were viewed with not much respect. Nurses were considered subordinate to men, as "hand-maidens to the physician." Hospital care was relegated to "uncommon women" — a group composed of prisoners, prostitutes and alcoholics.

Charles Dickens described Nurse Sairey Gamp as "a fat old woman, this Mrs. Gamp, with a husky voice and a moist eye....the face of Mrs. Gamp — the nose in particular — was somewhat red and swollen, and it was always difficult to enjoy her society without being conscious of the smell of spirits."

In more modern years the nurse has not always been treated too well. Nurse Diesel in the movie "High Anxiety" was portrayed as malevolent and sadistic. Nurse Ratched in "One Flew Over the Cuckoo's Nest" was tough and assertive — if she stood before her mirror and commanded her hair to part, it would part!

On the real-life and positive side, selfless and devoted work by nurses has raised their image. Sister Kenny's work with polio victims and Mother Theresa's tireless efforts with the poor are outstanding examples.

Health care today is too complex for physicians to do it all. A major reason for the public's greater respect for nurses is the increased acceptance of nurses by doctors as vital partners in their practice of medicine. Helping people get well is a team effort!

4 Robot Nurses of the Future

AS VALUABLE AND NECESSARY as nurses are, there are too few of them in America. This is a nationwide problem, particularly acute in metropolitan areas. In response to this problem, two remedies have been suggested.

One direction, recommended by the American Medical

Association, would create a new nursing category. Under this plan nursing assistants called "registered care technologists" would take over a major portion of the basic bedside nursing duties now handled by registered nurses.

The American Nursing Association has loudly protested that this would remove RNs from their traditional patient care relationship. The two organizations are working together toward a compromise.

An even more radical way to relieve registered nurses of some of their more mundane chores has been implemented at a number of hospitals: robots. In the late 1980s the Danbury, Connecticut Hospital was one of the first to experiment with the use of programmed, mobile robots. They currently have two in full-time use, each costing about $25,000. These ingenious machines quietly and willingly handle such simple chores as delivering food trays to patients who return to their room after mealtimes, because of tests or procedures; and whirring through the halls at night to deliver sterile supplies to nurses' stations. A spokesman for the hospital says they are very pleased with the robotic help, and have received no resistance from nurses.

But these robots surely can't soothe a fevered brow, or unclench a scared patient's white-knuckled fist. Will he/it drone a recorded message to the pre-operative patient or to the mother in labor? Heaven forbid that this Robbie the Robot, with his chilly metal digits, should ever give an enema to any patient of mine!

What a far cry is such mechanization of nursing from the picture of the proud RN of yesteryear, a lady in starched white, wearing her nurse's cap with great dignity, rendering tender loving care at the patient's bedside, or working with the physician as, yes, his "handmaiden."

The nurse of that era attained her degree through "training." During this period of hands-on learning, she lived in the student nurses' quarters adjacent to the hospital, and worked 12-hour shifts of floor duty as an unpaid nursing aide for the hospital. As an employee of the hospital, she was given food and lodging, and the laundering of her striped and bibbed student's uniform.

She was watched over by the piercing eyes of the old-time floor supervisor — and pity the poor girl who failed to snap to attention, giving a prim and prompt "Good Morning" to the head nurse as she made her hospital rounds.

Like Nurse Ratched of Ken Kesey's "One Flew Over the Cuckoo's Nest," at least on the surface, these mother hens had all the easy-going warmth and geniality of Marine drill sergeants. The students hated the tough head nurses then, but once out of training into the real world of nursing, they were grateful for having been taught the value of strict self-discipline.

That was then. Now, with the passing of only a few decades, nurse's "training" has become education, reflecting a dramatic change in a nurse's responsibilities. Today, young women — and men — study anatomy, chemistry and other quite literally "hard" sciences to prepare to be much more equal partners to physicians and to other medical care specialists. In their second year, they receive practical, clinical hands-on experience, not as employees of the hospital but as full-time students, eager to learn everything they can about the flesh and blood of medical and surgical care of their fellow human beings.

This welcome change in the status of the RN is partly due to the growing importance of sophisticated technology in patient care, which has engendered a new spirit of cooperation and inter-dependence between physicians and nurses. These complex new machines must be understood and adjusted, requiring specific skills for which nurses often are specially trained.

The nurse of today has been educated to take a much more active role in the medical management of the patient's status and recovery. But she or he has learned, sadly, that along with this increase in professional stature comes an increase in liability. Today even nurses are being taken to court in professional liability suits.

Today's registered nurse also has been loaded down by the immense amount of paperwork required by the government, Medicare, Medicaid and the insurance companies, to minutely detail the patient's record of care.

More to learn, more technology to handle, more paperwork to complete. And yet, to their credit, most RNs I know will try to steal a little time each day to go back to the bedside, to hold a hand and soothe a brow. Something no robot will ever be able to do.

5 Better Names for Aches and Pains

SOME PATIENTS ARE RELUCTANT to grouse about their aching rheumatiz, and maybe blame their sore kidneys on old age. It's no longer scientifically proper to complain of lumbago, sciatica or a hitch in your gitalong. To effect a cure they imagine we must use correct terminology.

For example, medical progress in rheumatology has brought us an amazing array of technical terms, all part of an effort to identify the underlying causes and to arrive at a specific diagnosis — and of course with a code number acceptable to Medicare and other third party payers.

Medically and technically, arthritis and rheumatism are virtually interchangeable terms. The two bone and joint disorders with which we are most familiar are osteo-arthritis and rheumatoid arthritis, separate and distinct clinical entities. Under a third general heading are a wide range of rheumatology problems, from gout to disc disease, from psoriasis to lupus, and including the so-called "collagen disease," fibrous connective tissue disorders resulting from inflammation of muscles, tendons, ligaments and bursas.

Things can get complicated in this third group. Here we deal with ailments both exotic and ordinary: spondylosis, bursitis, tendonitis, synovitis, polymyalgia rheumatica and ankylosing spondylitis. Tongue-twisting terms to be sure, but scientifically specific and accurate. It's important to make these distinctions, so that we can prescribe the most effective treatment regimens.

For example, it is vitally important to differentiate between the common form of arthritis, degenerative osteo-arthritis that affects older people, and the more worrisome rheumatoid arthritis that may strike young people.

Degenerative joint disease in the older age group affects mainly the weight-bearing joints — the hips, the knees and the spine. The basic cause is unknown, but a contributing factor is the continual abrasive wear and tear of long years of usage. Over time the smooth, gristle-like cartilaginous covering of the joint surface gradually wears down or flakes off, exposing rough bony surfaces. The result is pain, stiffness and swelling.

If you live long enough there's a good chance you'll be affected. Fortunately, the deterioration proceeds slowly, unless you're in a line of work which puts special stress on your joints — a ballet dancer or basketball player, for example. Football players are susceptible to knee and shoulder joint problems when they get older, because of repeated trauma when they were being pounded and pounding others for a living.

To confirm this condition, osteo-arthritic changes can be discovered by x-ray. Treatment early on consists of joint rest, heat, physical therapy, aspirin or one of the newer, more expensive anti-inflammatory medications. If these treatments don't work, injection of cortico-steroids between the joints may. If the degenerative process no longer responds to such conservative measures, joint replacement may be considered.

Rheumatoid arthritis, on the other hand, is a far different disease. Rather than being restricted to the joints, this disease may be a "systemic" disorder in which our own immune system may turn against the cells of our body, causing damage to the synovial lining of our joint spaces, resulting in pain, redness and swelling. In rare instances this disease may even attack blood vessels, the eyes and the heart.

RA is most often seen in the hands, wrists, knees and neck. Mis-shapen hands, with distorted alignment of the fingers, provide a tell-tale initial diagnosis. A definitive diagnosis can usually be made by blood tests, perhaps complemented by Magnetic Resonance Imaging.

Because this disease strikes younger people, even children, and because it may have an insidious onset with vague symptoms of tiredness, loss of weight and muscular pains, early diagnosis often is difficult.

The use of heat, rest, physical therapy, and immobilization of affected joints is an essential first step to treat the disease, along with aspirin and anti-inflammatory medications. More exotic treatments might include steroids, penicillamine, anti-malarial drugs, even gold. Methotrexate is a comparatively new drug that helps in some cases of rheumatoid arthritis. Late in the progress of this disease, surgical correction of the deformities may restore some function.

More difficult is the differential diagnosis of the hodgepodge of the other bone and joint disorders that come under the third heading of rheumatology. But there are a few ways we can categorize. For example, the sharp, shooting pain in your back could be a result of the pressure of a protruding intervertebral disc on a nerve.

The acute pain you feel in your shoulder when you have

difficulty combing your hair or putting on a belt can be a symptom of bursitis. The discomfort you feel in your forearm or elbow when you shake hands or try to twist open a stubborn jar lid can be an indication of inflamed tendons — the teno-synovitis of "tennis elbow."

The aching of "lumbago" in the middle and lower lumbar spine can be due to the wear and tear, the grinding down of the articulating surfaces of the bones of your spine. The excruciating pain of gouty arthritis is the result of the inflammation of joint (most often of your big toe) where prickly uric acid crystals have accumulated.

And so we go down the list to the more rare diseases and disorders with fancy names, such as spondylosis, spondylitis, spondylolithesis, spinal stenosis, often so difficult to diagnose and treat. Fortunately, in spite of the fact that not all these various forms of arthritis are curable, we usually can help patients obtain relief from the symptoms.

So don't just throw up your hands and put up with the aches and pains of growing old! And don't worry about the big words your doctor uses. Whatever the terminology, he or she may be able to help you with your sciatica, your lumbago, and the hitch in your gitalong.

6 *Healthful Alternatives To Traditional Medicine*

THE COUNTDOWN ENDED AND A LIGHTED SIGN FLASHED "On The Air." I was sitting in a television studio among a half dozen or so other "health care givers," part of a panel assembled to talk about "The Delivery of Health Care By Alternative Methods."

Put simply, the subject was healing by other than medical doctors, the traditional way, which I was there alone to represent. I might have felt defensive from the start, but I didn't. The alternative care-givers on the panel were a happy, self-confident group, looking forward to this public exposure.

First to be interviewed was a "reflexologist," a friendly young man who proudly related how he had learned his craft from a seminar put on by the International Institute of Reflexology in Florida. In this brief course he had learned to treat illness, real or imagined, by applying "acupressure" to certain "zones" in the foot. After his explanation, several of his satisfied clients rose to give testimony about how reflexology had brought them relief from ills ranging from dyspepsia to lumbago to mental problems. "Well, maybe," I mused. Everyone knows how great it feels to have someone massage your tired and aching feet.

Over the next fifty minutes (with time out for commercials), we heard in turn from a naturopath, a masseuse, a homeopath, an acupuncturist, a mid-wife and a chiropractor. All described their methods, and each had brought along a few satisfied clients.

Interwoven into all these presentations was this implied message: medical doctors are just pill-pushers, interested only in treating the disease, not the "whole person." Alternative care, by positive comparison, was more "holistic."

At least in this television studio setting, we "traditional" doctors were out-numbered, out-gunned and on the defensive. Needless to say, this was an uncomfortable experience for me.

Of course I had come to this panel discussion loaded with plenty of strong ammunition to defend the medical profession. I planned to relate how we medical doctors spend a dozen years or more in school before we can enter practice: four years of college, four years of medical school, and four or five years in postgraduate residency training.

How we are licensed and under the disciplinary control of the governor-appointed State Board of Medicine. And how we must be "accredited" each year to maintain the privilege of working as a member of the hospital staff.

I intended to tell the television audience how we MDs must attend a specified number of hours of formal postgraduate education each year. And that we must have our patient care records reviewed each month by hospital committees in a process called "peer review."

And finally I was quite prepared to state that the main concern we physicians have about "alternative care," whether it be squeezing a foot or giving high colonic flushings, is that they might simply temporarily relieve the symptoms of a much more serious illness. This could delay the diagnosis and treatment of a life-threatening organic condition, such as diabetes, heart disease or cancer.

But I never had a chance to make my points, because no time had been allowed for a presentation of the merits of "traditional" health care. Anyway, that probably wasn't what the TV audience had turned in to hear. As I drove home from the television station that evening, I reflected upon that experience, and what I might learn from it.

One lesson was a new sense of humility. Perhaps we "traditional" care-givers, with our batteries of fancy high-tech tests, our laser-powered surgical techniques, and our burgeoning array of magic medicines, simply were missing the boat.

Did we believe that our long years of training automatically assured superb patient care? My thoughts went back to a visit to the USSR where I'd observed relatively good health care being provided by "middle-educated doctors," vocationally trained right out of high school, working in villages and in urban clinics. And how on another trip I'd talked with "barefoot doctors" in China, who brought capable and caring health care to the people in the countryside.

Then I thought of another barefoot care-giver, born in

Bethlehem, the son of a humble carpenter, who two thousand years ago went about the countryside healing aches and pains of the heart and body, generally making folks feel better. He left behind untold generations of faithful followers.

Faith is, of course, the key to cure. People who have an ailment, real or imagined, organic or psychosomatic, desperately want to believe that the treatment — whatever it might be — will bring help.

The alternative care-givers on this TV program were honest and sincere in their practices, working within the law and within their areas of competence. They may not have received the long years of training in the science of medicine, or the degrees, the accreditation, the certification, the peer review, the postgraduate education. But they understood the art of healing.

And I, a "traditional" doctor, was once more reminded that the laying on of hands, the open and attentive ear, the compassionate heart, can be just as important to the ailing patient as all our modern technology.

7 Radiation Can Be Vital

IT'S VERY HUMAN TO FEAR THE UNKNOWN AND UNSEEN, which is why the terms "x-ray" and "nuclear" are particularly upsetting to many people. My patient Emma Anderson flatly refuses to have a mammogram because, as she so bluntly puts it, "I don't want no x-rays on my boobs — x-rays cause cancer." Of course, after leaving my office, on the way out to her car, Emma will light a cigarette. She'll feel its plump roundness, see the smoke and smell the fragrance. Surely anything that visible, that tangible, that pleasant should cause no fear.

In the same way, many of my patients are wary of being referred to the "Nuclear Medicine" department of our hospital, for fear they might get "irradiated." They should know that this department contains many magnificent tools to assist physicians in making a correct and accurate diagnosis, and to point the way toward a successful treatment plan. This excessive and unfounded fear of anything "nuclear" is why a diagnostic procedure first named "Nuclear Magnetic Resonance" now is known by the less terrifying "Magnetic Resonance Imaging," or MRI.

Recently the media have worried us about another invisible, intangible threat, radon. They warn that radon, a degradation product of plutonium, is right there in the soil beneath our homes, just waiting to seep up through the floors into where we live. Good heavens, even within the walls of our private castles we cannot escape the threat of irradiation! With all these evil elements surrounding us, we wonder how we ever got past puberty, let alone beyond the golden age of 65!

The Food and Drug Administration recently approved the irradiation of certain types of food to eliminate insects, bacteria and parasites. We now have evidence that irradiation kills trichina in pork, knocks out salmonella in fish and chicken, and reduces grain spoilage. The FDA has found that food so irradiated does not become radioactive, and it does not produce long-range ill effects.

A few years ago, First Lady Nancy Reagan sent a thrilling and courageous message to American women, in effect saying "I had a mammogram, I've had a mastectomy, I'm cured!" Take note, Emma Anderson: a mammogram requires about one tenth the amount of x-rays required for a chest picture, and the vital benefits of mammograms far outweigh any tiny risk they may pose.

It's ironic that we human beings willingly and even enthusiastically enjoy such hazardous recreational chemicals as nicotine and alcohol, while at the same time, because of an unrealistic fear of the unknown, deny the great good that can come to humanity through the use of x-rays and other forms of nuclear medicine.

8 Treat Computers With Healthy Respect — And Wariness

EVERY SO OFTEN WE'RE REMINDED OF HOW COMPUTERS have become such a fundamental — and sometimes fearful — part of our lives. When a hacking whiz kid can infect 6,000 computers in a research network with a "virus," sent for the fun of it a few years ago via electronic mail, we wonder about the privacy and vulnerability of these marvelous machines on which we've become so dependent.

My personal and professional concern is with maintaining confidentiality of medical records. Fortunately, safeguards also are built into the way these records are stored in hospital and medical insurer computers. The intent is to make it impossible for just anyone to punch a few computer keys to find out who has had mental problems, who has been treated for alcoholism, who has had an abortion, who has a sexually transmitted disease.

In the large and busy medical records department at our regional north Idaho hospital, there are eight computer terminals through which all patient records are processed. The specially trained and carefully screened operators at these work stations have been made fully aware of the responsibility they carry, inputting this very private information about patients admitted to the hospital.

Furthermore, each operator has been given their own personal "password," to give them and only them access to their computer. Furthermore, as an additional safeguard, these operators can put information into the system but they cannot retrieve it.

Moreover, all information is "coded," so that even if someone were able to retrieve the data, they would be unable to decipher the gobbledegook.

Sounds pretty safe, doesn't it? The medical records managers in our hospital, as I believe in all U.S. hospitals, have done everything humanly possible to make the medical records systems tamper proof.

Unfortunately, this protection is breached when the government gets involved. A patient who accepts health insurance coverage under Medicare or Medicaid automatically give the Feds the right to snoop into his or her medical records.

Under the guise of "Quality Assurance" — the government's euphemistic term for checking your doctor's diagnosis, and making sure your treatment was not a whit more than absolutely necessary — federal agents can come right into the hospital to review your confidential medical records. When the government gives, it also takes!

Private health insurance companies have been quick to follow. Many carriers now require you to consent to the release of all personal health records before they grant you coverage. They've gotcha!

The Oath of Hippocrates, sworn to by all physicians, requires that any information revealed by a patient be kept completely confidential by the doctor. Now, sad to say, computer technology has frayed this sacred pledge around the edges.

9 He Needs His Head Examined!

> *The mind in its own place, and in itself*
> *Can make a heaven of hell, or a hell of heaven.*
> — John Milton, "Paradise Lost"

BUT JUST WHAT IS THE MIND, how does it work, and how to fix it when it doesn't? For centuries, scientists have been frustrated in their search for quick and easy diagnoses of mental maladies. Now high-powered computers are helping answer these difficult questions.

When a patient presents his doctor with an unusual set of neurological, mental and emotional symptoms, the physician may be able to arrive at a diagnosis on the basis of the clinical history and the physical examination, determining whether the condition is psychologic or organic, and whether the patient is psychotic or just neurotic. With greater confidence than ever before, we can determine whether the complaining patient has a brain tumor or just a bad headache, whether he has had a serious stroke or a transient ischemic attack.

Usually these differentiations can be made by the primary physician — variously known as a family practitioner, a general practitioner or an internist. In the vast majority of cases, the headache, the dizzy spells, the transient weakness will be treatable and curable with medication and reassurance.

In those rare instances when a simple diagnosis is not possible, and all the therapeutic efforts have failed, your doctor may decide to use one of the more exotic (and costly) computer-driven diagnostic procedures.

Though you may not know just how it works, there's a good chance you've heard of CAT scans, an acronym for computerized axial tomography, often called CT scans. A few pages back I also referred to MRI, magnetic resonance imaging. And you may have read about one of the latest high-powered tests, nicknamed PET, for positron emission tomography. Each of these computerized diagnostic tests has certain advantages and fairly specific uses.

The CT scanner is the workhorse of the three, the one most commonly used. When being scanned by this machine the patient lies on a platform, while the x-ray emission tube moves in a circle around him, taking serial cross-section pictures of brain and body structures. A simple x-ray picture gives a single view, but the CT scanner gives a series of "moving pictures."

If you took high school science or physics you may have "illustrated" a magnetic field by placing iron filings on a sheet of paper or glass, then creating a pattern by moving a magnet beneath it. This is approximately how MRI works. Because our bodies are 80% water, and because water is composed of atoms of hydrogen and oxygen, some genius figured out that the hydrogen atoms inside your body could be made to dance in certain ways if they were magnetized. How they dance gives a picture of areas where everything is okay, or where there may be problems.

Once again, the patient undergoing an MRI diagnostic procedure lies on a platform, this time surrounded by a giant moving magnet. And here those hydrogen atoms we talked about are magnetized (like the steel filings) and made to dance around — the patient doesn't feel a thing, by the way. As the giant magnet moves, like a meat slicer at the butcher shop, it sends out pulses of magnetization, causing tiny hunks of nuclear substances inside the hydrogen atoms to send out weak radio signals. These radio waves are picked up by the scanner and electronically recorded by the computer as a photographic image.

Because different structures within the brain or the body are made up of varying amounts of water, these different tissues produce their particular identifying magnetic resonance image, which is how the MRI differential diagnosis is made. MRI's special advantage is that it can provide a somewhat better picture of "soft" tissue, the stuff of which tumors and stroke- and heart attack-inducing blood clots are made. Also MRIs do a better job of reaching certain areas at the base of the brain.

The third and most sophisticated scanning technology, positron emission tomography, is used mainly to study the physiology of the brain. As our brain functions it burns up sugar, and this metabolic action proceeds at varying rates in different areas. Taking advantage of this fact, the nuclear medicine specialists inject the brain with a sugar solution containing a mildly radioactive substance. Then, when the brain is photographed with the PET machine, the result is a a beautiful colored picture, demonstrating brain function.

The varying rates of metabolism of the sugar thus portrayed can differentiate tumors from normal brain tissue, and can — quite remarkably — assist in the diagnosis of schizophrenia, epilepsy, and perhaps even Alzheimer's disease

"That guy ought to have his head examined," is a common derogatory term. Will the day come when primary physicians will refer patients who are suffering from "mysterious maladies of the mind" to a computerized scanning machine, instead of to a neurologist or a psychiatrist?

That's highly unlikely, for several reasons. For one thing, the cost of these scanning procedures is prohibitively high, sometimes running into thousands of dollars. Moreover, PET tests are available only at a few medical centers equipped with a fancy contrivance called a "cyclotron." Finally, such high-tech tests are ordered only after every attempt has been made by the physician to arrive at an answer through the use of all appropriate standard diagnostic procedures, which are adequate in the vast majority of cases.

But when the doctor is stumped and concludes that

"that guy really needs to have his head examined," it's nice to know that by using sugar and water and magnetism, the mysterious maladies of his mind can be explored, computerized, and photographically recorded.

10 When A Death Can Give The Gift of Life

I RECENTLY OVERHEARD A COUPLE OF MY DOCTOR colleagues, Rich Langley and Gary Henson, shooting the breeze in the hospital lounge. As usual among such highly trained, serious professionals, these docs were talking about the surprisingly lopsided score in the Monday Night Football game, and the lousy duck hunting luck they were having so far this season.

Eventually their conversation did turn to their patients. Dr. Langley was was waiting for Mrs. Madeline Warnecke to get off the nest and produce her first offspring, while Dr. Henson had just asked the lab to cross-match a couple pints of blood for a worried stock broker with a bleeding ulcer.

About that time, Doctor Bob Alter, a senior attending physician, dropped by to hang up his coat before he went upstairs to make rounds. "Hey fellows," he called out, "have you heard the good news? Our hospital has been designated as an official Organ Retrieval Center for the Pacific Northwest."

I'd heard about this earlier in the day when the hospital administrator announced it to several of us with the statement "We're going to have visitors," referring to the surgeons from big hospitals in Seattle and Portland, even from as far away as San Francisco and and Salt Lake City, who we could expect to be flying up to our north Idaho hospital to pick up livers, kidneys, hearts and eyeballs to use in their transplant programs.

For some reason — maybe it's the mountain air and wide open spaces — our region has a high incidence of fatal automobile and motorcycle accidents. In a portion of these the victims suffer completely debilitating head injuries — they become "brain dead."

To be part of a cooperative organ transplant program seemed like a good idea to me, but Langley, an obstetrician, snorted that he thought it was going to be "pretty gross, having those super-docs jet in here to snatch organs — 'harvesting' they call it — and then zoom back to their fancy big city hospitals, leaving behind a disemboweled cadaver!"

That vivid image reminded me of the time on an African photo safari where my wife and I saw a zebra being feasted upon by vultures. Ugly black birds, swooping down out of the sky, squawking raucously as they attacked the carcass with their claws and their beaks.

Obviously something about organ transplantation had touched a sensitive nerve in Doctor Langley because he continued, getting a bit more agitated. "You know, I don't blame those nurses who refuse to scrub in on those 'harvesting' expeditions. They just can't bear to stand by while organs are being snatched out of a body while the heart is still beating."

"Oh come off it, Langley," retorted Dr. Henson, "all this organ retrieving is done with decency, and with careful consideration for the feelings of the family of the brain dead person, whose body and heart are being kept artificially alive for this purpose alone!" I wanted to jump in to say that the relatives have given their written consent to have organs removed because they understand that these donations are a gift of life. But before I could make this point, senior physician Alter added that, in his experience, "usually the parents or wife are actually relieved of some of their sadness. Though they've lost a loved one, in this way they can help someone to continue living, and to live better."

I couldn't stay out of this debate any longer, and I spoke from personal experience instead of my medical practice. I told them that I have two sons, and that both had some rather serious auto accidents in their young lives.

I explained that my eldest son totalled his car when he skidded into a tree after hitting some black ice. Fortunately he was wearing his seat belt, and so suffered only minor injuries. However, it happened that when he was younger we had discovered he had been born with only one functioning kidney. "Often since his accident," I told these three doctors, now listening to me as fathers, "I've been thankful his good kidney wasn't ruptured in that crash. If it had been, you can be sure I would have been hoping and praying that a kidney donation could have been found in the nick of time."

I went on to explain about the auto accident my younger son had had, skidding his open sports car on a gravelled country road to avoid a deer. He came to a stop upside down in a ditch, hanging from his seat belt, shaken but otherwise unhurt. "Yet what if his head had been crushed as he rolled over," I challenged them and myself, "and he had arrived at the hospital brain dead? Would I have wanted my strong young son to be an organ donor before being let die?" I could see they were relating this quandary to their own families and feelings. I quickly answered "You bet I would have."

Which is why each member of our family carries organ donor cards in our wallets. There's only the tiniest of chances they'll ever be used, but in that rare instance a death could give the gift of life.

11 New Hinges For Your Joints

ON THE OPERATING ROOM DOOR A LARGE, hand-lettered sign sternly discourages: "Do Not Enter." Beneath this an official-looking hospital sign explains why: "Total Hip Replacement Room."

While you might rightly imagine such major orthopedic surgery to be being mainly mechanical, it happens that bones and joints are extremely susceptible to bacterial infection. When old and worn out hips and knees, wrists and fingers are rejuvenated with replacements of steel, plastic and rubber, strict adherence to sterile technique is an absolute requirement.

"Do Not Enter" applies to everyone, doctors included, but today I'm allowed to pass through the swinging doors; I've scrubbed and donned sterile O.R. green, because my patient Elmer Cook is going to receive an artificial hip joint today, a prosthesis, and I'll be assisting the orthopedic surgeon.

I've been part of this operation dozens of times, but today I again marvel at how each member of the surgical team is moving smoothly, swiftly and methodically. Inside this sterile inner sanctum there is a no-nonsense atmosphere, and no wasted motion. Every step in the preparation for the surgery is quietly and methodically carried out.

First a large plastic sheet is hung as a barrier to isolate the operation area and the surgical crew from the less sterile side of the room — the anesthetic equipment, the computerized technological equipment, even the top half of patient Elmer himself.

The orthopedic surgeon, the bone doctor, sits facing Elmer's exposed hip, with access to it through an opening in the plastic drape. I sit beside him, and behind us stands the "scrub tech" who oversees the instrument table, laden with several thousand dollars worth of gleaming and sterilized chisels, hammers and screws, along with drills and saws driven by compressed air.

Then we begin. With his scalpel, the surgeon makes a slash in Elmer's upper thigh, carrying the incision through the fatty layer. The muscles are carefully divided in line with their fibers and then, after only a few minutes of cutting, the head of Elmer's thigh bone, his femur, is exposed.

The surgeon then swiftly and skillfully saws off the head of the femur, and dislodges it from its socket, the acetabulum. A quick glance at this chunk of bone reveals why Elmer had such pain walking, even with a cane: the articulating surface of the head has been completely worn away.

Next, the surgeon hollows out the marrow of Elmer's thigh bone, still in his leg, to receive the shaft of the steel ball. Then he roughens the acetabular space to accept the new plastic socket.

While he's doing this drilling and sanding, I'm mixing the epoxy-like glue that will hold the prosthetic devices in place, amazing stuff with the tongue-twisting name of methyl macrylate. I've carefully combined exact portions of separately packaged powder and liquid, and must steadily stir this creamy goop over a three-minute period, until I get it to exactly the right consistency.

"One minute" announces Alice the circulating nurse, as acrid fumes rise to insult my nostrils and irritate my eyes. "Two minutes," she sings out, and I see the gluey glob has become thicker, and can feel the stirring has become tougher.

Finally I'm relieved to hear "Three minutes," and I gladly hand the jar of glue over to the orthopod who then applies just the right amount to the shaft of the femur and to the acetabulum. Quickly and surely — the glue continues to stiffen as he works — he hammers the ball joint into the femur's shaft and then fits this "new and improved" thigh bone into the freshly-glued acetabular socket.

My brief summary makes this hip replacement operation

seem only a notch or two above repairing the leg of a chair or table. But I've neglected to include all the time spent by the surgeon with calipers and protractors and gauges, applied with skill and deftness gained from very specialized training and experience. The orthopedic surgeon's challenge is to make certain the weight distribution and bearing will be absolutely correct at the point where the steel ball meets the plastic socket.

The day after the surgery Elmer is out of bed with a little help from the nurses. On the second day the physiotherapist comes by to offer a little instruction, and to take him for a short and halting stroll. But soon Elmer is walking alone, gingerly but painlessly, and is just as proud as he can be. In a week he's at home, learning how to handle his new hip, how to climb stairs, perhaps even to dance.

These artificial replacement joints are wonderful all right, but are nothing compared to the originals. Consider the ball and socket joints of your hip and shoulder, the hinge joints of your knees and wrists, and the amazingly complex hinge and rotator joints of your ankles and elbows. Or the bending, stretching and twisting of the bones and joints of your spine.

Study these joints as you deliberately move them, and marvel at the ease and grace with which they function. We take for granted the body's remarkable system of pulleys and levers, our ligaments and tendons and muscles. Thinking about it now, as I watch my fingers flick across the computer keyboard, I have to admit that by comparison the movements of the most sophisticated robot are awkward and ungainly — and I only type using the "hunt & peck" method!

12 The Stress of Stress Tests

THE SIGN ABOVE THE DOOR flashed an ominous warning: "Anyone taking this space flight must be in good health, should have no back problems, and no heart condition."

As our line of soon-to-be extraterrestrial travelers inched slowly forward toward the blast-off area, the same sign appeared again and again, each repetition serving only to raise my apprehension. Would I qualify as a healthy male without back problems or a heart condition? Should I have had a cardiac stress test before venturing into outer space?

But it was too late to back out. My two earth-people companions, Sarah and Michael, ages 7 and 11, were eagerly looking forward to riding their space ship out of Space Mountain at Disneyworld USA.

Then we were aboard. After being tightly strapped in, we were warned to securely fasten all our loose belongings — glasses, caps, cameras and purses. We barely had time to lash down our possessions when, with an abrupt shoosh and roar, we were hurtled out into the black unknown, to endure what amounted to a 60-second stress test.

For what seemed instead like an eternity, my brain and body were twisted and tormented in ways both terrifying and exhilarating. Finally, and not soon enough, we were back down to good old terra firma, and I could be proud that I had passed my flight test.

As I caught my breath I asked myself, "What more would a formal stress test have told me?" I reflected on the many similarities of a stress test with what I'd just gone through, but thought also about the very important differences.

Heart tracings, electrocardiograms, ordinarily are administered while you are at rest. A stress test, on the other hand, is done during exercise or while the patient is under emotional stress, to determine how your heart functions at work, especially when called upon to work a little harder than usual. By increasing physical, mental and emotional stress, your doctor can evaluate your "cardiac reserve."

This test not only can demonstrate how much life-giving blood perfuses through your heart, it also can indicate to your physician if the major blood vessels of your heart, the coronary arteries, are beginning to show some narrowing. If the stress test reveals a diminished blood flow, this suggests an increased risk of heart attack.

Three different methods are used to obtain these evaluations: a Holter monitor test, a treadmill (or bicycle) test, or a thallium examination.

In the Holter test, the patient actually wears a portable heart tracing machine, which monitors and records how the heart functions throughout the varying stresses of daily living. This, then, gives your doctor a taped record of how your heart responds to the average day's activities.

The treadmill or bicycle test differs in that it challenges you to engage in gradually increasing physical exertion, to determine and record your activity tolerance. After being wired up to a battery of measurement machines you walk or ride at a steadily increasing pace, until you begin to show fatigue or exhaustion.

The thallium test goes one step further by producing a photographic record of the heart and its blood supply, telling us whether the circulation is providing sufficient oxygen in response to the stress of exertion. To make this picture-taking possible, a liquid radioisotope is injected into a blood vessel.

Stress, of course, can be everywhere; so should everyone — especially men who are over forty and engaged in a stressful occupation — trot down to the doctor's office and request a stress test?

A cardiologist colleague responded to my question in the

firm negative. It seems that this test may sometimes feed back some misinformation, "false positives." He advised that, rather than subjecting many concerned patients to such screening tests, heart specialists prefer to rely on the doctor's clinical judgment and evaluations of each individual case. Furthermore, these tests can be costly; the pricey thallium test can run eight hundred dollars or more.

In deciding which patients to urge to take a stress test, physicians balance a number of factors. These are the kinds of people whom I often suggest should have their cardiac reserve evaluated:

❦ The person who is at extreme risk because of his or her life style. This especially includes the obese adult who smokes and who fails to engage in regular, moderate exercise.

❦ Anyone who experiences "angina," chest pain in response to physical or emotional stress.

❦ The patient who has survived a previous heart attack, to evaluate the progress of his recovery.

❦ Those who have certain irregular heartbeats, called cardiac arrhythmias.

Even if you fall into one of these categories, your physician will advise you on the need or the advisability of your taking any of these tests.

On the other hand, if you'd like to engage in an informal and delightful (but not inexpensive, either) stress test on your own, without a doctor's advice, spend a few days in one of Walt Disney's theme parks with a couple of livewire grandkids!

13 Doctors Don't Know Everything

DOWN AT THE SERVICE STATION, Al poured out his complaints as he poured in the gas. "Why don't you doctors get your act together?" was his opening gripe. "Last month you prescribed a sleeping pill for my wife, then a couple days later I see a headline on the cover of Newsweek: 'Halcion — Is It Safe? The article says the stuff makes people lose their memories."

About all I could say to Al was, "Well, we try." It isn't always easy, either. We physicians carefully follow the guidelines laid down for us by the Food and Drug Administration when we prescribe a medication, and we depend on feedback from our patients. When Halcion was approved by the FDA, we had every reason to believe it was a safe, mild sedative which didn't give users a hangover and was quickly eliminated from the body. And before being approved by the U.S. government, Halcion already was being used by people in many other countries.

We now know that, yes, Halcion is a good sedative, but a drug to be used in the smallest possible dosages, especially when used by older people, and only for short periods of time.

Based on experience, it's sad but true that even though the FDA has approved a new drug based on laboratory and clinical trials, we physicians are wise to move cautiously until the medication has been used by a wider range of patients. Often, after longterm use out in everyday medical practice, we discover side effects not observed in the preliminary research trials. A good example of this are certain blood pressure medications that, after approval by the FDA, were found by physicians to cause coughing, constipation and even impotence.

We physicians may feel betrayed when the media seize on and sensationally publicize such medical mishaps. Certainly the pharmaceutical companies and the FDA are not pleased.

But there have been times when such disclosures were in the public interest.

Years ago there was an outcry against birth control pills. It was intimated that the oral contraceptive caused weight gain, skin changes, emotional upsets, depression, water retention, even cancer.

The pharmaceutical industry listened, went back to the research lab, and found most of these negative side effects could be eliminated by cutting the dose of the female hormone estrogen in half. Now we can tell our patients that not only does the lower dosage control fertility, it may also prevent cramps, anemia, PMS, even certain types of cancer. We learn.

Here is a more recent example of medical misinformation. Not long ago the drug Prozac was hailed as a blessing for the treatment of depression. The medication worked, and soon it was widely prescribed.

Unfortunately, several patients who were taking Prozac committed suicide. You don't need to be a medical doctor to know that depressed people may resort to suicide as a way out of their miseries, but a California cultist organization, the "Church of Scientology," twisted this information around to employ it in their ongoing campaign against drugs to treat depression.

As a consequence, although there is no scientific evidence that this medication could be the direct cause of suicide, physicians exercise extreme care and observe special precautions in caring for depressed patients who are on Prozac. Perhaps that's all to the good.

Today Americans are "cholesterol conscious," largely thanks to media publicity. This, too, is good, because a low fat diet just makes good common health sense. We know that reducing your intake of cholesterol not only protects your blood vessels, it may also lower your risk of getting breast or colon cancer.

The media render a service in bringing medical information to the public, yet sometimes they may do more harm than good. For example, an article in The New York Times scared the wits out of a lot of women who were proud possessors of breast implants, linking these prosthetic devices with cancer. Plastic surgeons in outstanding medical centers throughout the nation rose to the defense, stating emphatically that a careful statistical study had shown that among these thousands of women with implants there was not a single documented case where an implant caused cancer.

If any good came from this scare it was that more women who have breast implants had mammograms, since this still is the best protection against breast cancer.

What we read in the mass media today may be contradicted tomorrow. We've been informed repeatedly that coffee and caffeine are bad for us, and that we should use decaffeinated brands. Currently the word is out that coffee in limited quantities is really okay, but that decaf may have some hidden side-effects.

We are informed that aspirin is bad for us because it can cause your stomach to bleed. Not long after this we read an article encouraging us to take aspirin, even when we don't have a headache, as a way to help prevent heart attacks.

You're right, Al, we've got to work a little harder at getting our act together. Let me assure you that we physicians, the media, and the FDA are trying.

In the meantime, don't believe everything you see on "60 Minutes" or read in Newsweek.

14 Medications Are To Help Your Body Heal Itself

A FEW YEARS AGO Jim Henson, creator of The Muppets, died suddenly and tragically of Group A Streptococcus. Americans of many ages were shocked and saddened: Henson was a comparatively young man, and he died of pneumonia, a disease most of us take for granted as being curable in otherwise healthy people.

So much so that doctors chuckle at the story of the patient who complained that the prescribed antibiotics weren't curing his cold. His physician recommended his patient get pneumonia, "Because I can cure that!"

But you have to show up to be cured. Apparently Henson had not been feeling well, but was reluctant to take time out to go to a doctor.

Physicians and patients have come to rely on antibiotics to cure all our physical ills, from acne to asthma, from pneumonia to peritonitis. Just call the doctor and get a prescription. Indeed, in the short span of just four decades we have seen miraculous changes in the field of curing infectious diseases.

In the pre-antibiotic era, physicians had to rely on their wits and the "art" of medicine, as they struggled to cure or at least to control serious infections. Today many of these attempts seem almost ludicrous.

Not all that many years ago, purging with strong laxatives or high colonic irrigations were regularly used to rid the body of "poisons." Placing heated drinking glasses against the chest, called "cupping," was a common practice to "draw out infection." Blood-letting was practiced to eliminate "bad blood," and abscesses were allowed to proceed to "fluctuance," the indication that the time was right for making an incision to draw off the "laudable pus."

Surgical wards in hospitals in this century had an abundance of unhappy youngsters who suffered from a condition called "osteomylelitis," abscesses in their bones. Well-meaning surgeons often would place live maggots in these infected wounds, hoping these critters would "eat out the infection!"

As a teenager, I recall reading of the tragic death of the son of President Calvin Coolidge. The poor fellow got a blister from a pair of stiff tennis shoes, which led to fulminating "blood poisoning." White House doctors blamed a pair of colored socks, but now we know the young man had a serious staph infection, a bug today quickly controlled by antibiotics.

Then one day an investigator working in the laboratories of a dye factory in Germany noted that some of the white mice that had skin infections got better when he sprayed their coats with a red azo dye. This eventually led to the production of an azo drug called Prontosil, which subsequently became sulfanilamide, the parent of all the sulfa drugs that were to follow. Many of these medications remain in widespread use today for urinary tract infections, sinusitis and certain bowel disorders.

Chance and luck played a part in the discovery of another major antibiotic family, penicillin. A laboratory worker in London, Dr. Alexander Fleming, was growing different types of bacteria in culture tubes. He was having good and consistent success with his cultures, except in one corner of his lab. There the bacteria would start to grow, then suddenly up and die.

Searching for a reason, he remembered that nearby there was a forgotten loaf of moldy bread. The astute Doctor Fleming wondered if the spores from the penicillium mold on the bread had somehow interfered with with the growth of the bacteria. The rest, as they say, is history.

In the decades since these two breakthrough discoveries, a host of antibiotics have emerged from the experimental laboratories. Ways have been found to produce these infection fighters synthetically. By tinkering with the chemical structures of these drugs, a seemingly endless variety of antibiotics has been produced.

Now we use a bundle of off-shoots from the original penicillin, including ampicillin, amoxicillin and bicillin. And intensive research has produced a succession of other antibiotics: we have the mycins, the tetracyclines, the cephalosporins, the aminoglycocides, and now the newest kid on the block (and the most expensive, at three or four dollars a capsule), the quinolines.

In the real world marketplace, pharmaceutical companies are fighting a highly competitive battle, each one taking a million dollar gamble, hoping to bring out the next "wonder antibiotic." As the laboratories produce second, third and fourth generations of these medications, some hospitals and medical centers have designated antibiotic specialists to advise physicians on the optimum drug for a particular malady, balancing effectiveness, cost and side effects.

So far it seems that the research investigators are staying one jump ahead of various types of infection. As one drug begins to lose its effectiveness, or as one group of bacteria develop resistance, a new and more exotic antibiotic makes its appearance.

There is a limit. Antibiotics can't do it all. We must remember that the function of antibiotics is only to knock out the bacteria, to allow the patient's own immunity to bring about a cure. The case of Jim Henson was a sad example of this principle. He simply waited too long to see a doctor. By the time he did, his immune system was overwhelmed by the fulminating toxicity of the pneumococcus infection. With his own immunity depleted, the six different antibiotics the doctors pumped into him were of no avail.

15 Analgesia, Amnesia, Anesthesia

YESTERDAY A SUDDEN GUST OF WIND stabbed a sharp bit of dust into my eye, immediately inflicting excruciating pain. This real life experience abruptly and graphically illustrated my medical school textbook lesson, that such pain rivaled that of passing a kidney stone.

Of course this pain sent me scurrying to the eye doctor's office for help. After the opthamologist mercifully dripped a few drops of numbing medicine into my eye, my hurt was miraculously gone. Then he quickly removed the offending foreign body.

Not only did I immediately feel a lot better, this brief affliction reminded me of the importance of human compassion. We physicians have the privilege of relieving suffering through the use of pain medications, especially during obstetrical and surgical procedures. To put this in human perspective, it might be a good idea if every physician could, early in his or her training, undergo such a painful experience.

The modern science of pain control dates back a century and a half to the first uses of nitrous oxide, ether and chloroform. It all started in 1842 when Crawford Long, a rural physician in the town of Jefferson, Georgia, attended an "ether party." He observed that after inhaling this gas the party-goers would laugh and frolic, bumbling and tumbling about, completely oblivious to any pains from bumps or bruises they might sustain.

Two years later Horace Wells, a dentist in Hartford, Connecticut, recognized nitrous oxide for its anesthetic potential after he attended a "laughing gas" show. But the road to revelation is not always straight: when he botched up a demonstration of its use in a dental extraction, Wells was denounced as a fraud.

Another dentist, William Morton, learned of ether's numbing properties from a friend, Boston chemist Charles Jackson. Working together, in 1846 they convinced the chief surgeon at Massachusetts General Hospital to use ether for two operations, one for the removal of a large tumor of the neck and the other for the amputation of a leg. With the success of these surgeries the age of anesthesia was born.

With these humble beginnings, the science of anesthesiology progressed into the 20th century, and to its present high level of technology as we approach the 21st. Yet there were some early mishaps. Chloroform was found to be a superb "general" anesthetic, and was widely used in obstetrics. When it was discovered that chloroform could cause severe liver damage, its use was stopped.

"Twilight Sleep" found wide use as an analgesic/amnesic agent during labor and delivery. This combination of two potent drugs produced total amnesia in the mother, who would awaken the next day with no recollection of the birthing process. But, sadly, the baby might be born blue and listless, too often succumbing to respiratory failure.

Ether was for many years the standard general anesthetic, often used in combination with nitrous oxide, ethylene, or cyclopropane. But patients put to sleep with these gases often had terrifying dreams as they drifted off, and their post-operative recovery could be marred by excited pitching and tossing, nausea and vomiting. Plus, these anesthetics were highly explosive.

It wasn't always necessary for the patient to "go to sleep" to be operated on. For example it was possible to operate on the lower abdomen or the lower limbs by injecting numbing medicine into the spine. But early on "spinal" anesthesia got a bad name, when precipitous drops in blood pressure led to other complications. Today, with our refined techniques and improved medications, spinal anesthetic has become safe and sure for a number of surgical procedures.

For "topical" anesthesia physicians continue to rely on derivatives of much-maligned cocaine. Novocaine, a brand name of procaine, as well as other "caine" medications, have been used successfully in eye surgery and in other more superficial procedures.

One of the disadvantages of general anesthesia was the need to "deepen" the sleep when complete muscle relaxation was required. This was especially true when in abdominal surgery it became necessary to quiet down the squirming and bubbling of the bowels. To prevent this, today's anesthetist will inject the patient with a refined version of a poison called "curare," to temporarily paralyze the chest and abdominal muscles. This poison, an extract of the bark of a tropical tree, has been used for hundreds of years by South American Indians on the tips of their arrows, to immobilize both food and enemies.

If my description seems a bit barbaric, let me assure you that today "going under" is extremely safe, even pleasant. Usually the patient awakens gently, often asking "When will the operation start?"

16 Pain and Suffering

PAIN SPARES NO CULTURE, but various peoples deal with it differently. Some years ago I was part of a small group traveling to several hospitals and clinics in China, to study techniques used to relieve chronic pain. Ironically, bumping around the countryside on an ancient diesel bus at times made us quite mindful of our subject. The board-hard seats, limited leg room and rough roads gave the members of our troop assorted headaches, backaches, and pain in our derrieres.

Most uncomfortable was Mrs. Larry Chan, wife of Doctor Larry Chan, a Chinese-American physician based in California, fulfilling a dream of visiting the land of his ancestors. Unfortunately, Mrs. Chan suffered greatly from rheumatoid arthritis, and the rigors of this travel were taking their toll.

Our tour took us to urban and rural clinics and hospitals, where we were shown examples of native medicines used to control pain. These included opium, laudanum, senna and castor bean. Along with pulverized seeds, herbs and flowers, ground up bullfrogs and snakeskins.

One clinic we visited was noted for its success in treating pain with acupuncture. Of course, we would stop here long enough to allow Mrs. Chan to undergo acupuncture treatment for her rheumatic pain. After a gracious welcome, several Chinese doctors positioned her on a couch, and gave the introductory lecture, complete with charts of the human body, to explain how acupuncture works. Long needles would be inserted into certain acupuncture points in her skin. These needles would interrupt the life forces or *chi* that flow along the body's "meridians," the pathways through which pain travels.

The needles were inserted, and a hunk of incense smoldered in the hollow between the thumb and forefinger of Mrs. Chan's left hand. A half hour later she rejoined us, smiling and apparently pain-free, having been pleasantly punctured. Sadly, by that evening, the poorly padded seats and the bumpy byways brought back those painful "life forces." So out came the aspirin bottle — this bus trip must go on.

In China acupuncture has been used successfully as an anesthetic and in limited ways in the United States during dental procedures, minor operations, labor and delivery, even Cesarean sections. In the walk-in clinics of the ghettos of New York City, acupuncture has been used to relieve the excruciating pain addicts suffer during drug withdrawal.

A report in American Medical News explained how "the needles are inserted under the skin in areas the acupuncturists say correspond to key bodyparts, the central nervous system, and shen men, the 'spiritual center.'" According to the article, acupuncture works some of the time, for some of the addicts.

Down through the years, practitioners have continually searched for ways to relieve pain. In the 1700s an Austrian physician, Franz Mesmer, began using hypnosis to treat abnormal nervous conditions such as "hysteria." He "mesmerized" his patients into a trancelike period of altered awareness, during which he would give them messages of well-being that would carry over as post-hypnotic suggestions. Dr. Mesmer was able to report some "miraculous cures."

Hypnosis has attracted much popular interest, and also has been used for the relief of pain during surgical procedures. It has been tried for the relief of the psychological pain of smoking cessation, alcohol withdrawal, even weight reduction. Yet skepticism remains. Success has usually been limited to the person who is highly susceptible and who has a deep desire to gain relief. Some researchers suggest that the relief of pain during labor and delivery using the Lamaze "natural childbirth" method is a form of self-hypnosis.

Other less well-known methods to relieve chronic pain include a process with the acronym TENS, biofeedback and surgery. TENS stands for "Transcutaneous Electrical Nerve Stimulation," and is enabled by an ingenious battery-operated gadget that, when activated, sends tiny shocks to the nerve endings in the affected areas of the body. Even its promoters can't explain exactly just how and why it works, but they are convinced it does. One main hypothesis is that the electrical current stimulates the production of endorphins, the body's natural pain killers. Or the electrical zap may block the transmission of pain impulses to the spinal cord.

Biofeedback is another and entirely different approach to the relief of chronic pain. Under the assumption that pain often results from spasm and muscles contraction, biofeedback instructors teach patients internal relaxation techniques, often with good success.

Surgical intervention for the relief of chronic pain is the option of last resort, used most often to give some measure of comfort to terminally ill cancer patients. Here the technique is to sever the sensory nerves that transmit the unbearable pain sensations.

I've talked here so far about the relief of chronic pain without the use of medications. But we also do have a wide range of medicines for pain relief, including muscle relaxants, narcotics, tranquilizers, antidepressants, and anti-inflammatory medications. However, these are reserved for acute pain, with some exceptions.

Yet all the medicines and the methods of treatment have a common denominator — they achieve pain relief through their action on the central nervous system and the brain, either by blocking the transmission of the pain impulses along the sensory nerves, or by regulating the production of endorphins and of that mysterious brain chemical, serotonin, a substance that functions as a neurotransmitter producing the actual perception of pain.

When my 80-year-old patient, Hannah, complains of pain in her left foot, she forgets that several months ago her entire left leg was amputated because of gangrene. Now, for the relief of dear Hannah's "phantom pain" in her foot, we will actually be treating Hannah's brain.

17 Medicines Created From the Earth

IT WAS LATE AFTERNOON IN BEIJING, and we American physicians were weary after having spent a long day tramping through Chinese medical schools and hospitals. Our guide informed us that we would be making one more stop, at the hospital apothecary.

The Chinese pharmacist, Ching Lu, proved to be an enthusiastic lecturer, and we forgot our tired feet as he provided us with a rapid-fire presentation on the wonders of Chinese herbal medicine. Throughout his translated talk he referred to display boards on which were mounted flowers, seeds, and a variety of herbs, to demonstrate the magic that could be achieved with oriental medicine.

Perhaps it was the lateness of the hour or fatigue that prompted one of our group to ask, with a hint of condescension, whether Chinese doctors ever made use of modern pharmaceutical wonder drugs such as penicillin, sulfa, and the like.

Mr. Ching replied diplomatically that yes, of course, in instances of severe bacterial infection penicillin would be used. "We observe, doctor," he added, that penicillin had its origin in a living bread mold." He went on to say that 80% of the time Chinese medicaments — herbal teas, tinctures, powders and poultices — would very nicely bring about a cure.

Pharmacist Ching was especially proud of his flower and plant display. He reminded us that a number of "modern" medicines were derived from flowering plants. Among these are a heart medicine, digitalis; a mood-altering drug, rauwolfia; and a gout medicine, colchicine. He added that herbal medicines have been used by medicine men down through the ages, well before the birth of Christ, and that the use of plant derivations was mentioned in "your

Christian Bible." (I made a mental note to look that up when I got back home.)

Evening shadows were lengthening as our group of tourist doctors was bussed back to our Beijing hotel. Recalling the many flowers on the display board back in Ching's apothecary, I let my thoughts fly back halfway around the globe to my own flower beds. Could it be that I had a horticultural apothecary in my own back yard?

In a moist, shadowy corner of my north Idaho garden I grow an interesting plant called "Foxglove," which bears lovely, thimble-shaped blossoms. The leaves of this plant can be powdered up to produce the heart medicine, digitalis, that Ching had mentioned. Yet, the leaves are poisonous — chewing them can cause paralysis and death.

In sunnier areas I've planted a hardy perennial plant called yarrow, which grows like a weed and produces a profusion of yellow and white flower heads. The genus name for this flower is "achillea" from the Achilles in Homer's Iliad who is said to have used a poultice of ground-up achillea leaves to staunch the flow of blood from his vulnerable heel. The poor fellow died in spite of that.

In spring and fall, crocus flowers poke their pretty noses up through the soil, as the seasons change. These flowers have been used since ancient days as a source of medication to treat gout. The active ingredient, colchicine, is still being used by doctors to treat the gouty condition.

These naturally derived medicines are described in a magnificent book, "The Magic and Medicine of Plants," published recently by the Reader's Digest. It contains the stories, along with beautiful drawings, of 280 medicinal flowering plants.

In this day of modern biotechnology we have a pill or a shot or an ointment for every ailment, ache or itch, all of them produced synthetically. The thought of going back to the pre-penicillin days, or to sole reliance upon "natural" medicine is, of course, unthinkable to physicians or to their patients. We and they want quick and positive cures, strong medicines to fight disease. We can't be bothered to boil up teas, or to grind up herbs with mortar and pestle to mix with alcohol for a tincture or a tonic. We want health in a hurry.

Working in their sophisticated research laboratories, western pharmaceutical wizards can create seemingly magic medicines, "wonder drugs." Simply by changing a medicine's formulation, lopping off an oxygen ion here or adding a hydrogen ion there, they can create a new medication, one they hope will have greater therapeutic capabilities, fewer side effects, or a longer duration of action, requiring only one or two doses a day. Months and years later, by the time this new drug is available to the public, it will have passed through the strict surveillance of the U.S. Food and Drug Administration.

The capability to synthesize new and better medications in the laboratory need not belittle the wisdom of Ching Lu's reminder that the use of plant derivatives was even mentioned in "your Christian Bible." And, indeed, there it was in the Book of Ecclesiasticus: "The Lord created medicines from the Earth and a sensible man will not despise them."

The Family Doctor, Today and Tomorrow

Is the family doctor an endangered species? Let's hope not. I believe most people would prefer to have "their" doctor to go to — for regular checkups as well as when they're not feeling well. It's just human nature to be more comfortable and confident with someone who cares about your general physical and mental health, who knows you as an individual person, as someone who not only has a slightly abnormal electrocardiographic tracing, but a worried, aching heart, as well.

Yet fewer medical school graduates are choosing to become family doctors. At the end of 1991 there were 69,444 family doctors practicing in the United States, about 13% of all physicians providing care directly to patients. That same year only 7.7% of all new MDs concluded or completed a residency in family practice.

This drop in interest in family practice is consistent with recent trends. In the six years from 1986 to 1991, the number of graduating doctors electing to specialize in family practice dropped by nearly 10%, to 2,058.

Over the same period, interest increased in most other specialties, while the number of recognized specialties continued to grow. At least part of the allure of specialties for new physicians is the chance to use advanced biotechnology, wondrous medical machinery, and magnificent miracle drugs. Such "cutting edge" healing tools impart glamour to the specialist who uses them. By comparison, we see a diminished stature primary doctor who treats everyday backaches, stomachaches...and heartaches.

Not so many years ago, most all doctors were family doctors, who performed a wide range of services for their patients. Today "alternative" health care professionals, including nurse practitioners and physician's assistants, take medical histories, do physical exams, even order medications.

Chiropractors have learned to combine a caring bedside manner with massage and manipulation. Naturopaths, herbalists and accupuncturists are ready to fill the void left by the decreasing number of family physicians.

As I look ahead at the future of the family doctor, a Presidential task force is struggling to shape a program of health care reform. The details remain far from clear, but the need for change is there. Former Surgeon General C. Everett Koop, writing in his memoirs, observed that "the entire health care system in the United States has become desperately ill. It has grown inefficient, wasteful, even immoral." And Dr. Koop had to admit "there is no easy solution, no quick fix."

In this struggle to provide high quality and affordable health care to all Americans — and the quality of health care in the United States is by far the best in the world — the family doctor will be asked to play a leading role. A main cause of high medical costs is extremely expensive medical tests and procedures. Increased emphasis on primary health care is a way to reduce the frequency with which physicians and hospitals send very large bills to insurance companies, including to Medicare and Medicaid.

Indeed, with tongue in cheek Dr. Koop suggested it might not be a bad idea to return to some of the basic concepts of "horse-and-buggy medicine." It may well be that, in diagnosis and treatment, we physicians must increase our reliance on our eyes to observe, our ears to listen, and our hands to touch.

A fundamental question facing health planners is who in the medical arena has the wisdom, the experience and the judgment to strike an appropriate balance between cost and quality? I believe the length and breadth of experience of the primary physician best equips him or her for that responsibility. The family doctor generalist knows the patient and the patient's family and has provided continuity of care, often for many years. The specialist, a master of technology when it is called for, is trained and equipped to provide magnificent (and expensive) diagnostic and therapeutic care.

The family doctor has been trained in the care of the whole person; his or her exposure to medical knowledge has been broad, covering all of the specialties. And because the science and art of medicine continues to expand and develop, the family physician must continue to go back to school. Family practice is the only specialty that requires re-certification by examination at regular intervals.

Furthermore, because the generalist learns and practices in an office and community setting, in addition to in a hospital, he or she may be better able to see the whole picture. Most specialists, trained and practicing only within the walls of a hospital, will have a narrower range of understanding.

In many instances the family doctor cares for the patient from the cradle to the grave, from the delivery room to the nursing home. That experience provides a very special advantage of knowledge and understanding, essential to making sound ethical decisions, such as when to allow a person to die with dignity. Choices such as these can, of course, contribute directly to containing the overall cost of medical care.

The family doctor must also be a teacher, in the most basic sense of the word. If preventative medicine is to be a primary goal of our future health care system, then the family doctor must accept a teaching role.

It is my hope that the essays in this book may in some small way contribute to that very worthwhile aim.